Reviewing Research Evidence for Nursing Practice

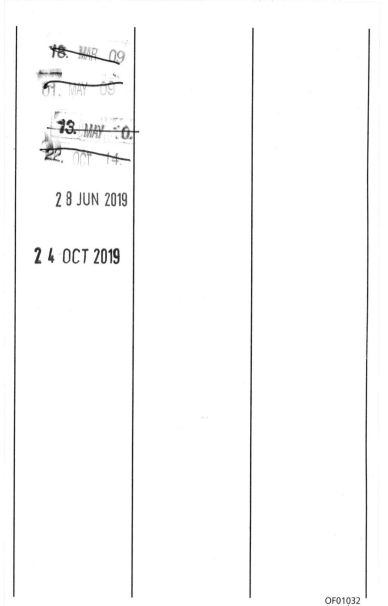

Reviewing Research Evidence for Nursing Practice: Systematic Reviews

Edited by

Christine Webb

Professor of Health Studies
Faculty of Health and Social Care, University of Plymouth, UK

and

Brenda Roe

Professor of Health Sciences
Institute of Health Research, Faculty of Health and Applied
Social Sciences, Liverpool John Moores University, UK

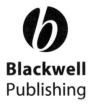

Blackwell
Publishing

Blackwell Publishing editorial offices:
Blackwell Publishing Ltd, 9600 Garsington Road, Oxford OX4 2DQ, UK
Tel: +44 (0)1865 776868
Blackwell Publishing Inc., 350 Main Street, Malden, MA 02148-5020, USA
Tel: +1 781 388 8250
Blackwell Publishing Asia Pty Ltd, 550 Swanston Street, Carlton, Victoria 3053, Australia
Tel: +61 (0)3 8359 1011

First published 2007 by Blackwell Publishing Ltd

ISBN: 978-1-4051-4423-0

Library of Congress Cataloging-in-Publication Data
Reviewing research evidence for nursing practice : systematic reviews / edited by
Christine Webb and Brenda Roe.
p. ; cm.
Includes bibliographical references and index.
ISBN-13: 978-1-4051-4423-0 (pbk. : alk. paper)
1. Nursing—Research—Methodology. 2. Systematic reviews (Medical
research) 3. Evidence-based nursing. I. Webb, Christine. II. Roe, Brenda H.
[DNLM: 1. Clinical Nursing Research. 2. Review Literature. 3.
Meta-Analysis. WY 20.5 R454 2007]
RT81.5.R488 2007
610.73072—dc22
2007010023

A catalogue record for this title is available from the British Library

Set in 9.5/11.5pt Palatino
by Graphicraft Limited, Hong Kong
Printed and bound in Singapore
by Fabulous Printers Pte Ltd

For further information on Blackwell Publishing, visit our website:
www.blackwellnursing.com

Contents

Contributors

Donna Ciliska is Professor in the School of Nursing at McMaster University and has an appointment as a nursing consultant with Hamilton Public Health. She is editor of the journal *Evidence-Based Nursing*, and has contributed as a co-editor to two evidence-based nursing texts. Her research interests include community health, obesity, eating disorders and knowledge translation.

Mike Clarke is Director of the UK Cochrane Centre, which provides training and support to systematic reviewers in the UK. He is Professor of Clinical Epidemiology at the University of Oxford, working on systematic reviews of individual patient data. These include the breast cancer overview, which brings together data on more than 300 000 women in 400 randomised trials. He works on more than a dozen other systematic reviews across health care and on trials in pre-eclampsia, subarachnoid haemorrhage, breast cancer and poisoning – which are the world's largest randomised trials in each condition.

Maureen Dobbins is an associate professor in the School of Nursing at McMaster University and has an appointment as a nursing consultant with the City of Hamilton Public Health Services. She holds a career scientist award with the Ontario Ministry of Health and Long-Term Care. Her research interests include knowledge transfer and exchange, evidence-informed decision-making, community health, healthy body weight, physical activity and chronic disease prevention.

Chantale L. Dumoulin is an assistant professor at the School of Physical and Occupational Therapy, Faculty of Medicine, University of Montreal, Canada. Her research interests include psychometric evaluation of measuring instruments, conservative interventions for urinary incontinence in women, service delivery and research dissemination.

David Evans is Senior Lecturer in the Division of Health Sciences at the School of Nursing and Midwifery, University of South Australia. His areas of interest include all aspects of acute care nursing, evidence-based practice, safety and quality issues and practice evaluation.

Beverley French is a senior research fellow at the University of Central Lancashire. Her experience of quantitative systematic review is mainly in Cochrane reviews of interventions in stroke rehabilitation. She is currently involved in a number of syntheses of wider evidence sources relating to mental health advocacy, and community development and engagement.

E. Jean C. Hay-Smith is a lecturer in the Rehabilitation Teaching and Research Unit at the Wellington School of Medicine and Health Sciences, University of Otago, New Zealand. She is an editor of the Cochrane Incontinence Review Group. Her research interests include the conservative management of urinary incontinence (particularly pelvic floor muscle training), self-efficacy and treatment adherence.

Peter Herbison works in the Department of Preventive and Social Medicine at the University of Otago in Dunedin, New Zealand, providing statistical help for researchers.

Myfanwy Lloyd Jones is a senior research fellow in the Health Economics and Decision Science Section of the University of Sheffield School of Health and Related Research (ScHARR). A specialist in systematic reviewing, she is a member of the ScHARR Technology Assessment Group (ScHARR-TAG), and has contributed to a number of technology assessments within the NHS Health Technology Assessment Programme.

Rachel McNamara is a research fellow in the Department of General Practice, Cardiff University, UK.

Lynn Nicholls is Lecturer in Midwifery at the University of Plymouth in Taunton, UK.

Christine Norton is Nurse Consultant (Bowel Continence) at St Mark's Hospital in Harrow and Burdett Professor of Gastrointestinal Nursing, King's College London, UK. She is an editor for the Cochrane incontinence group, chairs the Royal College of Nursing Gastroenterology and Stoma Care Forum and is associate editor of *Gastrointestinal Nursing.*

Beverly O'Connell holds the Inaugural Chair in Nursing at the Deakin-Southern Health Nursing Research Centre. Previously she held the positions of Chair in Nursing, Cabrini Health; Nursing Research Director, Sir Charles Gairdner Hospital; and Director of Nursing Research and Development, Curtin University, Australia. Her research interests include aged care, quality and safety, incontinence care and carer support.

Joan Ostaszkiewicz is a research fellow and PhD candidate at the School of Nursing at Deakin University. She holds a joint appointment with the Southern Health Network and Deakin University. Her research interests are ageing and the integration of research with practice.

Barbara L. Paterson holds a Tier 1 Canada Research Chair in Chronic Illness and is a professor at the University of New Brunswick in Canada. She is widely published in the fields of chronic illness and qualitative research.

Brenda Roe is Professor of Health Sciences at Liverpool John Moores University. She has a background in nursing, health visiting, primary care, public health, gerontology, health services research and management. She is a Fellow of the Queen's Nursing Institute and Fellow of the Royal Society for the Promotion of Health.

Margarete Sandelowski is Cary C. Boshamer Professor in the School of Nursing at the University of North Carolina at Chapel Hill, USA. She is Director of the Annual Summer Institutes in Qualitative Research, and of the new Certificate Program in Qualitative Research, both offered at the School of Nursing. She has published widely in nursing and social science anthologies and journals in the areas of technology and gender, especially reproductive technology and technology in nursing, and of qualitative methods. Her latest book, co-authored with Julie Barroso, is *Handbook for Synthesizing Qualitative Research* (Springer, New York, 2007).

Chris Shaw is Reader in Nursing Research in the School of Care Sciences at the University of Glamorgan, South Wales, UK. Her research interests focus on chronic disease management and health behaviours such as self-care and help-seeking. She has a background in nursing and midwifery and is a chartered health psychologist.

Helen Thomas is an Associate Professor in the School of Nursing, McMaster University and a Clinical Consultant with the Public Health Research, Education and Development Program, Hamilton, Ontario, Canada, where she is Project Leader of the Effective Public Health Practice Project.

Lois Thomas is Senior Research Fellow in the Department of Nursing at the University of Central Lancashire. Her research interests include stroke nursing, particularly urinary incontinence after stroke, and the effectiveness of clinical guidelines in nursing and allied health professions.

Christine Webb is Professor of Health Studies at the University of Plymouth, UK, Executive Editor of *Journal of Advanced Nursing*, and Editor of *Nurse Author & Editor*. Her initial clinical specialism was women's health, but more recently she has focused on nurse education as a manager and researcher. She is a Fellow of the Royal College of Nursing (UK).

Robin Whittemore is Associate Professor at the Yale School of Nursing in New Haven CT, USA. Her research interests include lifestyle change, nurse-coaching, type 2 diabetes, psychosocial adjustment to chronic illness, nursing intervention research, and nursing theory development.

Preface

We know from many research studies that practising nurses and other healthcare professionals do not always have the time, confidence or skills to carry out research or systematic reviews for themselves. Therefore they rely on reviews by other people when considering innovations and developments in their practice.

Our aim for this book, therefore, is to present readers with the issues arising from conducting systematic reviews and thereby to help them understand reviews that they identify and read when considering developing their health policy, services and clinical practice.

It is not solely a 'how to do a systematic review' book – as other examples of that have already been published. Rather, we have presented how a selection of reviews has been carried out in a range of specialist areas related to health policy, service development and clinical practice. This will help readers to critically appraise the reviews they read and judge how useful they are for changing practice and service development. A particular novel and groundbreaking feature of this book is that it includes examples of all types of review – quantitative, qualitative and integrative or mixed-method reviews which include both qualitative and quantitative empirical studies – whereas other books are limited to only one of these types. By bringing all these approaches together in one book, we hope to offer a reader-friendly and economical volume for nurses, healthcare professionals and health-services researchers.

The book will be of interest to nurses and healthcare professionals in practice, people following an MSc or taught doctorate programme in advanced or specialist practice or postgraduate study, as well as academic researchers and research doctorate students.

Introduction

Brenda Roe and Christine Webb

From the early 1990s systematic review as a method of establishing the evidence of effectiveness of healthcare interventions has developed apace – most notably, with the development of the international Cochrane Collaboration and the Cochrane Library for the electronic dissemination of systematic reviews. These reviews focus on quantitative evidence from randomised controlled trials and meta-analyses. Parallel developments, but not on the large international scale of the Cochrane Collaboration, have also evolved looking at the meta-study and meta-synthesis of qualitative research evidence. Methods, handbooks, critical appraisal and quality criteria are available and are described in this book. More recently, integrative reviews are being developed to combine the evidence from quantitative research and qualitative research on clinical topics, management and policy, as undertaken by the Joanna Briggs Foundation. It is acknowledged that the methodology and methods for systematic reviews are developing and increasingly need to take account of diverse sources of evidence (Popay, 2006), along with the recognition and development of terms and definitions (Sander & Kitcher, 2006).

The purpose of this book is to present the issues arising when conducting systematic reviews and to provide a 'how to' of the methods used, based on reviewers' experiences of undertaking published systematic reviews. It provides a selection of reviews carried out in a range of specialist areas related to clinical practice, along with recommendations for practice and future research. Not only does the book inform people wishing to undertake systematic reviews themselves, but also clinicians who may wish to appraise the reviews they read with a view to incorporating their recommendations into practice. It is known from many research studies that practising clinicians do not have the time, confidence or skills to carry out research and they rely on reviews undertaken by others when considering innovations and developments in their clinical practice.

The book is novel and is the only one of its kind to include systematic reviews of quantitative research, qualitative research, and integrative reviews incorporating both quantitative evidence and qualitative evidence. The methods for systematic reviews are continuing to evolve and this book provides an indication of this evolution in one volume. The book is primarily intended for nurses and nursing, but is of relevance to medical and health services researchers and clinicians as well as those from the professions allied to medicine.

The book is in four parts. Part 1 covers Systematic Reviews and Meta-Analysis of Quantitative Research and predominantly cites as examples reviews undertaken as part of the Cochrane Collaboration involving randomised controlled trials. Part 2, entitled Meta-synthesis and Meta-study of

Qualitative Research, includes systematic reviews of qualitative evidence and studies, while Part 3 includes Integrative Reviews of Quantitative and Qualitative Research. Finally, Part 4 looks at the Application and Uses of Reviews in health services as well as offering reflections on the past, present and future of systematic reviews.

Each of the chapters begins with an Introduction to set the clinical context and concludes with implications for practice and future research. In Part 1, Chapter 1, an Overview of Methods by Mike Clarke, gives an overview of systematic review methods for quantitative studies, notably randomised controlled trials, and includes methods for locating, appraising and combining independent studies that are transparent and minimise bias. Such reviews place research in context and ensure that new research is developed and implemented appropriately. Systematic reviews are increasingly more common, as exemplified by the endeavours of the Cochrane Collaboration and the Cochrane Library based on a global effort established in 1993. Clarke's chapter looks at question formulation, study identification, appraisal of studies for inclusion, data collection, statistical analysis, updating of reviews and appraising and using systematic reviews. He concludes that systematic reviews offer the best way to ensure that evidence is available on which to make decisions.

Chapter 2 is by Brenda Roe and includes Key Stages and Considerations when Undertaking a Systematic Review. The Cochrane systematic review on bladder training for the management of urinary incontinence in adults is used as an example and sections of the chapter include guidelines, developing a protocol and necessary steps, literature searching, publication bias, inclusion and exclusion criteria, quality assessment, data extraction, outcomes, review methods, presentation, and combining and interpretation of results, along with statistical outcome measures and combined effect estimates. The chapter is supported with figures and tables as examples that can be used by people wishing to undertake future systematic reviews, and concludes with sections on writing up and disseminating reviews.

Chapter 3, entitled Prevention and Treatment of Urinary Incontinence After Stroke in Adults: Experiences, is based on a systematic review for the Cochrane Collaboration by Lois Thomas and Beverley French. It provides an overview of the methods used and the reviewers' conclusions, followed by sections on issues that arose when carrying out the review, designing the protocol, designing the search, retrieval of potential studies for inclusion, data extraction and assessment of study quality. Sections on extraction of outcome data, data analysis and synthesis are followed by valuable learning points which are of direct benefit for people wishing to undertake future systematic reviews. The chapter concludes not only with implications for practice but also with lessons for future similar reviews.

Chapter 4, like Chapters 2 and 3, also focuses on a Cochrane systematic review on urinary incontinence as an example. It is entitled Pelvic Floor Muscle Training for Urinary Incontinence in Women and is by Jean Hay-Smith, Chantale Dumoulin and Peter Herbison. An overview of the review is provided, along with conventional subject headings followed by a discussion and the issues that arose when carrying out the review. These include sections on methodological heterogeneity, other sources of heterogeneity, and choice and reporting of outcome measures. Their chapter illustrates the evolving nature and complexity of randomised controlled trials designs and methods.

Chapter 5, the last chapter in Part 1, is by Christine Norton and also includes a Cochrane systematic review by way of example, entitled Biofeedback and Anal Sphincter Exercises for Faecal Incontinence in Adults. Faecal incontinence, biofeedback and exercises are set in context, followed by an overview of the review and its methods, results and conclusions. Issues that arose while carrying out the review included randomised versus non-randomised evidence, outcome measures, international relevance and translating the evidence into clinical recommendations. The chapter concludes by discussing the relationship of the review with other systematic reviews on the subject and with reflections for future reviews.

Part 2 is a section on Meta-study and Meta-synthesis of Qualitative Research, with Myfanwy Lloyd Jones in Chapter 6 including an Overview of the Methods in which both meta-study and meta-synthesis are defined. She provides a brief history and then goes on to cover key methodological aspects, such as the focus of the study, inclusion and exclusion criteria and theoretical framework.

This is followed by sections on study identification and selection, summary, analysis and synthesis of findings. The chapter is completed by presenting the interpretation of results and dissemination of findings, along with assessing the quality of meta-syntheses.

Chapter 7 looks at Coming Out as Ill: Understanding Self-Disclosure in Chronic Illness from a meta-synthesis of qualitative research by Barbara L. Paterson. The chapter includes primary research and deals with sample characteristics, preparing for the meta-study, analytic components, meta-synthesis, challenges in meta-study projects, conducting a meta-study alone and issues of selecting the primary research to be included.

Chapter 8 is entitled From Meta-synthesis to Method: Appraising the Qualitative Research Synthesis Report and is written by Margarete Sandelowski. She looks at the components of the qualitative research synthesis report and evaluation criteria and methods, using her study of prenatal diagnosis as an example. Qualitative research synthesis is contrasted with narrative overview, synthesis of quantitative research findings, secondary analysis, within-study and within-programme research synthesis and meta-study, and this is followed by consideration of results and discussion of the synthesis produced.

Chapter 9 completes Part 2 and is by Myfanwy Lloyd Jones, who presents her study on Role Development in Acute Hospital Settings: A Systematic Review and Meta-synthesis. She gives an overview of the methods used and aim of the study, which looked at innovative roles of nurses, and barriers and facilitators, and used Paterson's meta-study methodology (see Chapter 7). Conventional section headings of methods, results and findings are included, followed by discussion of issues that arose while carrying out the review, identifying potentially relevant studies and retrieving them, data extraction and study appraisal. Sections on meta-data-analysis and meta-synthesis follow, and the chapter concludes with consideration of interpretation of the results and limitations.

Part 3 is particularly novel and covers Integrative Reviews of Quantitative and Qualitative Research. Chapter 10 by David Evans provides an Overview of Methods and looks at rigour in integrative reviews, systematic methods, problem and purpose, literature searching and data collection.

He continues with sections on evaluation of the quality of primary research, evidence of critical appraisal, and transparency, and concludes by considering quality in integrative reviews.

Chapter 11, entitled Rigour in Integrative Reviews, by Robin Whittemore develops some of these themes. She starts by considering what are integrative reviews, their purpose, the review protocol, problem identification and location of studies. She provides details about evaluating studies, data collection and analysis – specifically descriptive data synthesis, statistical data synthesis and qualitative data synthesis – along with a section on the integrative review report.

Chapter 12 is by Joan Ostaszkiewicz and Beverly O'Connell and looks at Habit Retraining for Urinary Incontinence in Adults. It builds on a Cochrane systematic review of quantitative evidence from randomised controlled trials and synthesises evidence from other study designs to provide an integrative review on the topic. As well as conventional method sections and related considerations, they include discussion of the dilemmas they encountered in implementing the Cochrane systematic review criteria, in limiting the review to one form of evidence, as well as with critical appraisal and establishing levels of quality. They go on to detail managing and integrating evidence from mixed design studies, using habit retraining as the example.

Chapter 13 addresses the question What Makes a Good Midwife? and is by Lynn Nicholls and Christine Webb, who undertook an integrative review to answer this question. They give an overview of the methods, protocol and search methods, appraisal of studies, analysis of findings as well as discussing methodological issues. The chapter is completed with a summary of the main findings, aspects of conducting an integrative review and issues that arose.

In Chapter 14, Rachel McNamara and Chris Shaw present an integrative review investigating Older People and Respite Care. They address the questions of who are carers and what impact their role has on them, and then go on to consider respite care and evidence of its effectiveness. They provide an overview of the research aims, methodology and methodological issues. They consider how to devise an appropriate search strategy to capture both quantitative and qualitative evidence, along with assessment of study quality – which for quantitative studies is more established than for qualitative studies (see chapters in Parts 1 and 2). The identification of studies, data extraction, analysis plan and data synthesis are considered, along with lessons for future reviews.

Part 3 concludes with Chapter 15 by David Evans, which presents an integrative review on the Use of Physical Restraint. As well as methodological considerations, he provides a synthesis of results and lessons learned on use of physical restraint, characteristics of restrained people, reasons for restraining people, injury and physical restraint, the experience of physical restraint and restraint minimisation.

Finally, Part 4 considers the Applications and Uses of Reviews, with Chapter 16 providing steps, methods and considerations for Using Systematic Reviews in Health Services; this chapter is written by Donna Ciliska, Maureen Dobbins and Helen Thomas. They look at how systematic reviews have been used to inform clinical practice, management and policy development by critically appraising reviews using explanation and application of criteria to existing systematic reviews and clinical scenarios with a public health and health promotion focus. The clinical scenarios include teenage suicides and type 2 diabetes mellitus, and include sections on finding the evidence and critical appraisal.

Chapter 17 by Christine Webb and Brenda Roe concludes the volume by summarising the chapters and offering Reflections on the Past, Present and Future of Systematic Reviews. It sets systematic reviews in historical context, from the evolution of systematic reviews for quantitative evidence, then the synthesis of qualitative evidence, followed more recently by integrative reviews which combine analysis and synthesis of both types of evidence in a review. Finally, the possibility of undertaking synopses of a number of related systematic reviews using meta-study techniques is suggested.

Contributors are drawn from a variety of professional disciplines and countries around the globe, reflecting the interdisciplinary nature of systematic reviewing and the international collaborations and networks that have been formed. We are indebted to and would like to thank our contributing authors, who are not only pioneers in their fields but generous individuals willing to communicate effectively and share their expertise with the wider community, despite having busy schedules and workloads.

References

Popay, J. (ed.) (2006) *Moving Beyond Effectiveness in Evidence Synthesis: Methodological Issues in the Synthesis of Diverse Sources of Evidence.* National Institute for Health and Clinical Excellence, London. (NICE website www.nice.org.uk)

Sander, L. & Kitcher, H. (2006) *Systematic and Other Reviews: Terms and Definitions Used by UK Organisations and Selected Databases. Systematic Review and Delphi Survey.* National Institute for Health and Clinical Excellence, London. (NICE website www.nice.org.uk)

Part 1

Systematic Reviews and Meta-Analysis of Quantitative Research

1 Overview of Methods

Mike Clarke

Introduction

Systematic reviews are both scientific research and the application of common sense. They serve to identify studies relevant to a particular question, to appraise and assess the eligibility of these studies, and to summarise them, using statistical techniques to combine their results, if feasible and appropriate. Without systematic reviews, we are faced with an ever-increasing number of individual studies. There may be many, sometimes hundreds, on the same question. If this research is to be used to make well-informed decisions, we need to be confident that the effects of both bias and chance are minimised. These effects must be minimised not only within the individual studies but also in the process of bringing them together in a review.

This is where systematic reviews are especially helpful. Regardless of whether the underlying research comprises randomised trials assessing the relative effects of different interventions, studies of test accuracy to determine which is the best technique to diagnose an illness, cohort studies to estimate the prognosis of patients with different characteristics, or qualitative research to understand better the ways in which people make choices, systematic reviews of the research appropriate to answer a question will provide someone making decisions with a more reliable basis for doing so than an individual study.

Systematic reviews are pieces of research, which aim to identify, appraise and summarise studies of relevance to a particular topic. Such a review uses a predefined, explicit methodology, setting out the objectives, eligibility criteria and methods for the review. These methods should be chosen so as to minimise bias in all aspects of the conduct and reporting of the review; including study identification, assessment of eligibility, collection of data, analyses and interpretation. A systematic review does not need to combine the results of the studies to provide an average estimate but, if it does so, this should also be done in a way that minimises bias, with a clear separation between hypothesis testing and hypothesis generating results. This chapter outlines some of these key features of systematic reviews, setting the scene for the more detailed discussion and examples that follow.

Background

Most individual pieces of research are too small on their own to answer reliably all the questions addressed by the research or of relevance to a person wishing to use the research when making a decision about health care. Individual studies may be subject to biases in regard to their availability and might not contain a sufficiently large number or range of participants. Chance effects may lead to an overestimate or underestimate of the true effect in any scientific investigation. For example, even the best-conducted randomised trial is not immune to the effects of chance and there is no way of knowing whether chance has caused its result to be better or worse than it should be. To minimise the effects of chance, the results of similar studies can be combined – in a meta-analysis – to produce a statistically more reliable result. To minimise the effects of bias, as many as possible of the eligible studies need to be identified and their quality and relevance need to be assessed.

The narrative review article has long been a feature of the healthcare literature, but systematic reviews represent an important departure from these. In a systematic review, the methods used to locate, appraise and, where appropriate, combine independent studies are clearly described. These methods should be transparent and should minimise the possibility of bias.

Systematic reviews are needed both to place research in context and also to ensure that new research is designed and implemented in the most appropriate way (Clarke, 2004). They are increasingly common, not least through the work of The Cochrane Collaboration. This global effort was established in 1993 (Chalmers, 1993) and more than 14 000 people in 100 countries are now involved in its efforts to prepare, maintain and promote the accessibility of systematic reviews of the effects of healthcare interventions (www.cochrane.org). Through this work, the *Cochrane Database of Systematic Reviews (CDSR)* now contains the full text for more than 3000 Cochrane systematic reviews, with protocols for 1600 more that are in progress also published in *CDSR*, which is available in *The Cochrane Library* (www.thecochranelibrary.com). There are also several thousand other systematic reviews of the effects of healthcare interventions in the literature; as well as a small, but growing, number of systematic reviews of other aspects of health.

Question formulation and study identification for a systematic review

A systematic review would usually aim to identify and include all research relevant to the question for the review. This objective might be driven by a desire to provide as precise an estimate as possible of the relative effects of two treatments. But it might also be driven by a desire to bring together as much relevant research as possible so as to describe what has already been done, to help ensure that new research learns from the successes and failures of the past, and to identify gaps in the research base (Alderson & Roberts, 2000). Whichever type of review is to be done, the most important first step is the same as that for any research – decide upon the objectives and the questions to be tackled by the systematic review. This will have an impact on the inclusion and exclusion criteria for the review. These might be set out by describing the types of study design, participants, interventions and outcome measures that would be relevant.

When this has been decided, the systematic process for identifying relevant studies begins. Collecting all studies – irrespective of their results – will remove any biases that would be introduced if research with positive results, or which agrees most closely with the opinions and prejudices of the person doing the review, was sought preferentially over other research. Finding and using the results of all relevant studies will minimise chance effects by maximising the amount of data available for analysis and, hence, improve the precision of the estimate in the meta-analyses.

The ideal systematic review is one in which all the relevant studies have been identified before their results could influence decisions about their inclusion. This would overcome the problem of publication bias and of other biases where prior knowledge of the results of a study might influence the reviewer's decision on whether it should be included in her review. However, it needs to be remembered that systematic reviews are, by their nature, a form of retrospective research. The reviewers might already know of some of the potentially eligible studies, and their results. If the systematic review is transparent about the choices made when it was done and strived to find studies beyond those that were already known to the reviewer, users of their review can be more confident that its conduct was not overly influenced or biased by this prior knowledge.

The problem of publication bias makes the search for relevant studies especially difficult, and it will only be overcome through initiatives such as prospective registration of studies at inception (Dickersin et al., 1992). Publication bias usually arises because studies are more likely to be written up and published if they have statistically significant positive results. A more general rule is that whether or not a trial is published might be influenced by its results. This means that the results of published and unpublished trials might be systematically different. Therefore, unless all trials are sought regardless of their publication status, the systematic review may contain a biased set of studies. In such a case, regardless of the data collection and statistical methods used, a meta-analysis based on these studies may be mathematically precise but clinically wrong. Therefore, unpublished research and studies published only as abstracts or in journals that are difficult to obtain must be sought. This may require extensive searching of relevant bibliographic databases and of journals and conference proceedings (Hopewell et al., 2002), with attention also being given to strategies to find studies published in languages other than English (Pilkington et al., 2005).

The ease of finding randomised trials for systematic reviews has increased throughout the past decade. This is largely through the work of members of The Cochrane Collaboration who have hand searched journals and conference abstracts from cover to cover, looking for reports of randomised trials, and have conducted extensive electronic searching of bibliographic databases. In 1993, fewer than 20 000 reports of randomised trials could be found easily in MEDLINE, even though that database alone contained several tens of thousands more such reports. The Cochrane Collaboration's efforts to identify and make accessible information on reports of trials that might be suitable for inclusion in Cochrane reviews have led to the re-indexing of many of these reports in MEDLINE. Furthermore, the Collaboration, with coordination by the US Cochrane Center, built the *Cochrane Central Register of Controlled Trials* (*CENTRAL*) as a repository of records relating to controlled trials. These include records from MEDLINE and EMBASE and also tens of thousands of records that are in neither database. *CENTRAL* is, therefore, a unique resource for reviewers searching for randomised trials (Dickersin et al., 2002). Unfortunately, reviewers for whom other types of study would be eligible for their review are not so fortunate and still need to rely on their own extensive searches of databases, journals, conference proceedings, etc.

Appraising studies for inclusion in a systematic review

Assessing the eligibility of studies for a systematic review is a key step in determining that the studies meet the inclusion criteria and are of appropriate quality. Many tools are available for assessing the quality of randomised trials but caution is needed in using these. As Juni and colleagues have shown, different quality instruments can give widely different findings (Juni et al., 1999). Rather, it may be preferable for the reviewers to decide upon the key aspects of quality for studies in their review and then to appraise and describe each study on this basis. In randomised trials, these aspects might relate to the generation and concealment of the randomisation schedule, blinding or masking of the interventions, and loss to follow-up. Tools and means to assess the quality of non-randomised trials have also been developed, and some of these have been identified as particularly suitable for use in systematic reviews (Deeks et al., 2003). The distinction between being able to assess the quality of a report, rather than the quality of the underlying study, also needs to be kept in mind (Soares et al., 2004).

Whichever technique is used to assess the quality of the studies in the review, reviewers should also consider how they will use their conclusions about study quality in their review (Detsky et al., 1992). For example, if a systematic review is designed to generate as reliable an estimate as possible of the effects of an intervention, poor-quality studies might be excluded from this calculation. Whereas, if the review seeks to map out what is good and bad about prior research, the inclusion of poor-quality studies would add to the richness of this discussion.

Collection of data

Having decided on the studies that are eligible for the review, the reviewer then needs to gather together information and data on these studies. Even if there is no intention to do a meta-analysis, this information will help to highlight differences and similarities between the studies and will also make it easier to summarise each study and its findings in a standardised way. This should make it easier for the user of the review to compare and contrast these studies. The reviewer needs to decide how much or how little information to extract for each study, and what sources will be used if the published reports contain insufficient information (Clarke & Stewart, 1994). In compiling as complete a dataset as feasible and sensible, the principles of minimising systematic biases and chance effects must be applied. All relevant trials should be included in the meta-analysis and, if this is not possible, any trials that do not contribute data must not be so numerous or atypical that they introduce important bias to the result of the meta-analysis. If the results of a study have not been published or have only been published in part, the reviewer will need to contact the researchers responsible to try to obtain the necessary data. This can take time and there is no guarantee of success. However, without these data, there is a risk that publication bias will dominate the estimate obtained from the review and make it unreliable. Even if a study has been published in full, this is no guarantee that its results can be incorporated directly into a meta-analysis without additional information. For example, the reviewer might need to supplement the published data with extra detail on subgroups of participants, further follow-up or the re-inclusion of data from participants mistakenly excluded by the original researcher.

The results to be sought from the original researchers might be aggregate data (for example, by asking them to fill in a table), or data at the level of individual participants. Collection of data from the researchers might make the dataset available for the review more complete, up-to-date and accurate than anything that has been published. It should also facilitate the conduct of standardised analyses across the studies. The collection of individual patient data will provide much greater flexibility for the analyses and, if done in a collaborative way with full participation from the original researchers, such reviews might also benefit from a more rounded interpretation and endorsement of the findings (Stewart & Clarke, 1995).

Statistical analysis

A variety of techniques for combining results from separate studies in meta-analyses are available to the reviewer (Cooper & Rosenthal, 1980; Deeks,

2002). The overriding principle should be that each study is analysed separately and the overall result for the review comes from combining these results from the individual statistics. In this way, participants in one study are only directly compared with others in the same study. By showing the results of the meta-analysis as a forest plot, the relative contribution of each study can be clearly seen, and exploration of differences among the results of studies are made easier (Lewis & Clarke, 2001; Glasziou & Sanders, 2002; Higgins et al., 2003).

In planning and conducting statistical analyses for any review, careful consideration needs to be given to subgroup analyses. One of the rationales for doing a systematic review is to bring together more data than are available for any individual study and it is then tempting to break these data apart again into new subgroups. Caution is needed when doing this because of the possibility that spurious, chance results will be obtained; which will be misinterpreted as being of importance in making decisions about health care (Counsell et al., 1994; Clarke & Halsey, 2001).

Even if there is an a priori reason to expect a subgroup analysis to show something different to the overall result, this is no guarantee that a statistically significant difference is reliable clinically. This is because the more analyses are done, the more likely it is that statistically significant results will be found, even when there is truly no difference between the subgroups. Subgroup analyses in a systematic review should be regarded as a way of showing that the direction of effect is the same across different types of patient or as a generator of a hypothesis for testing in future research. Regardless of whether subgroup analyses are done, it is often more reliable to assume that the overall result is as good, if not a better, estimate of the relative effects of treatments in the particular type of patient than that obtained by looking at the results for just these types of patient in the review. This is because the effect of chance will be smaller for the overall result than it would be on the result in any subgroup.

Systematic reviews might also include sensitivity analyses, which ideally should also be planned in advance. A sensitivity analysis is used to determine how sensitive the results of the systematic review are to the decisions that the reviewer took about how the review was done. They are particularly useful where there is uncertainty about the choices that a reviewer needs to make. For example, sensitivity analyses could be used to determine the effect of including studies published in languages other than English, of using data from studies assessed to be of poor quality or of choosing one statistical technique over another.

Updating systematic reviews

The intention for Cochrane reviews is that these will be updated at least every 2 years or would be annotated to explain why this has not been done. This desire to keep reviews up to date reflects the fact that they are retrospective research seeking to influence current decisions. Thus, the ideal is that the review includes all relevant research available at the time that it is being used to inform a decision. This is clearly impractical without a process for continually updating reviews as new evidence emerges. Instead, mechanisms for periodic updating are needed, in which new research is sought, appraised and added to the review, if appropriate. The updating process might also serve to maintain the contemporary relevance of the review. This may be especially important if the review uses information that changes over time, such as economic costs, the organisational structures for delivering health care or the processes by which decisions are made about health care.

Appraising and using systematic reviews

Before using a systematic review, those factors that are most important when doing one can be considered in order to assess whether the review is fit for purpose. In some cases, the published review might not contain sufficient information to allow it to be appraised fully but, by bearing these issues in mind, the user of a review should be able to identify whether caution needs to be exercised in its interpretation. One particular reason for the need for caution in interpreting systematic reviews is, as noted above, their retrospective nature. They all rely on factors that are quite often out of the control of the reviewers, since they depend on the research done by other people, in other places and at other times.

The foremost of the potential difficulties is that the review is only possible if the appropriate research has been done. Even if there is a wide consensus that a particular question needs to be addressed in a systematic review, the findings of such a review will be dependent on whether, at some time in the past, other researchers felt likewise and actually did the studies (Alderson & Roberts, 2000). If the studies have been done, then the reviewer would ideally hope to find all of these and to be able to include information and data from them in the review, but this will not always be achievable.

Conclusion

Decisions about health care should be based on the best available evidence. This evidence should be of sufficient quality to be fit for purpose. The evidence needs to be robust against the effects of bias and chance. Systematic reviews, in which as much as possible of the relevant research is sought, appraised, summarised and, if appropriate, meta-analysed, provide the best way to ensure that the necessary evidence is available to people at the time they are making decisions (Tharyan et al., 2005). However, as with all scientific research, whether or not the relevant systematic reviews are available and whether studies are available for these will depend upon the prioritisation of the studies and of the reviews (Chinnock et al., 2005).

References

Alderson, P. & Roberts, I. (2000) Should journals publish systematic reviews that find no evidence to guide practice? Examples from injury research. *British Medical Journal*, 320, 376–7.

Chalmers, I. (1993) The Cochrane Collaboration: preparing, maintaining, and disseminating systematic reviews of the effects of health care. *Annals of the New York Academy of Sciences*, 703, 156–65.

Chinnock, P., Siegfried, N. & Clarke, M. (2005) Is evidence-based medicine relevant to the developing world? Systematic reviews have yet to achieve their potential as a resource for practitioners in developing countries. *PLoS Medicine*, 2 (5), 367–9.

Clarke, M. (2004) Doing new research? Don't forget the old: nobody should do a trial without reviewing what is known. *PLoS Medicine*, 1, 100–2.

Clarke, M. & Halsey, J. (2001) DICE 2: a further investigation of the effects of chance in life, death and subgroup analyses. *International Journal of Clinical Practice*, 55, 240–2.

Clarke, M.J. & Stewart, L.A. (1994) Systematic Reviews: Obtaining data from randomised controlled trials: how much do we need for reliable and informative meta-analyses? *British Medical Journal*, 309, 1007–10.

Cooper, H.M. & Rosenthal, R. (1980) Statistical versus traditional procedures for summarizing research findings. *Psychological Bulletin*, 87, 442–9.

Counsell, C.E., Clarke, M.J., Slattery, J. & Sandercock, P.A.G. (1994) The miracle of DICE therapy for acute stroke: fact or fictional product of subgroup analysis? *Britsh Medical Journal*, 309, 1677–81.

Deeks, J.J. (2002) Issues in the selection of a summary statistic for meta-analysis of clinical trials with binary outcomes. *Statistics in Medicine*, 21, 1575–600.

Deeks, J.J., Dinnes, J., D'Amico, R. et al. (2003) Evaluating non-randomised intervention studies. *Health Technology Assessment*, 7 (27), 1–183.

Detsky, A.S., Naylor, C.D., O'Rourke, K., McGeer, A.J. & L'Abbe, K.A. (1992) Incorporating variations in the quality of individual randomized trials into metaanalysis. *Journal of Clinical Epidemiology*, 45, 255–65.

Dickersin, K., Min, Y.I. & Meinert, C.L. (1992) Factors influencing publication of research results. Follow-up of applications submitted to two institutional review boards. *Journal of the American Medical Association*, 267, 374–8.

Dickersin, K., Manheimer, E., Wieland, S., Robinson, K.A., Lefebvre, C. & McDonald, S. (2002) Development of the Cochrane Collaboration's CENTRAL Register of controlled clinical trials. *Evaluation and the Health Professions*, 25, 38–64.

Glasziou, P.P. & Sanders, S.L. (2002) Investigating causes of heterogeneity in systematic reviews. *Statistics in Medicine*, 21, 1503–11.

Higgins, J.P.T., Thompson, S.G., Deeks, J.J. & Altman, D.G. (2003) Measuring inconsistency in meta-analyses. *British Medical Journal*, 327, 557–60.

Hopewell, S., Clarke, M., Lusher, A., Lefebvre, C. & Westby, M. (2002) A comparison of handsearching versus MEDLINE searching to identify reports of randomized controlled trials. *Statistics in Medicine*, 21, 1625–34.

Juni, P., Witschi, A., Bloch, R. & Egger, M. (1999) The hazards of scoring the quality of clinical trials for meta-analysis. *Journal of the American Medical Association*, 282, 1054–60.

Lewis, S. & Clarke, M. (2001) Forest plots: trying to see the wood and the trees. *British Medical Journal*, 322, 1479–80.

Pilkington, K., Boshnakova, A., Clarke, M. & Richardson, J. (2005) 'No language restrictions' in database searches: what does this really mean? *Journal of Alternative and Complementary Medicine*, 11, 205–7.

Soares, H.P., Daniels, S., Kumar, A. et al.; Radiation Therapy Oncology Group (2004) Bad reporting does not mean bad methods for randomised trials: observational study of randomised controlled trials performed by the Radiation Therapy Oncology Group. *British Medical Journal*, 328, 22–4.

Stewart, L., Clarke, M., for the Cochrane Collaboration Working Group on meta-analyses using individual patient data (1995) Practical methodology of meta-analyses (overviews) using updated individual patient data. *Statistics in Medicine*, 14, 2057–9.

Tharyan, P., Clarke, M. & Green, S. (2005) How The Cochrane Collaboration is responding to the Asian Tsunami. *PLoS Medicine*, 2 (6), e169.

2

Key Stages and Considerations when Undertaking a Systematic Review: Bladder Training for the Management of Urinary Incontinence

Brenda Roe

Introduction

Systematic reviews are a valuable source of information and help policy makers and clinicians appraise the evidence on which to make decisions. This chapter deals with the systematic identification, appraisal and synthesis of quantitative evidence, notably that from randomised controlled trials (RCTs), and draws on the methods of the Cochrane Collaboration (Green & Higgins, 2005) and others (CRD, 2001; Egger & Davey Smith, 2005), using a systematic review of bladder training for the management of urinary incontinence in adults (Wallace et al., 2004) by way of illustration.

Systematic reviews follow a strict protocol to ensure that as many of the research studies as possible have been considered and original primary studies or trials and papers arising from them are appraised and synthesised in a valid way. The purpose of these systematic methods of review is to minimise bias, provide transparency and enable replication (CRD, 2006). More than one reviewer is involved in independent study inclusion decisions, quality assessment and data extraction, with agreement and consensus reached to avoid individual bias.

Systematic reviews undertaken as part of the Cochrane Collaboration include RCTs, which are recognised as the 'gold standard'. Their reviews adopt an established format and are developed from an initial title and protocol, which are registered

with a relevant Cochrane Review Group (CRG). The key stages, procedures and policies are published in each of the CRG websites. Key aspects of Cochrane systematic reviews are that they involve consumers in their production, as well as undergoing scientific and statistical peer review, and are produced according to guidelines in the *Cochrane Handbook for Systematic Reviews of Interventions* (Green & Higgins, 2005). The reviews are published electronically in the Cochrane Library and are disseminated widely via the internet. All reviews are regularly updated.

The Cochrane Incontinence Review Group was established in 1996 and can be accessed via the Cochrane Collaboration website (Grant et al., 2006a). The bladder training review was first published in 1998 (Roe et al., 1998), and two updates have been undertaken (Roe et al., 2000; Wallace et al., 2004). The bladder training review is referred to in this chapter by way of example, but all Cochrane systematic reviews follow the same format and provide an example of robust methods for systematically reviewing quantitative data from RCTs.

Guidelines for undertaking systematic reviews

Textbooks and chapters (Sindhu, 1998; Glasziou et al., 2001; Egger et al., 2005), as well as handbooks

(CRD, 2001; Green & Higgins, 2005), are available as guidance for undertaking a systematic review, and support is provided by Cochrane Review Groups across the globe (see Cochrane Collaboration website for contacts and locations).

Developing a protocol

Developing a protocol is the first step in undertaking a systematic review, as it is with any research endeavour or inquiry. Before a Cochrane systematic review can be undertaken a title needs to be registered and then a protocol developed according to specific criteria; the protocol is then published in the library, having been reviewed by a CRG (see Cochrane Library for examples of protocols). The Cochrane Collaboration runs workshops on 'How to develop a protocol', and these are available for anyone to attend. Irrespective of whether a systematic review is aimed at publication in an academic journal or the Cochrane Library, the protocol formulated needs to include the same considerations and steps (CRD, 2001; Egger & Davey Smith, 2005; Green & Higgins, 2005). According to Egger & Davey Smith (2005), the protocol needs to include seven steps, which relate to:

(1) the research question
(2) inclusion and exclusion criteria
(3) locating studies
(4) selecting studies
(5) assessing the quality of studies
(6) extracting the data
(7) potential analysis and presentation of results.

Steps (4)–(6) all require more than one reviewer to undertake independent assessment and extraction activities and make comparisons to reach agreement and consensus, as required by the systematic review methods of the Cochrane Collaboration to reduce individual bias (Green & Higgins 2005). The systematic review on *Bladder Training for the Management of Urinary Incontinence in Adults* (Wallace et al., 2004) had its protocol first published in 1997 (Roe et al., 1997). This included the background and justification, objectives and hypotheses to be tested, criteria for considering studies (types of studies, participants, interventions, outcome measures), search strategy for identification of studies, inclusion and exclusion criteria for studies, methods for assessment

of quality and appropriateness, data extraction, tables of comparisons and analysis.

The objectives and hypotheses tested for the bladder training review on urinary incontinence (whether defined by symptom classification or urodynamic study as indicated by the trialists) are explicit and are measurable (Wallace et al., 2004) (Box 2.1).

Literature searching

The search strategy for identifying relevant studies (trials) should be explicit and included in the methods of the systematic review. Search strategies for identifying controlled trials have developed over recent years, with terms to index RCTs being introduced into the bibliographic databases of MEDLINE and EMBASE. For this purpose, the Cochrane Collaboration examined around 300 000 MEDLINE and EMBASE titles and abstracts, which were then retagged as clinical trials if appropriate. Both databases were examined, as their overlap of journals was around 34% (Smith et al., 1992). The majority of journals in MEDLINE are published in the United States of America, while EMBASE has better coverage of European journals. The retagging of trials in these databases continues, supplemented by manual or hand searches of journals, conference proceedings, other sources and specialised databases. The results of retagging and hand searches have been included in The Cochrane Controlled Trials Register in the Cochrane Library, which includes over 250 000 trials and is the best single source of published studies. Searches of MEDLINE and EMBASE are still recommended, along with other specialised databases, conference abstracts, monographs and references in review articles. Hand searching is also recommended as part of the search strategy, as is identifying unpublished studies by contacting lead investigators in order to remove publication bias.

Each CRG has explicit search strategies and those for incontinence are available on the Cochrane Incontinence Review Group website (Grant et al., 2006a), and include electronic searches of the Cochrane Central Register of controlled trials (CENTRAL), MEDLINE and the Cumulative Index of Nursing and Allied Health Literature (CINAHL), and hand searching of journals and conference

Box 2.1   Objectives and hypotheses tested by the Cochrane review on bladder training for urinary incontinence in adults (reproduced from Wallace et al. (2004) with permission from J. Wiley & Sons, Chichester and Sheila Wallace).

Objectives

To assess the effects of bladder training on urinary incontinence, however the diagnosis is made.
   The following hypotheses were tested:

(1)   Bladder training is better than no bladder training for the management of urinary incontinence.
(2)   Bladder training is better than other treatments (such as conservative or pharmacological) for the management of urinary incontinence. This hypothesis will be tested by looking at the following comparisons:
  (a)   bladder training compared with anticholinergic drugs;
  (b)   bladder training compared with adrenergic agonist drugs;
  (c)   bladder training compared with other drugs (non-anticholinergic, non-adrenergic agonist drugs);
  (d)   bladder training compared with other behavioural /physical/psychological treatments;
  (e)   bladder training compared with surgical management;
  (f)   bladder training compared with medical devices;
  (g)   bladder training compared with other intervention.
(3)   Combining bladder training with another treatment (such as conservative or pharmacological) is better than the other treatment alone. This hypothesis will be tested by looking at the following comparisons:
  (a)   bladder training combined with pharmacological treatment compared with that of pharmacological treatment alone;
  (b)   bladder training combined with a non-pharmacological treatment compared with that of non-pharmacological treatment alone.

proceedings to identify published and unpublished trials. There is also an attempt to hand search journals that are not in English. Topic specific search terms for urinary incontinence were combined (with the Boolean operator AND) with the randomised controlled trials methodology terms. The revised CRG design methodology search strategy for randomised controlled trials in PubMed is shown in Box 2.2, while search terms specific to bladder training are given in Box 2.3. It is advisable when developing a search strategy to consider electronic and hand searching, and the Medical Subject Heading (MeSH) terms and keywords to be used.

   Initial development, testing and refinement are important unless 'standardised' searching according to Cochrane and a CRG are used. It is advisable to finalise the search strategy with a librarian or information scientist. The search strategy for identification of studies is a standard entry in all Cochrane reviews. For the bladder training review extra specific searches also included reference lists of relevant articles and contact with investigators for information on other possible trials that were

published or unpublished, and no year or language limits were set (Wallace et al., 2004).

Publication bias

Historically, there was a tendency for only trials that found statistically significant findings to be published (Sindhu, 1998). There is also evidence that authors from high-prestige organisations are more likely to have their studies published than those from lower-prestige organisations (Peters & Ceci, 1982; Egger et al., 2005). These publication policies can influence what studies are published and represent publication bias. Publication bias can threaten the validity of the meta-analysis within systematic reviews as not all results or findings are available or known about and can be compared, and this can distort the results. In order to reduce publication bias, every effort needs to be made to locate all trials on a particular subject when undertaking a systematic review. This can be addressed by hand searching or electronic searching of conference

---

Box 2.2   Cochrane highly sensitive search strategy for identifying reports of randomised controlled trials in PubMed (2005 revision) (source: Glanville et al., 2006, permission for reproduction granted by Carol Lefebvre of the Cochrane Collaboration and colleagues and the Medical Library Association).

1.   clinical trial [pt] need to explode in OVID as automatic in PubMed
2.   randomized [tiab]*
3.   placebo [tiab]
4.   dt [sh]*
5.   randomly [tiab]
6.   trial [tiab]
7.   groups [tiab]
8.   #1 OR #2 OR #3 OR #4 OR #5 OR #6 OR #7
9.   animals [mh]
10. humans [mh]
11. #9 NOT (#9 AND #10)
12. #8 NOT #11

*[pt] denotes Publication Type; [mh] denotes Medical Subject Heading (MeSH); [tiab] denotes a word in the title or abstract; [sh] denotes a subheading.
   Sets 9 to 11 of the strategy capture animal studies that are also not human studies, and allow these records to be safely excluded from the search, while returning records that are not indexed as either human or animal studies, as these may be relevant.

Box 2.3   Cochrane Incontinence Review Group keyword system search terms for bladder training for use in the Cochrane Central Register for Controlled Trials (CENTRAL) (reproduced with permission from Sheila Wallace, Search Coordinator for the Cochrane Incontinence Review Group).

Search terms for CENTRAL

Bladder NEAR/2 (train or retrain* or educat* or re-educat* or drill) in All Fields in The Cochrane Central Register of Controlled Trials (CENTRAL)

Key: * = truncation symbol; NEAR/2 = search for terms within two words of bladder.

---

proceedings, and contacting directly principal investigators and organisations known to fund work in the related area or that have an interest in the particular subject. Another way to address this is for all trials to be entered on a register when they commence. Registers have been set up and can be accessed via the Cochrane Collaboration's Register of Registers. Others can be accessed via the internet, such as the metaRegister of Controlled Trials published by *Current Science* (Lefebvre & Clarke, 2005).

Inclusion criteria

Explicit inclusion criteria for studies that are to be included in a systematic review are required at the start. However, decisions to include or exclude studies are to a certain extent subjective, despite having explicit criteria. Methods for undertaking systematic reviews recommend using two observers to check the eligibility of studies for inclusion, with discussion and consensus as to those that should be included. If agreement is not possible, then a third reviewer can also be involved (Egger & Davey Smith, 2005). Systematic reviews should involve more than one reviewer, which is a requirement for Cochrane reviews, and ideally reviewers should have a variety of multidisciplinary backgrounds and international perspectives.

In the bladder training review, inclusion criteria were pre-specified for types of studies, participants and interventions (Wallace et al., 2004). Studies included all randomised or quasi-randomised controlled trials that included bladder training for the treatment of urinary incontinence. Urinary incontinence was defined and diagnosed by the trialists either by symptom classification or by urodynamics. Subjects were all adult men and women with urinary incontinence, and the term adult was accepted as defined by the trialists. Studies that were eligible also had to include at least one trial group receiving bladder training, even if explicit descriptions of bladder training were not described. As long as the term 'bladder training' was stated, studies that fulfilled the above criteria were eligible. Bladder drill, bladder re-training and bladder re-education were accepted as being synonymous with bladder training. Studies were included if the following specific terms were not used but they comprised the intervention:

- Mandatory schedule or a self-schedule which increased the time interval between voids, as a minimum, and
- Participant education, and
- Positive reinforcement and follow-up

If the intervention was unclear, then trialists were contacted for clarification. No restrictions were set for where bladder training took place and this could include out-patient, in-patient or home settings, although these locations were not compared as to their effectiveness and nor was bladder training being undertaken by different healthcare professionals (Wallace et al., 2004).

Exclusion criteria

Studies excluded from a systematic review and the reasons why are also explicit and are published within individual reviews in the Cochrane Library. Exclusion criteria are also stated in advance in

the protocol and are adhered to. For instance, in relation to the bladder training review, studies that did not fulfil the above inclusion criteria were excluded. Those that also described bladder training as it related to the clamping or removal of urinary catheters were excluded. If trials did not include mention of a mandatory or self-schedule, they too were excluded. If an additional intervention was added to supplement bladder training, such as pelvic floor muscle exercise training (PFMT) compared to no treatment, 'usual care' or bladder training alone, these trials were also excluded as it is not possible to assess the direct effects of bladder training (Wallace et al., 2004). This illustrates the importance of having exclusion criteria as well as inclusion criteria for studies when undertaking a rigorous systematic review, and having a minimum of two reviewers or observers to assess which studies are included and excluded by consensus.

Quality assessment

Once studies have been selected for inclusion, an assessment is made about the quality of their design in relation to randomisation and blinding of subjects, people undertaking the intervention and those measuring outcomes. More than one reviewer should undertake assessment of the quality of each included study independently, with agreement reached by consensus. Although randomised controlled trials are the gold standard and provide the best evidence for efficacy of interventions, they are still vulnerable to bias. The quality of a trial can influence the effect size (Egger & Davey Smith, 2005). Inadequate concealment or blinding of randomisation and group allocation can lead to larger treatment effects. Treatment effects can be overestimated when 'intention to treat' analyses are not undertaken and subjects withdrawing or not adhering to the intervention are not included in the analysis. However, there is a divergent view within the Cochrane Collaboration that intention to treat analysis should only include those who received and completed the treatment and exclude those that withdrew (S. Wallace, personal communication). Based on the bladder training review, it is apparent that the older trials did not include sufficient detail of how random allocation was undertaken and whether concealment was achieved.

Also, 'intention to treat' analysis was rare, as were reasons for withdrawal from the study (see Wallace et al., 2004). While concealment of random allocation and treatment group are preferable, along with outcome assessment, it is not always possible with healthcare interventions to blind subjects, since they know what treatment they are receiving, as do the professionals administering the intervention, as is the case with bladder training. However, it may be possible to blind those people undertaking the outcomes assessment, and this needs to be borne in mind in future trial designs. The debate surrounding the assessment of methodological quality continues to evolve, as do designs and methods for trials (Egger & Davey Smith, 2005). Quality assessment checklists have been developed (see Figure 2.1 for the quality assessment checklist used in the bladder training review). Such checklists are useful for summarising information about quality assessment for the trials included in the systematic review and can provide description, but an overall quality score may not be so useful (Egger & Davey Smith, 2005). Techniques for blinding the reviewers as to the authors and locations of the trials they are assessing can be undertaken, but the effort to achieve this may outweigh the benefits.

ASSESSMENT OF QUALITY OF TRIAL METHODOLOGY FOR THE COCHRANE INCONTINENCE GROUP

TITLE:
FIRST AUTHOR:
JOURNAL:
YEAR:
VOLUME/NUMBER:
PAGES:

Name of review:

Name of reviewer:

To be completed by the reviewer

Is the study relevant to the above review?
Yes
No (please send it back to the editorial base – sorry!)

Is the study a randomised or quasi-randomised trial? (quasi-randomised = alternation, day of week, etc.)
Yes (include in study)
Unclear (seek author clarification)
No (reject but give reason in review)

Was there a clear description of inclusion and exclusion criteria?
Yes
No

1. Potential for selection bias at trial entry (quality of random allocation concealment)

A = Adequate
good attempt at concealment, method should not allow disclosure of
assignment (telephone, third-party involvement in allocation procedure, etc.)

B = Unclear
states random allocation but no description given

Figure 2.1   Quality assessment checklist used by the Cochrane Incontinence Review Group. Update June 2006. Source: Grant et al. (2006b), reproduced with permission from the Cochrane Incontinence Review Group.

C = Inadequate
definitely not concealed (open random numbers tables or quasi-randomised, e.g. day of week, date of birth, alternation) or an attempt at concealment but real chance of disclosure of assignment prior to formal entry (envelopes without third-party involvement, 'random numbers table' but procedure not described).

2. Potential for bias around time of treatment or during outcome assessment (blinding)

2.1 Were participants 'blind' to treatment status?
A = action taken to blind participants to treatment likely to be effective (e.g. placebo)
B = blinding stated but no description given
C = attempt at blinding participants to intervention but reason to think it may not have been successful (e.g. placebo smells different)
D = no mention of blinding
E = not blinded

2.2 Were healthcare providers 'blind' to treatment status?
A = action taken to blind healthcare providers to treatment likely to be effective (e.g. placebo)
B = blinding stated but no description given
C = attempt at blinding healthcare providers to intervention but reason to think it may not have been successful (e.g. placebo smells differently)
D = no mention of blinding
E = not blinded

2.3 Were outcome assessors 'blind' to treatment status?
A = action taken to blind outcome assessors as to treatment likely to be effective (e.g. placebo)
B = blinding stated but no description given
C = attempt at blinding outcome assessors to intervention but reason to think it may not have been successful (e.g. assessor involved in trial allocation or treatment)
D = no mention of blinding
E = not blinded

2.4 Were the groups treated identically other than for the named interventions?
Yes
Unclear
No

3. Potential for selection bias in analysis

3.1 Was there a description of withdrawals, dropouts and those lost to follow-up?
A = states numbers and reasons for withdrawals
B = states numbers of withdrawals only (no reason given)
C = states withdrawals but no number given
D = not mentioned

3.2 Was the analysis on intention to treat (or is it possible to do so on available data)? i.e.

A) Are results reported for everyone who entered the trial?
Yes
Unclear
No

B) Are participants analysed in the groups they were originally allocated to?
Yes
Unclear
No

If yes to both A and B intention to treat analysis has been performed.

Figure 2.1   *Continued*

Data extraction

Data from individual studies are extracted independently by two reviewers and agreement reached by consensus. A minimum of two reviewers is required to avoid errors. A standardised form can be used for this activity. As with any data collection this should be well-designed, piloted and revised if required. Figure 2.2 is an example of a data extraction form used for the bladder training review. Electronic forms can be developed and they have the advantage of combining data abstraction with data entry. They can also detect errors in data entry between observers, but their development and revision can involve a great deal of work (Egger & Davey Smith, 2005).

Interventions Group I: Bladder training. Referenced   Trial ref:
        Scheduled voiding:
        Participant education:
        Relaxation and distraction techniques:
        Self-monitoring or charting:
        Positive reinforcement:
        Other:
        Treatment duration:
        Bladder training provided by:
        Group II:
        Compliance
        Co-interventions:
Notes:
Allocation concealment code:
Participants
Number of participants randomised: Total =   ; Group I =   ; Group II =
Number of participants followed up: Total =   ; Group I =   ; Group II =
Gender:

Age: based on   , mean years (SD   ).
Inclusion criteria:

Exclusion criteria;
Diagnostic groups: n =   ; urge incontinence =   ; stress incontinence =   ; mixed incontinence =
Baseline measurement:
Baseline comparability:
Menopausal status:

Methods Design:
    Blinding:
    Setting – place:
    Setting – time:
    Intention to treat analysis
    Length of follow up:
      At end of treatment phase:
      At any other follow-up point months:
    Power calculation:
    Funding:

Figure 2.2   Data extraction form developed for the Cochrane Bladder Training Review (developed by, and reproduced with permission of, Sheila Wallace, Search Coordinator for the Cochrane Incontinence Review Group).

Outcomes

The outcomes of interest for a systematic review are pre-determined and form part of the protocol. Five primary outcomes were pre-specified for the bladder training review:

- Participant's perception of cure of urinary incontinence
- Participant's perception of improvement of urinary incontinence
- Number of incontinent episodes
- Number of micturitions, and
- Quality of life measures (QoL) (Wallace et al., 2004)

The outcomes were based on those suggested by the International Continence Society (Lose et al., 1998). Adverse events were also a pre-specified outcome, and secondary outcomes were captured by 'other outcomes'.

Perception of symptoms, cure or improvement were as reported by participants or as marked on a visual analogue scale. Quantification of symptoms was generally derived from a self-completed diary, ideally over 7 days. Health status measures related to QoL and could include the Severity of Incontinence Index score (slight, moderate and severe) (Sandvik et al., 1993); impact of incontinence, such as the Incontinence Impact Questionnaire (IIQ); the Urogenital Distress Inventory (UDI) (Shumaker et al., 1994); psychological measures, such as the Crown Crisp Experiential Index (1979) (Crown & Crisp, 1979); and general health status, for example the Short Form (SF36) (Ware, 1993). Adverse events that were reported could also be documented, along with health economics matters, such as the costs of intervention or resource use, and 'other outcomes' not pre-specified but judged important (Wallace et al., 2004). Figure 2.3 provides an example of the outcomes data extraction form developed for the bladder training review. If there are more than two intervention groups in a study, then additional columns can be introduced on the right-hand side. Data from the initial treatment and subsequent follow-ups can also be captured. As part of good methods, two reviewers extract the outcome data independently and then reach agreement by consensus.

Methods of the review

Once all the data have been extracted and agreed, then writing the text can begin; this includes 'Characteristics of Included Studies' (see Figure 2.4 for headings). For systematic reviews that are ultimately published in the Cochrane Library, then Review Manager software is used to undertake this (see Cochrane Collaboration website, Review Manager Software RevMan 4.2.8). This is useful software for undertaking systematic reviews but it is not essential to use it if the review is not being published in the Cochrane Library. It is, however, useful because it is 'tried and tested' and is continually evolving and being maintained. Also, it can handle the table of comparisons for the outcome data and perform the statistical meta-analyses required if sufficient data are available.

The 'Methods of the Review' section includes information on the description of the studies, including settings and locations, participants, age, diagnosis, description of interventions and compliance or adherence. The 'Characteristics of Included Studies' table can then be described according to the groupings for each of the objectives or hypotheses being tested, for example using the following headings (see Wallace et al., 2004):

- *Bladder training compared with 'no treatment'*
- *Bladder training compared with anti-cholinergic drug treatment*
- *Bladder training compared with adrenergic agonist drug treatment*
- *Bladder training compared with other drugs (non-anticholinergic non-adrenergic agonist)*
- *Bladder training compared with other behavioural/physical/psychological interventions*
- *Bladder training plus pharmacological intervention compared with pharmacological intervention alone*
- *Bladder training plus non-pharmacological intervention compared with non-pharmacological interventions alone*

A section follows these on 'Description of Outcomes', where narrative summative descriptions are included but reference is made to individual trials. The 'Description of Outcomes' includes sections on all the pre-specified outcomes, along with adverse events and 'other' outcomes of importance. The Cochrane Library has a referencing system that cites one surname (that of the principal investigator

FU	Intervention Group 1			Intervention Group 2		
	1st	2nd	3rd	1st	2nd	3rd
Participants' perception of cure						
Participants' perception of improvement (includes cured and improved)						
Number of incontinent episodes per:..............						
Number of micturitions per:..............						
QoL instrument used:.............						
Other outcomes						

Figure 2.3   Outcomes data extraction form developed for the Cochrane Bladder Training Review (developed by, and reproduced with permission of, Sheila Wallace, Search Coordinator for the Cochrane Incontinence Review Group). FU, follow-up; QoL, quality of life.

Study	Methods	Participants	Interventions	Outcomes	Notes
Colombo 1995					
Dougherty 1998					
Fantl 1991					
etc.					

Figure 2.4   Headings used in the Cochrane Systematic Review table of Characteristics of Included Studies (see Wallace et al., 2004, 'Characteristics of Included Studies' for further details).

for the trial whenever first published) and the date (e.g. Fantl, 1991; Jarvis, 1980); however, in the reference section all names of investigators are cited according to referencing convention and alphabetical order (see Green & Higgins, 2005). This format allows for the fact there may be a number of publications arising from a trial which are tagged to the original trial publication (see Box 2.4).

Box 2.4   Example of the referencing system used in Cochrane systematic reviews.

Fantl 1991

Fantl A., Wyman JF., McCLish DK., Harkins SW., Elswick RK., Taylor JR et al. Efficacy of bladder training in older women
    with urinary incontinence. Journal of the American Medical Association 1991; 265(5) 609–613.
Fantl JA., Wyman JF, Harkins SW & Taylor JR. Bladder training in women with urinary incontinence (Abstract). Neuro-
    urology and Urodynamics 1988; 7(3) 276–277.
McLish DK., Fantl JA, Wyman JF., Pisani G & Bump RC. Bladder training in older women with urinary incontinence: relation-
    ship between outcome and changes in urodynamic observations. Obstetrics and Gynecology 1991; 77(2) 281–286.
Wyman JF., Fantl JA., McClish DK., Harkins SW, Uebersax JS & Ory MG. Quality of life following bladder training in older
    women with urinary incontinence. International Urogynecology Journal 1997; 8(40) 223–229.
Wyman JF., McClish DK., Ory MG & Fantl JA. Changes in quality of life following bladder training in older women with
    urinary incontinence (Abstract). Neurourology and Urodynamics 1992;11(40) 426–427.

Jarvis 1981

Jarvis GJ. A controlled trial of bladder drill and drug therapy in the management of detrusor instability. British Journal of
    Urology 1981; 53(6) 565–566.
Jarvis GJ. The unstable bladder – a psychosomatic disease? (Abstract) Proceedings of the International Continence Society
    (ICS), 11th Annual Meeting; 1981; 45–46.

A section on 'Methodological Quality of Included
Studies' follows, with summative narrative on:

- *Quality of allocation concealment;*
- *Stratification/minimisation;*
- *Blinding;*
- *Intention to treat analysis;*
- *Length of follow up;*
- *Withdrawal/drop outs to follow with reasons why;*
- *Follow up beyond the treatment phase;*
- *Baseline measurement and comparability;*
- *Other aspects of trial designs.*

Characteristics of excluded studies are also
included in a table, along with a description of why
the studies were excluded.

Results

Presentation, combining and interpretation

Once all data have been extracted this information
is entered into a tabular format (see Figure 2.4) so
that comparison across studies can be undertaken,
and descriptive summative text is written in which
results are combined and interpreted. This comprises the 'Results' section of the systematic review
(see 'Results section', Wallace et al., 2004). Once

again, the layout can conform to the headings which
comprise each of the hypotheses being tested and
objectives (see above).

Tables of comparisons

The tables of comparisons for data are standardised
and systematically compare data available for all
studies that are 'pooled', compared and analysed
for each objective or hypothesis under test (7 at
this level), for each of the pre-specified and other
outcomes (a further 7 at this next level down)
subdivided again. In the example of the bladder
training review (Wallace et al., 2004), this was done
according to type of incontinence – urge, stress,
mixed and other, where other is two or more types
combined (a further 4 comparisons at this lowest
level). This gives the potential for comparison of
data in 196 instances, and can make for extremely
long tables of comparison. They are, however, systematic as well as comprehensive.

Standardised outcome measure and combined effect estimate

The data extraction and outcome measures are
standardised across all of the studies, which allows

comparisons to be made. Where the endpoint of outcomes is in binary format (for example, incontinent versus cured/not incontinent; or improved versus not improved), then relative risks (RR) or odds ratios (OR) can be calculated. OR allows combination of data to establish the overall effect in terms of statistical significance. The OR and RR may differ where the outcome is common (see Egger & Davey Smith, 2005). Where outcomes are continuous and measurements are from a scale, then mean differences between treatment groups and control are used. Data are displayed graphically using a 'forest plot', so that data are presented either side of a mid-line which indicates the direction of effect either positively or negatively. This graphical display allows quick and easy reference to see whether the outcomes from treatment or intervention from individual studies are favourable or effective when compared to the outcomes for the control (Egger & Davey Smith, 2005).

Meta-analysis

Meta-analysis is the last step in analysing data from studies and consists of estimating an overall effect by combining or pooling all the data for each outcome from all of the individual studies. Often there is insufficient or varying data from studies to be able to do this. Tests for statistical homogeneity have to be applied for individual study results to see if they reflect a single underlying effect, in which case a meta-analysis may be indicated. It is beyond the scope of this chapter to go into such statistical details but further reading is available (Deeks et al., 2005; Deeks & Altman, 2005; Egger & Davey Smith, 2005; Thompson, 2005).

In the bladder training review, RR could be calculated for some of the outcome data but there was insufficient data for meta-analysis. There were only 10 trials, which were predominantly small, with only 1366 subjects included (Wallace et al., 2004).

Writing up a systematic review

As with any research study, a systematic review is written up according to the recognised convention with headings and subheadings for the introduction and background, methods, results, discussion and conclusion. All systematic reviews published in the Cochrane Library have adopted a consistent format. The results and findings of the review are discussed and the reviewers' conclusions are presented on the implications for practice and further research.

In the case of the bladder training review on implications for practice, the evidence was inconclusive in terms of judging the short- and long-term effects; however, results from the trials reviewed, although having too few data for reliability, appeared to favour bladder training (Wallace et al., 2004). Data were too few to make choices among bladder training, drug treatment or other conservative therapies, or whether adding bladder training to any of these other treatments was of benefit. Trials were small and of variable quality. It was also not possible to assess the magnitude of resource implications.

Conclusions for the design of future research were also included and related to larger, more fully reported trials with long-term follow-up so that the benefits of bladder training for the management of urinary incontinence can be reliably determined. Some of the trials included people with symptoms of an overactive bladder but who were not incontinent, and it was recommended that future trials specific to the management of overactive bladder are warranted. The benefits of bladder training alone or in conjunction with other treatments, drugs in particular, are also warranted (Wallace et al., 2004).

Within the write-up of the review, acknowledgement is made of additional people and organisations who have been involved or have provided assistance, as are any sources of funding received and potential conflict of interest. Such an approach assures transparency and demonstrates adherence to research governance.

Finally, at the beginning of the review a synopsis is provided which can be considered as an abstract, along with the comment or view of a consumer; this is usually a comment from a lay person or member of the public, so that the meaning and interpretation can be communicated as widely as possible. Individual consumer and consumer organisation views on systematic reviews are obtained at the protocol development stage, particularly on whether the outcomes assessed are relevant, and again once the review is completed.

Dissemination of systematic reviews

Systematic reviews undertaken on behalf of the Cochrane Collaboration are disseminated electronically, via the Cochrane Library. Systematic reviews are also published as reports and as papers in academic journals. A requirement of the Cochrane Collaboration is that systematic reviews are regularly updated. This has been the case for the bladder training review, which has been updated twice since it was first published, with an additional lead reviewer to the original review team; it is in the process of being updated again (Roe et al., 1998, 2000; Wallace et al., 2004). Updating of reviews does have resource implications, which is a factor that needs consideration not only by reviewers but also funding organisations. Updating existing reviews contributes to the continued development of the body of knowledge and evidence on which nurses and healthcare professionals can base their practice.

Conclusion

The methods for undertaking systematic reviews of randomised controlled trials, in particular, are well established and continue being developed. Key stages and considerations for undertaking a systematic review have been presented in this chapter. Systematic reviews can provide the evidence on which to base practice, as well as making recommendations for future research. Systematic reviews of randomised controlled trials and meta-analyses can, where data are available, provide robust evidence for effectiveness and 'cause and effect'. Systematic reviews as a research design and method may be an end in their own right; however, the skills and techniques required can also be used for reviewing the research evidence in projects that go on to answer other research questions or undertake interventions.

References

CRD (2001) *Undertaking Systematic Reviews of Research on Effectiveness*. CRD Report 4 (2nd edition). Centre for Reviews and Dissemination, University of York. http://www.york.ac.uk/isnt/crd/report4.htm (accessed 5 April 2006).

CRD (2006) *What is a systematic review and how is it different from a literature review?* Centre for Reviews and Dissemination, University of York. http://www.york.ac.uk/inst/crd/faq1.htm (accessed 5 April 2006).

Crown, S. & Crisp, A.H. (1979) *Crown-Crisp Experiential Index*. Hodder and Stoughton Educational, London.

Deeks, J.J. & Altman, D.G. (2005) Effect measures for meta-analysis of trials with binary outcomes. In: *Systematic Reviews in Health Care. Meta-Analysis in Context* (Egger, M., Davey Smith, G. & Altman, D.G., eds), pp. 313–35. BMJ Publishing. London.

Deeks, J.J., Altman, D.G. & Bradburn, M.J. (2005) Statistical methods for examining heterogeneity and combining results from several studies in meta-analysis. In: *Systematic Reviews in Health Care. Meta-Analysis in Context* (Egger, M., Davey Smith, G. & Altman, D.G., eds), pp. 285–312. BMJ Publishing, London.

Egger, M. & Davey Smith, G. (2005) Principles and procedures for systematic reviews. In: *Systematic Reviews in Health Care. Meta-Analysis in Context* (Egger, M., Davey Smith, G. & Altman, D.G., eds), pp. 23–42. BMJ Publishing, London.

Egger, M., Davey Smith, G. & Altman, D.G. (eds) (2005) *Systematic Reviews in Health Care. Meta-Analysis in Context*. BMJ Publishing, London.

Glanville, J.M., Lefebvre, C., Miles, J.N. & Camosso-Stefinovic, J. (2006) How to identify randomised controlled trials in MEDLINE: ten years on. *Journal of the Medical Library Association*, 94 (2), 130–6 (erratum: Figure 2 (p. 135) should be replaced by figure in erratum *Journal of the Medical Library Association*, 94(3), 354).

Glasziou, P., Irwig, L., Bain, C. & Colditz, G. (2001) *Systematic Reviews in Health Care. A Practical Guide*. Cambridge University Press, Cambridge.

Grant, A.M., Cody, D.J., Glazener, C.M.A., et al. (eds) (2006a) Incontinence Group. About The Cochrane Collaboration (Cochrane Review Groups (CRGs)) 2000, Issue 4. http://www.mrw.interscience.wiley.com/cochrane/clabout/articles/INCONT/frame.html (accessed 2 May 2006).

Grant, A.M., Cody, D.J., Glazener, C.M.A., et al. (eds) (2006b) Additional Information. Assessment of Quality of Trial Methodology for the Cochrane Incontinence Group. Incontinence Group. About The Cochrane Collaboration (Cochrane Review Groups (CRGs)) 2000, Issue 4. http://www.mrw.interscience.wiley.com/cochrane/clabout/articles/INCONT/frame.html (accessed 26 April 2006).

Green, S. & Higgins, J. (eds) (2005) Cochrane Handbook for Systematic Reviews of Interventions 4.2.5. (updated May 2005). http://www.cochrane.dk/cochrane/handbook/handbook.htm (accessed 26 April 2006).

Lefebvre, C. & Clarke, M.J. (2005) Identifying randomised controlled trials. In: *Systematic Reviews in Health Care.*

Meta-Analysis in Context (Egger, M., Davey Smith, G. & Altman, D.G. eds), pp. 69–86. BMJ Publishing, London.

Lose, G., Fantl, J.A., Victor, A., et al. (1998) Outcome measures for research in adult women with symptoms of lower urinary tract dysfunction. *Neurourology and Urodynamics*, 17, 255–62.

Peters, D. & Ceci, S. (1982) Peer-review practices of psychological journals. The fate of published articles, submitted again. *Behavioural and Brain Sciences*, 5, 187–225.

Roe, B., Williams, K. & Palmer, M. (1997) *Bladder Training for the Treatment of Urinary Urge Incontinence (Protocol)*. The Cochrane Library, Issue 3. Update Software, Oxford.

Roe, B., Williams, K. & Palmer, M. (1998) *Bladder Training for the Treatment of Urinary Urge Incontinence (Cochrane Review)*. The Cochrane Library, Issue 4. Update Software, Oxford.

Roe, B., Williams, K. & Palmer, M. (2000) *Bladder Training for the Treatment of Urinary Urge Incontinence (Cochrane Review Update)*. The Cochrane Library, Issue 1. Update Software, Oxford.

Sandvik, H., Hunskaar, S., Seim, A., Hermstead, R., Vanik, A. & Bratt, H. (1993) Validation of a severity index in female urinary incontinence and its implementation in an epidemiological survey. *Journal of Epidemiology and Community Health*, 47, 497–9.

Shumaker, S.A., Wyman, J.F., Uebersax, J.S., McClish, D. & Fantl, J.A. (1994) Health related quality of life measures for women with urinary incontinence: the Incontinence Impact Questionnaire and the Urogenital Distress Inventory. *Quality of Life Research*, 3, 291–306.

Sindhu, F. (1998) Meta-analyses and systematic reviews of the literature. In: *Research and Development in Clinical Nursing Practice* (Roe, B. & Webb, C., eds), pp. 84–111. Whurr Publishers, London.

Smith, B.J., Darzins, P.J., Quinn, M. & Heller, R.F. (1992) Modern methods of searching the medical literature. *Medical Journal of Australia*, 157, 603–11.

Thompson, S.G. (2005) Why and how sources of heterogeneity should be investigated. In: *Systematic Reviews in Health Care. Meta-analysis in Context* (Egger, M., Davey Smith, G. & Altman, D.G., eds), pp. 157–75. BMJ Publishing, London.

Wallace, S., Roe, B., Williams, K. & Palmer, M. (2004) *Bladder Training for Urinary Incontinence in Adults (Cochrane Review)*. The Cochrane Library, Issue 1. John Wiley & Sons Ltd, Chichester.

Ware, J.E. (1993) Measuring patients' view: the optimum outcome measure. SF36: a valid, reliable assessment of health from the patient's point of view. *British Medical Journal*, 306, 1429–30.

3 Prevention and Treatment of Urinary Incontinence after Stroke in Adults: Experiences from a Systematic Review for the Cochrane Collaboration

Lois Thomas and Beverley French

In this chapter, we describe our experiences of conducting a systematic review for the Cochrane Collaboration Incontinence Review Group (Thomas et al., 2005). Throughout the chapter, we highlight learning points and the more 'messy' features of systematic reviewing which are often not obvious from reading published reviews or methodological literature on systematic reviewing. We begin the chapter with an overview of the origins and the content of the review, followed by an examination of each stage of the review process.

Introduction

The incidence and prevalence of urinary incontinence after stroke is high, affecting 40–60% of people admitted to hospital after a stroke, with 25% still having problems on hospital discharge and around 15% remaining incontinent at 1 year (Barrett, 2001). One of the review collaborators, L.T., was particularly interested in the role health professionals play in helping overcome the potentially numerous effects of stroke impacting on patients' continence status, such as limb weakness and communication problems. Anecdotal evidence suggests that helping patients to retain or regain continence is not top of the list of competing priorities with this patient group, and guidance

regarding best practice was, at the time the review was instigated, too vague to guide practice (Royal College of Physicians, 2000). While stroke care in general has risen up the policy, research and practice agendas in recent years, fuelled by the Stroke Trialists' Collaboration's seminal review of stroke units (2001), our perception was that the management of continence has remained relatively under-researched and overlooked. To begin moving continence after stroke up the agenda, a group of national experts with an interest in continence and stroke was convened, one of whom (Professor Adrian Grant) was the coordinating editor of the Cochrane Incontinence Review Group. The group were in agreement that the ideal foundation for future research would be a systematic review of the evidence so far, echoing the view of Clarke and Langhorne (2001) that systematic reviews 'should precede and conclude the design and conduct of all new studies'.

Overview of the review

Objectives

The objective of the review was to determine the optimal methods for prevention and treatment of urinary incontinence after stroke in adults.

Search strategy

We searched the Cochrane Incontinence and Stroke Groups specialised registers (searched 15 December 2004 and 26 October 2004, respectively), the Cumulative Index of Nursing and Allied Health Literature (CINAHL) (January 1982 to November 2004), national and international trial databases for unpublished data, and the reference lists of relevant articles.

Selection criteria

Randomised or quasi-randomised controlled trials evaluating the effects of interventions designed to promote continence in people after stroke.

Data collection and analysis

Data extraction and quality assessment were undertaken by two reviewers working independently. Disagreements were resolved by a third reviewer.

Main results

Seven trials with a total of 399 participants were included in the review. Participants were from a mixture of settings, age groups and phases of stroke recovery. No two trials addressed the same comparison.

Four trials tested an intervention against usual care, including acupuncture, timed voiding, and two types of specialist professional intervention. One cross-over trial tested an intervention (oestrogen) against placebo (Judge, 1969). One trial tested a specific intervention (oxybutynin) against another intervention (timed voiding) (Gelber & Swords, 1997a), and one trial tested a combined intervention (sensory–motor biofeedback plus timed voiding) against a single-component intervention (timed voiding alone) (Gelber & Swords, 1997b).

Reported data were insufficient to evaluate acupuncture or timed voiding versus usual care, oxybutynin versus timed voiding, or sensory-motor biofeedback plus timed voiding versus usual care. Evidence from a single small trial (Wikander et al., 1998) suggested that structured assessment and management of care in early rehabilitation may reduce the number of people with incontinence at hospital discharge (1/21 versus 10/13; relative risk (RR) 0.06, 95% confidence interval (CI) 0.01 to 0.43), and have other benefits. Evidence from another trial (Brittain & Potter, 2000) suggested that assessment and management of care by continence nurse practitioners in a community setting may reduce the number of urinary symptoms (48/89 versus 38/54; RR 0.77, 95% CI 0.59 to 0.99) and increase satisfaction with care.

Reviewers' conclusions

There was evidence to suggest that specialist professional input through structured assessment and management of care and specialist continence nursing may reduce urinary incontinence after stroke. Data from trials of other physical, behavioural, complementary and anticholinergic drug interventions are insufficient to guide continence care of adults after stroke.

Issues that arose when carrying out the review

Designing the review protocol – early decisions

Type of review There is a difference between scoping (or 'fishing') reviews which collate existing material relating to all interventions, and reviews of the effectiveness of a single intervention, for example habit retraining (Ostaszkiewicz et al., 2004) or prompted voiding (Eustice et al., 2000; Higgins & Green, 2005). Our decision to undertake the former was influenced by our perception, based on our knowledge of the literature and evidence from practice (for example from the North West Stroke Task Force), that the evidence base was small: while several interventions had been tested with stroke patients, we considered that a review focusing on particular interventions would be unlikely to yield many studies for inclusion.

Type of intervention There is a difference between the prevention and management of incontinence, and the promotion of continence. We stated in our protocol for the Cochrane Collaboration that one arm of the trial must include an intervention to promote continence; however, during the review there were disagreements about whether the primary intention of some interventions was to promote continence specifically, or independence more generally. For example, the trial by Wikander et al. (1998) evaluates the effectiveness of structured assessment and management of care. While this trial has measurement of continence as a primary outcome, one reviewer argued that the intervention was not specific and should not be included. Two other reviewers disagreed, so the decision was taken to include it in the review.

Type of client   We planned to exclude trials of interventions for conditions causing urinary incontinence unrelated to stroke (e.g. prostatectomy), or trials where patients were incontinent prior to the stroke. However, this proved difficult to determine in practice, as studies frequently did not report whether patients did have pre-existing continence problems. For example, the largest trial testing the effectiveness of a nurse practitioner in the community (Brittain & Potter, 2000) did not differentiate between patients who did and did not have urinary incontinence prior to stroke. Some trials tested interventions for specific conditions, for example pelvic floor muscle weakness in women after stroke (Tibaek et al., 2004), but whether the incontinence was related to or the result of stroke is a moot point.

Furthermore, we initially planned to include only studies where patients had had a stroke within the past 12 months, as this is the time when there is most potential for improvement (Jorgensen et al., 1995). This plan was abandoned, as studies often did not report time since stroke.

Type of outcome: definition of incontinence   We started with the definition of incontinence specified by the International Continence Society (Abrams et al., 1988), but we then came across a study that used a broader but much more specific definition of incontinence, encompassing the symptoms of urinary incontinence such as urgency and nocturia (Brittain & Potter, 2000).

Type of outcome: specification of continence as primary outcome   A number of studies that tested interventions were excluded because they measured proxy or intermediate outcomes, for example residual volumes of urine. In reality, interventions in stroke in clinical practice are sequential and time-related and happen in a cascade towards the final outcome. Some trials might offer useful information about safety (e.g. of catheter removal) or about usefulness of assessment (e.g. bladder scanning), which were not included in our review.

Learning points

A scoping review provides different information to a review of the effectiveness of a single intervention. This type of review tells us what kind of interventions have been tested, with what client groups and in which settings. We only found single trials for each of the different types of intervention, and a whole range of types of intervention, for example pharmacological, physical, behavioural and environmental. There is usually not enough evidence in this type of review to suggest best practice, but reviews of this type are useful for identifying which interventions may justify further research. It is important also to look carefully at the definitions, inclusions and exclusions when relating review findings to your own clinical practice: all reviews have parameters and it is important not to assume the review covers everything.

Designing a search

Once the protocol has gone through the peer review process, the Cochrane review group administrators provide reviewers with all the randomised controlled trials on the topic that they have already collated. The Cochrane Collaboration argue that providing this information *before* the protocol is written may bias decisions made at this stage and may lead to available trials dictating the review question, rather than choosing a question that is clinically relevant. Each review group maintains their own searches and specialised registers of trials in their topic, and the extent of the coverage depends on how long the review group has been going, and its focus. Our topic tapped into two different review groups. The search developed by the Stroke Review Group is extensive and covers a large range of sources, while the Continence Review Group search is newer and less extensive.

Box 3.1   Some of the descriptors in the Cumulative Index of Nursing and Allied Health Literature (CINAHL) for catheterisation, which were added for searching.

- Catheters Urinary
- Catheter Care Urinary
- Urinary Catheterisation
- Urinary Bladder Irrigation
- Catheter Irrigation Urinary
- Incontinence Aids

In theory, relying on both together should have been more than adequate, but we made the decision to do some extra searching in addition to Cochrane because nursing databases, topics and studies may not be as well indexed – both in terms of the nursing slant and the study type. Both of these issues were pertinent to our review.

- The Cochrane search strategy for incontinence is very comprehensive (at 162 lines long!), but it is shaped mainly by the more medically driven interventions and outcomes. Catheterisation, more nursing driven, was not covered. Box 3.1 illustrates some of the descriptors in CINAHL for catheterisation, which were added for searching. No new randomised controlled trials were identified through this searching, but it did identify other types of studies and facilitated contacts with other researchers.
- We also chose to do some searching on databases less specific to health care, e.g. Web of Knowledge (covering the science and social science literatures), which is not yet included in the Continence Review Group search strategy. We used a broad search without the filters for randomised controlled trial study type used by Cochrane (Higgins & Green, 2005). This identified one new trial which was not indexed on MEDLINE and had nothing in the keywords to indicate that it was a trial. Our policy was to retrieve all studies, which could not be excluded by title and abstract, and this trial was only identified as such after retrieval.

Once a search had been built for CINAHL, it was sent to the Cochrane search coordinator for checking. She identified a small mistake of syntax on a crucial line way down in the search, which made the end results of the search more or less invalid!

It is important, therefore, to validate searches, and in nursing to search less specifically but more widely. The normal Cochrane search strategy of highly sensitive searching resulting in large numbers of references, with the number then made manageable by the addition of filters for study type, may need to be adapted for nursing-related topics.

Learning points

Clinicians may not have the skills to check a search, but they will be able to see if keywords they know about are included, and to look at how searches have been checked. It is important not to assume that the searches are right, and readers are urged to inform the reviewers if they know about relevant studies that have been missed.

Retrieval of potential studies for inclusion

This stage sounds easy – but it is not necessarily so.

- Eighteen studies only came in the form of an abstract with not enough detail to assess eligibility; therefore we needed to trace the authors. This involved tracking down the authors' contact details, which for some studies were not given in the database. There followed a great deal of internet searching, emailing, letter writing, and phone calls at odd hours of the day, which was very time consuming and needed some creative thinking. For example, to trace the authors of a Korean study, we contacted the Korean Nurses Association. We had to do this in English, and hope that someone there could speak English. Luckily, they did.
- For studies conducted more than 10 years ago, some authors had moved institutions. We had a

chance of tracing them from later publications if they had continued to work in the same field, but for some of our studies we could not trace the authors, and had to rely on the inadequate information in the abstract.

- Twenty-four studies were in languages other than English (two Italian, two German, one French, 18 Japanese and one Korean). All had to be translated in enough depth to determine whether to include them. We managed by using students and colleagues for most of the studies, but it was important that these translators had clinical knowledge. Non-clinical people did not have the understanding to be able to make decisions about, for example, whether incontinence had been measured. It proved more difficult to obtain a translation of the Korean trial. The Cochrane Review Group trials search coordinator finally managed to obtain a translation by virtue of the fact that the most recent International Continence Society conference had been held in Korea, but if that had not been the case, commercial translation would have been very expensive. Consequences of this for the review were that trials not in English were checked for inclusion by only one person (i.e. the translator), and therefore not strictly as per the protocol.

Learning points

There are issues of generalisability when considering trials from countries with different healthcare systems, and also older trials. In our review, one older trial tested oestrogen, which is no longer used. Another trial from China used scalp acupuncture, which might not even be premised on the same model as Western acupuncture, let alone be considered a feasible intervention in usual clinical practice.

Data extraction and assessment of study quality

This part of the review posed few problems, as only a small number of trials were included and coordinating the team of reviewers was relatively straightforward. However, one aspect not mentioned much in the formal reports or textbooks on reviewing is maintaining the paperwork of a review. It is important to record all the decisions taken in the form of an audit trail. Even for a small review such as ours, there were 700 abstracts to be considered and decisions recorded, 127 data inclusion decision forms completed independently by two people and final decisions recorded. For each of the 47 studies retrieved there were copies of emails, letters, phone calls and the results of author tracing. For the 12 studies which progressed to data extraction there were two or three copies of data extraction forms, and a master copy of discussion, arbitration and final decisions with feedback to reviewers. Some studies had multiple publications. Then there were the records of Advisory Group meetings, finance, communication with Cochrane, setting up the software needed, and responses to requests for information from practitioners from all over the world. Systems for managing this volume of data are important and the most helpful guide was a book by Williamson et al. (2002).

Assessment of study quality

It is standard practice in all Cochrane reviews to appraise study quality in terms of the extent to which findings are potentially influenced by four types of bias: selection (relating to the way comparison groups are assembled), performance (systematic differences in the care provided to participants in the comparison groups other than the study intervention being investigated), detection (systematic differences between comparison groups in outcome assessment) and attrition (systematic differences between comparison groups in the loss of participants from the study) (Higgins & Green, 2005). Typically, however, this appraisal is not taken into account in the interpretation of study findings (Moja et al., 2005). In our review, our final conclusions did take into account the effect of study quality, but this was prompted by our editor, Professor Adrian Grant, who suggested we modify our conclusions to give greater consideration to the impact of the (often poor) quality of our included studies.

Extracting outcome data

These were collected in the form they were reported and transformed subsequently.

- We had missing data, and data not reported in the original trial in a form that could be transformed. For example, Brittain & Potter (2000) provided mean differences but we did not know the numbers in each arm of the trial at certain time points and so could not use these data.
- Some outcomes included in the trials were not included in the review, for example global dependency scores. We were primarily interested in incontinence as a final outcome, whereas some studies may be taking a wider global functional perspective, with incontinence only one of the outcomes measured.

Learning points

A review is composed of hundreds of little decisions with varying shades of grey, each of which should be checked and a record made of what was done and why. But mistakes can happen and it is fine to ask a reviewer if you see something that does not look right. You should be able to see the decision made, for example about study quality, and the justification for the decision. Olsen et al. (2001), in their assessment of the quality of Cochrane reviews published in 1998, found that in nine (17%) reviews the conclusions presented the intervention in a more favourable light than was warranted. Also, it is important not to assume that a review includes everything that is in the original study.

Data analysis and synthesis

Decisions about what comparisons will be made are taken at the protocol stage of the review. For example, a study that measures an intervention against standard care cannot be compared (or combined) with one that compares an intervention against a placebo, because the expected magnitude of the differences between intervention and control versus intervention and placebo will be different. We therefore began with four comparison groups:

(1) intervention versus no intervention/usual care;
(2) intervention versus placebo;
(3) specific intervention versus another intervention;
(4) combined intervention versus single intervention.

The next step involves considering sensible subgroupings of comparisons, based on the topic. Decisions might be based on the type of intervention, for example the results of drug trials cannot be synthesised with trials of habit training because they work on different mechanisms of action. It might also not be sensible to combine interventions that are designed for different time periods, such as interventions that might be appropriate in early rehabilitation versus later rehabilitation, when patterns of incontinence might be more established. Also, trials measuring the outcome of an intervention 3 months after a stroke cannot be compared with trials measuring outcome at 6 months, or at the end of treatment, given the nature of spontaneous recovery within the first 3 months after stroke (Jorgensen et al., 1995).

To take the example of our first comparison group, intervention versus no intervention/usual care, we found four studies making this comparison:

(1) a special intervention programme based on assessment using the functional independence measure (FIM) versus usual rehabilitation care (Wikander, 1998);
(2) care from a continence nurse practitioner (CNP) versus usual care provided by the general practitioner (GP) (Brittain & Potter, 2000);
(3) scalp acupuncture versus no scalp acupuncture (Chu & Feng, 1997);
(4) timed voiding versus void on request (Gelber & Swords, 1997b).

However, due to the diversity of interventions, settings, client groups and outcomes, it did not make sense to combine these trials. A corollary of this is the difficulty of writing a narrative review that is fair to the underlying evidence. Our discovery of two trials of specialised professional input (Wikander et al., 1998; Brittain & Potter, 2000), both with some findings favouring the intervention, led us initially to overstate the effectiveness of this type of intervention. Our peer reviewers, however, urged us to 'tone down' this view, arguing that while Wikander et al. (1998) did indeed report a range of positive findings, these need to be treated with caution because of methodological weaknesses such as a small sample size and unblinded outcome measurement. The study by Brittain & Potter (2000), while much larger and of better methodological quality, found far fewer outcomes favouring the intervention, with outcomes from nurse continence advisor and usual care groups similar at all data points, with the exception of the number of people cured of all urinary symptoms at 6 months and satisfaction with the service at 3 months. Our Cochrane editor therefore advised us to revise our wording, using statements such as 'provide some evidence' and 'may improve some outcomes'.

Learning points

The implications are that, because our review included such a diverse array of interventions, client groups and outcomes, our comparisons and results are really useful more as an initial attempt to make some order out of the available trials and to suggest a structure for future trials and the data that need to be collected to ensure comparability across studies, rather than providing answers for what to do in clinical practice. This is more a function of the state of the underlying evidence, rather than of the review process, but narrative review is a skilled, not a mechanical, process involving interpretation of the data (Dixon-Woods et al., 2005). Olsen et al. (2001) suggest that readers of Cochrane reviews should subject them to critical appraisal, rather than assuming there is only one set of conclusions to be made from the data available. However, Cochrane reviews compare favourably with non-Cochrane reviews, for example those on the Database of Reviews of Effectiveness (DARE), of which up to half have been shown to present misleading conclusions (Petticrew et al., 2000).

Lessons for future similar reviews

- Scoping reviews usually do not provide enough evidence to suggest best practice, but are useful for identifying which interventions may justify further research
- There are issues of generalisability when considering trials from countries with different healthcare systems, and also older trials whose findings may have been superseded
- Systems need to be in place for managing the volume of paperwork generated by the review, as does an audit trail of key decisions

Conclusion

Implications for practice

There is very little evidence from stroke-specific studies to guide practice. The lack of trials testing the same category of intervention means that recommendations for practice are based on the results of single, usually small, trials. Two trials provide some evidence to suggest that specialised professional input using systematic methods to assess and manage continence problems may improve some outcomes. The limited evidence suggests that the greatest impact on urinary incontinence may be in the acute phase of rehabilitation after stroke. However, specialist input and individualised care management may improve the number of symptoms of urinary incontinence even in the longer term.

Implications for research

There is a need for larger trials, in particular the use of individualised assessment and goal setting to tailor interventions to neurological and functional problems.

As well as the need for trials of methods to promote continence, methods of managing continuing urinary incontinence such as intermittent catheterisation or the use of catheter valves are also needed.

There is a need for more well-designed studies. Further research should, for example, use standardised definitions and classification systems to record details of the type and severity of stroke, and the type and severity of urinary incontinence. Specific details of structured assessment and intervention protocols need to be given, with standardisation of treatment, measures of between groups contamination or differences, and tailoring of intervention to the early or later phases of rehabilitation. Outcome measures of urinary incontinence and of urinary symptoms should be standardised, with attention to their validity and reliability and the blinding of outcome assessment. The time periods for review should be standardised for the acute, early and later phases of rehabilitation. Lastly, sample size calculations and securely concealed randomisation at either the cluster or individual patient level should be used appropriately and reported accordingly.

Implications for review consumers

It is important also to look carefully at the definitions, inclusions and exclusions when relating review findings to your own clinical practice: all reviews have parameters and it is important not to assume reviews cover everything. Readers need to adopt a critical approach to reviews, for example by examining search strategies for potentially omitted key words and assessing if conclusions are justified by the evidence.

References

Abrams, P., Blaivas, J.G., Stanton, S. & Andersen, J.T. (1988) The standardisation of terminology of lower urinary tract function. *Neurourology and Urodynamics*, 7, 403–26.

Barrett, J.A. (2001) Bladder and bowel problems after a stroke. *Reviews in Clinical Gerontology*, 12, 253–67.

Brittain, K.R. & Potter, J.F. (2000) *The Treatment of Urinary Incontinence in Stroke Survivors*. Report for NHS R&D Programme on Cardiovascular Disease and Stroke Project. Division of Medicine for the Elderly, Department of Medicine, University of Leicester, in collaboration with the MRC Incontinence Study.

Chu, M. & Feng, J. (1997) Discussion on treating frequent urine due to multiple cerebral embolism with scalp acupuncture (translation from Chinese). *Information on Traditional Chinese Medicine*, 5, 42.

Clarke, M. & Langhorne, P. (2001) Revisiting the Cochrane Collaboration. *British Medical Journal*, 323, 821.

Dixon-Woods, M., Agarwal, S., Jones, D.R., Young, B. & Sutton, A.J. (2005) Synthesising qualitative and quantitative evidence: a review of methods. *Journal of Health Services Research and Policy*, 10, 45–53.

Eustice, S., Roe, B. & Paterson, J. (2000) *Prompted Voiding for the Management of Urinary Incontinence in Adults*. The Cochrane Database of Systematic Reviews, Issue 2. Art. No. CD002113. John Wiley & Sons, Chichester.

Gelber, D.A. & Swords, L. (1997a) Treatment of post-stroke urinary incontinence (abstract). *Journal of Neurologic Rehabilitation*, 11, 131.

Gelber, D.A. & Swords, L. (1997b) Treatment of post-stroke urinary incontinence (abstract). *Journal of Neurologic Rehabilitation*, 11 (2), 131.

Higgins, J.P.T. & Green, S. (eds) (2005) *Cochrane Handbook for Systematic Reviews of Interventions 4.2.5* (updated May 2005). The Cochrane Library, Issue 3. John Wiley & Sons Ltd, Chichester.

Jorgensen, H.S., Nakayama, H., Raaschou, H.O., Vive-Larsen, J., Stoier, M. & Olsen, T.S. (1995) Outcome and time course of recovery in stroke. Part II: Time course of recovery. The Copenhagen Stroke Study. *Archives of Physical Medicine and Rehabilitation*, 76, 406–12.

Judge, T.G. (1969) The use of quinestradol in elderly incontinent women, a preliminary report. *Gerontologica Clinica*, 11, 159–64.

Moja, L.P., Telaro, E., D'Amico, R., Moschetti, I., Coe, L., Liberati, A. and on behalf of the Metaquality Study Group (2005) Assessment of the methodological quality of primary studies by systematic reviews: results of the metaquality cross sectional study. *British Medical Journal*, 330, 1053–7.

Olsen, O., Middleton, P., Ezzo, J., et al. (2001) Quality of Cochrane reviews: assessment of a sample from 1998. *British Medical Journal*, 323, 829–32.

Ostaszkiewicz, J., Johnston, L. & Roe, B. (2004) *Habit Retraining for the Management of Urinary Incontinence in Adults*. The Cochrane Database of Systematic Reviews, Issue 2. Art. No. CD002801. John Wiley & Sons, Chichester.

Pettigrew, M., Song, F., Wilson, P. & Wright, K. (2000) The DARE database of abstracts of reviews of effectiveness: a summary and analysis. *International Journal of Technology Assessment in Health Care*, 15, 671–8.

Royal College of Physicians (2000) *Stroke: National Clinical Guidelines*. Royal College of Physicians, London.

Stroke Unit Trialists' Collaboration (2001) *Organised Inpatient (Stroke Unit) Care for Stroke*. The Cochrane Database of Systematic Reviews, Issue 3. Art. No. CD000197. John Wiley & Sons, Chichester.

Thomas, L.H., Barrett, J., Cross, S., et al. (2005) *Prevention and Treatment of Urinary Incontinence after Stroke in Adults*. The Cochrane Database of Systematic Reviews, Issue 3. Art. No. CD004462. John Wiley & Sons, Chichester.

Tibaek, S., Jensen, R., Lindskov, G. & Jensen, M. (2004) Can quality of life be improved by pelvic floor muscle training in women with urinary incontinence after ischaemic stroke? A randomised, controlled and blinded study. *International Urogynaecological Journal*, 15, 117–23.

Wikander, B., Ekelund, P. & Milsom, I. (1998) An evaluation of multidisciplinary intervention governed by functional independence measure (FIMSM) in incontinent stroke patients. *Scandinavian Journal of Rehabilitation Medicine*, 30 (1), 15–21.

Williamson, J.W., Weir, C.R., Turner, C.W., Lincoln, M.J. & Cofrin, K.M.W. (2002) *Healthcare Informatics and Information Synthesis: Developing and Applying Clinical Knowledge to Improve Outcomes*. Sage, Thousand Oaks, California.

4 Pelvic Floor Muscle Training for Urinary Incontinence in Women

E. Jean C. Hay-Smith, Chantale L. Dumoulin and Peter Herbison

This paper is based on a Cochrane review published in The Cochrane Library 2006, Issue 1 (see www.thecochranelibrary.com *for information*). *Cochrane reviews are regularly updated as new evidence emerges and in response to feedback, and* The Cochrane Library *should be consulted for the most recent version of the review.*

Introduction

In an ideal world, authors of a systematic review would be able to draw on multiple well-designed and well-conducted randomised controlled trials addressing a similar question, in similar (but not identical) samples. There would be similarity in the interventions used in each trial, and the interventions would be well defined and could be widely implemented if effective and affordable. The included trials would also have measured outcomes important to patients and used the same validated and reliable instruments.

Systematic reviews of non-drug complex interventions in relatively new areas of research rarely have the luxury of the ideal. Because nursing, physiotherapy and occupational therapy, for example, commonly provide complex interventions and are 'young' in research terms, systematic reviewers in these areas often face a number of difficulties that are frustrating for reviewers and readers alike. In this chapter, a systematic review of pelvic floor muscle training (PFMT) for urinary incontinence in women is used to illustrate two specific and common problems, namely: heterogeneity and the choice and reporting of outcome measures.

Overview of the review

The full version of this systematic review was published by Hay-Smith & Dumoulin (2006) in The Cochrane Library (Hay-Smith & Dumoulin, 2006). All parts of the review have been abbreviated for the purposes of this chapter.

Introduction review objectives

Urinary incontinence is a common problem amongst adults living in the community. It is more frequent in women, increases with age, and is particularly common among those in residential care (Hunskaar et al., 2002). Estimates of the prevalence of urinary incontinence in women vary between 10 and 40% (Hunskaar et al., 2002). The two most common types of urine leakage in women are stress or urge urinary incontinence. It is possible to have both, and this is called mixed urinary incontinence.

If a woman reports involuntary urine leakage with physical exertion, this is called stress urinary incontinence (SUI). Urodynamic (a physiological test) stress incontinence is demonstrated by involuntary urine loss during increased intra-abdominal pressure, in the absence of detrusor muscle (bladder smooth muscle) contraction. SUI is associated with anatomical defects in the structures that support the bladder and urethra, resulting in suboptimal positioning of these structures at rest or on exertion, or dysfunction of the neuromuscular components that help control urethral pressure, or both. As a result, the urethra is not closed properly during exertion and leakage occurs.

The classic symptom of urge urinary incontinence (UUI) is involuntary leakage associated with, or immediately preceded by, a sudden and compelling need to void (i.e. urgency). UUI usually results from an increase in bladder pressure due to an involuntary contraction of the detrusor muscle. When urodynamic investigations show this, then it is called detrusor overactivity incontinence.

One of the most common conservative treatments offered to women with stress, urge or mixed incontinence is pelvic floor muscle training (PFMT). The use of PFMT is based on two functions of pelvic floor muscle: support of the pelvic organs, and a contribution to the sphincteric closure mechanism of the urethra. For SUI, the aims of PFMT are to improve pelvic organ support (particularly of the bladder, bladder neck and urethra) and increase intraurethral pressure during exertion. The biological rationale for the use of PFMT for UUI is less clear, but a reflex inhibition of detrusor contraction has been demonstrated with an electrically stimulated contraction of the pelvic floor muscles (Godec et al., 1975). It has also been suggested that reflex inhibition of detrusor contraction may accompany repeated voluntary pelvic floor muscle contractions (Polden & Mantle, 1990).

Review objective

The objective of the review was to determine the effects of PFMT in the management of female urinary (stress, urge and mixed) incontinence. The review tested the hypothesis that pelvic floor muscle training is better than no treatment, placebo, sham, or any other form of inactive control treatment.

Methods

Eligibility of studies for inclusion in the review was based on the following a priori criteria:

- Randomised and quasi-randomised (e.g. allocation by alternation) controlled trials were eligible. Other forms of controlled clinical trial were excluded.
- Eligible studies included those of women with stress, urge or mixed urinary incontinence; there were no restrictions by method of diagnosis. Excluded studies were those that recruited antenatal or postnatal women up to 3 months from delivery, women whose leakage might be due to significant factors outside the urinary tract (e.g. neurological disorders), or women with nocturnal enuresis.
- Trials had to compare a PFMT programme with no treatment, placebo treatment, sham treatment (e.g. sham electrical stimulation), or an inactive control (e.g. advice on use of pads). PFMT was defined as a programme of repeated voluntary pelvic floor muscle contractions taught and supervised by a healthcare professional.

Although eligibility was not determined by the outcomes measured, the a priori primary outcomes of interest were patient-reported symptomatic cure or improvement and incontinence-specific quality of life.

Relevant trials were identified by searching the Cochrane Incontinence Group Specialised Trials Register in December 2004. The Register contains trials identified from the Cochrane Central Register of Controlled Trials (CENTRAL), MEDLINE, the Cumulative Index of Nursing and Allied Health Literature (CINAHL) and hand searching of journals and conference proceedings. There was no restriction on language of publication. The date of the last search was December 2004.

Two researchers evaluated all potentially eligible studies, and any disagreements regarding study eligibility were resolved by discussion. Similarly, two researchers assessed methodological quality (using the Cochrane Incontinence Group criteria) and extracted data independently, and any disagreements or discrepancies were again resolved by discussion.

All included data were processed as described in the *Cochrane Collaboration Handbook for Systematic*

Reviews of Interventions (Higgins & Green, 2005). For categorical outcomes, the numbers reporting an outcome were related to the numbers at risk in each group to derive a relative risk. For continuous variables, means and standard deviations were used to derive mean differences. A formal meta-analysis was planned, but was not performed because of heterogeneity amongst the studies. The extent of heterogeneity was assessed in three ways: visual inspection of data plots, chi-square test for heterogeneity and the I^2 statistic.

Subgroup analysis was used to address the effect of type of incontinence on outcome. Because the rationale for PFMT is different for the two main types of urinary incontinence (stress and urge), it is plausible to expect a difference in the outcome of PFMT on the basis of diagnosis. It is commonly believed that PFMT is most effective for SUI women and that it may be effective, in combination with behavioural interventions, for women with mixed urinary incontinence. PFMT has rarely been the first-choice treatment for women with UUI alone. The four pre-specified diagnostic (whether based on symptoms, signs or urodynamics) subgroups were trials that recruited women with (1) only SUI; (2) only UUI; (3) only mixed urinary incontinence; or (4) a range of diagnoses.

Sensitivity analysis by trial quality was planned, but there were too few trials and too many other potential causes of heterogeneity to make this useful. Similarly, formal analysis of publication bias was not possible because there were insufficient trials in any comparison to make this useful.

Description of included studies

Sixteen trials were identified, and three excluded. The 13 included trials are summarised in Table 4.1. *All included trials are cited using the first author and year of the trial publication.*

Ten studies recruited women with SUI only (Henalla et al., 1989, 1990; Hofbauer et al., 1990; Ramsay & Thou, 1990; Lagro-Janssen et al., 1991; Miller et al., 1998; Bø et al., 1999; Bidmead et al., 2002; Aksac et al., 2003; Schagen van Leeuwen et al., 2004). Because nearly all the women (91%) in the study by Burns had SUI only, this study was analysed with the SUI studies (Burns et al., 1993). The two remaining studies recruited women with a range of diagnoses (Burgio et al., 1998; Yoon et al., 2003).

The PFMT programmes used are described in Table 4.2. Unfortunately, four studies (three of which were abstracts) gave no details of the PFMT programme. A PFMT programme may be prescribed to increase strength (the maximum force generated by a muscle in a single contraction), to increase endurance (ability to contract repetitively, or sustain a single contraction), for coordination of muscle activity, to suppress urge, or a combination of these. Based on the descriptions of training, one study clearly targeted coordination (Miller 1998) and two, strength training (Ramsay 1990, Bø 1999). It was more difficult to categorise the other trials because they used either a mixed PFMT programme (e.g. strength and endurance) or did not give sufficient information about the programme to be sure what its purpose was.

It was difficult to assess the methodological quality of the four trials that were published as conference abstracts, due to brevity of reporting (Henalla 1990, Ramsay 1990, Bidmead 2002, Schagen van Leeuwen 2004). To assess methodological quality, random allocation and allocation concealment, description of dropouts and withdrawals, analysis by intention to treat, and blinding during treatment and at outcome assessment were considered (see Table 4.1).

Results

Thirteen randomised or quasi-randomised trials compared PFMT (375 women) with no treatment, placebo, sham or other non-active control treatments (339 women). Only six trials contributed to the analysis of primary outcomes (Ramsay 1990, Lagro-Janssen 1991, Burns 1993, Burgio 1998, Bø 1999, Yoon 2003).

Patient-reported 'cure' or 'improvement'

Two trials reported data on cure: women reported '100% perceived improvement (that is dry)' (Burgio 1998), or that the participant's incontinence was now 'unproblematic' (Bø 1999). Both found that PFMT women were statistically significantly more likely to report that they were cured. The estimated size of treatment effect was quite different in the

Table 4.1 Description of included studies.

Study	Method	Participants	Interventions	Outcomes	Notes
Aksac 2003	3 arm RCT, parallel design. Not clear if adequate allocation concealment. Not clear if blinded outcome assessment	50 women with urodynamic SUI. No further inclusion or exclusion criteria stated. Median age, years: PFMT 52.5 (SD 7.9), control 54.7 (SD 7.8). Single centre, Turkey	(1) PFMT ($n = 20$). Use of digital palpation to teach VPFMC with abdominal and buttock muscle relaxation. Weekly clinic visits for 8 weeks. Details of PFMT programme in Data Table 01.03. (2) Control ($n = 10$). No PFMT. (3) PFMT with biofeedback ($n = 20$)	Primary outcome: not stated. Other outcomes: pad test cure (weight gain of 1 g or less), pad test improvement (50% or greater reduction in pad weight), vaginal squeeze pressure, digital palpation score, incontinence frequency (four point ordinal scale), Social Activity Index	Post-treatment evaluation at 8 weeks, no longer-term follow-up. Dropouts: not stated
Bidmead 2002	4 arm RCT, parallel design (after treatment period control patients crossed over into group 3). Not clear if adequate random allocation concealment. Blinded outcome assessment. Primary analysis by intention to treat	Women with urodynamic SUI (number recruited not clear, 170 or 173?). Inclusion: new diagnosis of SUI or no treatment for SUI in previous 6 months. Exclusion: no further criteria reported. Mean age, years: PFMT 46.2 (SD 8.5), control 47.5 (SD 11.5). Single centre, UK	(1) PFMT ($n = 40$). Conventional PFMT supervised by physiotherapist. Individually tailored lifestyle advice. Five clinic visits in 14 weeks (weeks 1, 3, 6, 10 and 14). (2) Control ($n = 20$). No treatment for 14 weeks. Thereafter crossed over into group 3. (3) PFMT with electrical stimulation ($n = ?$). (4) PFMT with sham electrical stimulation ($n = 42$)	Primary outcome measure: not stated. Other outcome measures: pad test, King's Health Questionnaire	Post-treatment evaluation at 14 weeks, no longer-term follow-up. Dropouts: 10/40 PFMT, 7/20 control, 15/? PFMT + electrical stimulation, 12/42 PFMT + sham stimulation

Study	Methods	Participants	Interventions	Outcomes	Notes
Burgio 1998	3-arm RCT, parallel design. Stratified by type (UUI, MUI) and severity of incontinence (number of leakage episodes). Not clear if adequate allocation concealment. Blinded outcome assessment. Primary analysis by intention-to-treat	197 women, with DO with or without urodynamic SUI. Inclusion: community dwelling women aged 55 years or more, 2 or more urge accidents per week, urge incontinence predominant pattern. Exclusion: continual leakage, uterine prolapse past introitus, unstable angina, decompensated heart failure, history of malignant arrhythmias, impaired mental status (MMSE < 20). Mean age, years: PFMT 67.3 (SD 7.6), control 67.6 (SD 7.6). Mean duration symptoms, years: 9.4 (10.8), control 12.7 (15.9). More than 10 leakage episodes per week: PFMT 52%, control 54%. Diagnosis: 96 UUI only (49%), 101 MUI (51%). Single centre, USA	(1) PFMT ($n = 65$). Use of anorectal biofeedback to teach VPFMC with abdominal muscle relaxation. Response to urge (pause, sit, relax, repeated VPFMC to suppress urge). Use of bladder-sphincter biofeedback at third visit for those with <50% reduction in leakage episodes to teach VPFMC against increasing fluid volume and urge. Fortnightly clinic visit with nurse practitioner, 8 weeks. Details of PFMT programme in Data Table 01.03. (2) Controls ($n = 65$). Placebo drug, three times a day, for 8 weeks. Capsule contained 500 mg riboflavin phosphate marker. Fortnightly clinic visit with nurse practitioner. (3) Drug ($n = 67$)	Primary outcome: change in leakage frequency (2 week urinary diary). Secondary outcomes: Hopkins Symptom checklist for psychological distress, self report (worse to much better), satisfaction with progress (not at all to completely), perceived improvement (none or 0% to dry or 100%), willingness to continue PFMT, desire for other treatment, leakage episodes (2 week urinary diary), cystometry (for 105/197)	Post-treatment evaluation at 10 weeks, no longer-term follow-up. Dropouts: 4/65 PFMT, 12/65 control, 12/67 drug. ITTA: for primary outcome, most recent urinary diary data carried forward

Table continues

Table 4.1 continued

Study	Method	Participants	Interventions	Outcomes	Notes
Burns 1993	3 arm RCT, parallel design. Not clear if adequate allocation concealment. Blinded outcome assessment	135 women, with urodynamic SUI with or without DO. Inclusion: women with SUI or MUI, 55 years or older, minimum of 3 leakage episodes per week, demonstrates leakage with stress manoeuvres during physical examination, MMSE > 23, absence of glycosuria or pyuria, post void residual < 50 ml, maximum uroflow > 15 ml/s. Exclusion: no additional criteria reported. Mean age, years: PFMT 63 (SD 6), control 63 (5). Mean leakage episodes 24 hours: PFMT 2.6 (SD 2.1), control 2.6 (2.6). Diagnosis: 123 urodynamic SUI (91%), 12 MUI (9%). Single centre, USA	(1) PFMT (n = 43, after dropouts). Booklet explaining anatomy, PFMT, and completion of exercise and urinary diaries. Videotape describing exercise protocol. Weekly exercise reminder cards mailed between visits. Weekly clinic visits with nurse, 8 weeks. Details of PFMT programme in Data Table 01.03. (2) Control (n = 40, after dropouts). No treatment. (3) PFMT with weekly clinic biofeedback (n = 40, after dropouts)	Primary outcome: leakage episodes (2-week urinary diary). Secondary outcomes: incontinence severity (based on number of leakage episodes from diary), pelvic floor muscle EMG, cystometry	Post-treatment evaluation at 8 weeks, with longer-term follow-up at 12 weeks and 6 months. Dropouts: 10/135 and 2/135 excluded from analysis (no urinary diary); group not specified

Table continues

| Bø 1999 | 4 arm RCT, parallel design. Stratified by severity of leakage on pad test. Adequate allocation concealment. Blinded outcome assessment. Secondary analysis by intention to treat. A priori power calculation | 122 women, with urodynamic SUI. Inclusion: women with a history of SUI, waiting for surgery or recruited through advertising, >4 g leakage on pad test with standardised bladder volume. Exclusion: other types of incontinence, DO on urodynamics, residual urine >50 ml, maximum uroflow <15 ml/s, previous surgery for urodynamic SUI, neurological or psychiatric disease, ongoing urinary tract infection, other disease that could interfere with participation, use of concomitant treatments during trial, inability to understand instructions given in Norwegian. Mean age, years: PFMT 49.6 (SD 10.0), control 51.7 (SD 8.8). Mean duration symptoms, years: PFMT 10.2 (SD 7.7), control 9.9 (SD 7.8). Mean leakage episodes 24 hours: PFMT 0.9 (SD 0.6), control 1.0 (SD 1.0). Diagnosis: 122 urodynamic SUI (100%). 5 centres, Norway | (1) PFMT (n = 29). Explanation of anatomy, physiology, and continence mechanism by physiotherapist. Audiotape of home training programme. Weekly 45 min exercise class to PFMT in a variety of body positions, and back, abdominal, buttock and thigh muscle exercises. Monthly clinic visit with physiotherapist, 6 months. Details of PFMT programme in Data Table 01.03. (2) Controls (n = 32). Explanation of anatomy, physiology, and continence mechanism. Correct VPFMC confirmed by palpation. No clinic visits. Offered instruction in use of the Continence Guard (14 accepted). (3) Electrical stimulation (n = 32). (4) Vaginal cones (n = 29) | Primary outcomes: 60 second pad test with standardised bladder volume, self-report (very problematic to unproblematic). Secondary outcomes: Norwegian Quality of Life Scale, Bristol Female Lower Urinary Tract Symptoms Questionnaire, Leakage Index, Social Activity Index, leakage episodes (3 day urinary diary), 24 hour pad test, vaginal squeeze pressure | Post-treatment evaluation at 6 months, no longer-term follow-up. Dropouts: 4/29 PFMT, 2/32 controls, 7/32 electrical stimulation, 2/29 vaginal cones. ITTA: baseline values used for losses to follow-up |

Table 4.1 continued

Study	Method	Participants	Interventions	Outcomes	Notes
Henalla 1989	4-arm RCT, parallel design. Not clear if adequate random allocation concealment. Not clear if blinded outcome assessment	100 women with urodynamic SUI. Exclusion: fistula, more than one surgical procedure for incontinence, major degree of prolapse, absolute contraindication to oestrogens. Single centre, UK	(1) PFMT (n = 26). Correct VPFMC taught by physiotherapist. Weekly clinic visit for 12 weeks. Details of PFMT programme in Data Table 01.03. (2) Control (n = 25). No treatment. (3) Electrical stimulation (n = 25). (4) Drug (n = 24). Oestrogen	Primary outcome measure: not stated. Other outcome measures: pad test cure (negative following positive result), pad test improvement (50% or greater reduction in pad weight), cystometry	Post-treatment evaluation at 12 weeks, with longer-term follow-up at 9 months (questionnaire). Dropouts: none at 12 weeks?
Henalla 1990	3 arm RCT, parallel design. Not clear if adequate random allocation concealment. Not clear if blinded outcome assessment	26 women with urodynamic SUI. Inclusion: postmenopausal. Exclusion: no further criteria stated. Mean age, years: 54 (range 49–64). Single centre, UK	(1) PFMT (n = 8). No detail given. (2) Control (n = 7). No treatment. (3) Drug (n = 11). Oestrogen	Primary outcome: not stated. Other outcome measures: pad test cure or improved (not defined), vaginal pH, vaginal cytology, anal EMG	Post-treatment evaluation at 6 weeks, no longer-term follow-up. Dropouts: none?
Hofbauer 1990	4 arm RCT, parallel design. Not clear if adequate random allocation concealment. Not clear if blinded outcome assessment	43 women with urodynamic SUI. Exclusion: urge incontinence. Mean age, years: 57.5 (SD 12). Grade 3 incontinence: 4 PFMT, 2 control Single centre, Austria	(1) PFMT (n = 11). Exercise programme including PFMT, abdominal and hip adductor exercise, twice a week for 20 minutes with therapist, and daily home programme. (2) Control (n = 10). Sham electrical stimulation. (3) PFMT + electrical stimulation (n = 11). (4) Electrical stimulation (n = 11)	Primary outcome: not stated. Other outcome measures: incontinence scale (? symptom scale, not defined), leakage episodes (urinary diary), cystometry	Not clear when post-treatment evaluation performed. Further follow-up at 6 months. Dropouts: none?

| Lagro-Janssen 1991 | 2 arm RCT, parallel design. Stratified by type and severity of incontinence. Inadequate allocation concealment. Blinded outcome assessment | 110 women, with urodynamic SUI with or without DO. Inclusion: women between 20 and 65 years of age reporting 2 or more leakage episodes per month. Exclusion: previous incontinence surgery, neurological causes of incontinence, urinary tract infection, temporary cause of incontinence. Mean age, years: PFMT 46.1 (SD 10.1), controls 44.6 (SD 8.2). Symptoms for more than 5 years: PFMT 55%, control 33%. Mean leakage episodes 24 hours: PFMT 2.5 (SD 2.0), control 3.3 (SD 2.2). Diagnosis: 66 urodynamic SUI (60%), 20 MUI (18%), 18 UUI (16%), 6 other (6%). NB: only data from urodynamic SUI women are included in the review, because women with other diagnoses also had bladder training. 13 general practices, The Netherlands | (1) PFMT (n = 54, but 33 with urodynamic SUI only). Advice about incontinence pads from practice assistant. Information on PFM function and how to contract by family doctor. PFMT for 12 weeks. Details of PFMT programme in Data Table 01.03. (2) Control (n = 56, but 33 with urodynamic SUI only). Advice about incontinence pads only. Offered treatment after 12 weeks | Primary outcome: not stated. Other outcomes: incontinence severity (12 point score), subjective assessment, health locus of control questionnaire, general health questionnaire, leakage episodes (7 day diary), self-reported treatment adherence | Post-treatment evaluation at 12 weeks, with longer-term follow-up at 6 months, 12 months and 5 years. Dropouts: 1/54 PFMT, 3/56 control |

Table continues

Table 4.1 continued

Study	Method	Participants	Interventions	Outcomes	Notes
Miller 1998	2 arm RCT, parallel design (after 1 month controls cross over into treatment group). Not clear if adequate allocation concealment. Blinded outcome assessment	27 women with symptoms and signs of SUI. Inclusion: community dwelling women, mild to moderate SUI (at least one and up to 5 leaks per day), 60 years or more, direct visualisation of urine loss on cough with 100 ml or more voided after stress test. Exclusion: systemic neuromuscular disease, previous bladder surgery, active urinary tract infection, delayed leakage after cough, more than moderate leakage with cough, inability to do a VPFMC, prolapse below hymenal ring. Mean age, years: 68.4 (SD 5.5). Mean number leakage episodes per day: 1.4 (SD 1.4). Single centre, USA	(1) PFMT (n = 13). Education on basic physiology and function of pelvic floor muscles, digital palpation to teach VPFMC. Taught 'The Knack', i.e. VPFMC prior to hard cough maintained throughout cough until abdominal wall relaxed. Practice at home for one week. (2) Control (n = 14). No treatment for one week, then cross over to treatment group at one month	Primary outcome measure: Paper towel test. Secondary outcome measures: digital palpation	Post-treatment evaluation: one week, no longer-term follow-up. Dropouts: none
Ramsay 1990	2 arm RCT, parallel design. Not clear if adequate allocation concealment. Blinded participants	44 women, with symptoms of SUI. Inclusion: women whose only symptom was SUI. Exclusion: no additional criteria reported. Diagnosis: 44 SUI (100%). Single centre, Scotland	(1) PFMT (n = 22). Taught by physiotherapist. PFMT for 2 weeks. Details of PFMT programme in Data Table 01.03. (2) Controls (n = 22). As above, but with sham PFMT programme comprising hip abductor muscle contraction with feet crossed at the ankles	Primary outcome: not stated. Other outcomes: self-reported severity (worse to improved), pad test, vaginal squeeze pressure	Post-treatment evaluation at 12 weeks, with no longer-term follow-up. Dropouts: none. ITTA: data for all participants

Study	Methods	Participants	Interventions	Outcomes	Notes
Schagen van Leeuwen 2004	RCT, 2 × 2 design. Not clear if adequate random allocation concealment. Blinded for drug but not PFMT components of intervention? Intention to treat analysis	201 women with urodynamic SUI or positive cough test. Inclusion: women aged 18–75 years with two or more stress leakage episodes per day and normal voiding frequency. Exclusion: enuresis, urge incontinence. Five centres, 3 countries (The Netherlands, UK, USA)	(1) PFMT + placebo drug (n = 50). (2) Control (n = 47). Imitation PFMT (not defined) and placebo drug. (3) PFMT + drug (n = 52). Duloxetine. (4) Imitation PFMT + drug (n = 52)	Primary outcome: percent change in incontinence episode frequency. Secondary outcomes: change in Incontinence Quality of Life (I-QoL), percent change in pad use	Post-treatment evaluation at 12 weeks, no longer-term follow-up. Dropouts: yes, but no data given
Yoon 2003	3-arm RCT, parallel design. Not clear if adequate allocation concealment. Blinded outcome assessment	50 women with urinary incontinence. Inclusion: urine loss >1 g on 30 min pad test, 14 voids or more in 48 h. Exclusion: women under 35 and over 55 years of age, urinary tract infection, previous surgery for urinary incontinence, hormonal or other drug therapy for incontinence. Mean voids per day: PFMT 15.1 (SD 1.6), control 16.3 (1.8). Diagnosis: urinary incontinence (100%). Single centre, Korea	(1) PFMT (n = 15). 20 min weekly session of EMG biofeedback with nurse, 8 weeks. Details of PFMT programme in Data Table 01.03. (2) Control (n = 14). No treatment or clinic contact	Primary outcome: not stated. Other outcomes: urinary incontinence score (severity based on leakage with 18 activities), leakage episodes and frequency (2 day diary), 30 min pad test, vaginal squeeze pressure	Post-treatment evaluation at 8 weeks, with no longer-term follow-up. Dropouts: 2/15 PFMT, 2/21 Bladder training, 2/14 controls

DO, detrusor overactivity; EMG, electromyography; ITTA, intention-to-treat analysis; MMSE, mini mental state examination; MUI, mixed urinary incontinence; PFMT, pelvic floor muscle training; SD, standard deviation; SUI, stress urinary incontinence; RCT, randomised controlled trial; USI, urodynamic stress urinary incontinence; UUI, urge urinary incontinence; VPFMC, voluntary pelvic floor muscle contraction.

Table 4.2 Description of voluntary pelvic floor muscle training (VPFMC) programmes.

Study	VPFMC confirmed	Description	VPFMC per day	Training	Supervision
Aksac 2003	VPFMC confirmed by palpation. Relaxation of abdominal and buttock muscles	Set: 10 VPFMC, with 5 second hold and 10 second rest. Progressed at 2 weeks to 10 second hold and 20 second rest. Sets per day: 3	30	8 weeks	Weekly clinic visits
Burgio 1998	Anorectal biofeedback for teaching selective contraction and relaxation of pelvic floor muscles, while keeping abdominal muscles relaxed	Set: 15 VPFMC, with 10 seconds hold. Sets per day: 3. Body position: lying, sitting, standing. Use of VPFMC to prevent leakage (the Knack), and to suppress urge. Interrupt urine stream once per day. 45.8 weeks. Fortnightly clinic visit with nurse practitioner	45	8 weeks	Fortnightly clinic visit with nurse practitioner
Burns 1993		Set: 10 VPFMC with 3 second hold, and 10 VPFMC with 10 second hold. Progressed by 10 per set to daily maximum of 200. Sets per day: 4. Videotape describing exercise protocol	200	8 weeks	Weekly exercise reminder cards mailed between visits. Weekly clinic visits with nurse
Bø 1999	VPFMC confirmed by palpation	Set: 8 to 12 high intensity (close to maximal) VPFMC, with 6–8 second hold and 3–4 fast contractions added at the end of each hold, 6 second rest between contractions. Sets per day: 3. Body position: included lying, kneeling, sitting, standing; all with legs apart. Women used preferred position. Audiotape of home training programme. Weekly 45 min exercise class to music, with PFMT in a variety of body positions, and back, abdominal, buttock and thigh muscle exercises	36	6 months	Weekly 45 min exercise class. Monthly clinic visit with physiotherapist
Henalla 1989	Correct VPFMC taught by physiotherapist	Set: 5 VPFMC, with 5 second hold. Sets per day: 1 set per hour	Approximately 80	12 weeks	Weekly clinic visit
Lagro-Janssen 1991	Teaching from family doctor	Set: 10 VPFMC, with 6 seconds hold. Sets per day: 5–10	50–100	12 weeks	
Ramsay 1990	Taught by physiotherapist	Set: 4 maximum isometric VPFMC, with 4 second hold and 10 second rest. Sets per day: 1 set every waking hour	Approximately 64	12 weeks	
Yoon 2003	Weekly surface electromyography biofeedback with nurse	Set: not stated. Sets per day: 30 VPFMC for strength and endurance per day (not clear if 30 total or 30 each), taking 15–20 min/day. Strength: burst of intense activity lasting a few seconds. Endurance: 6 second holds progressed by 1 second per week to 12 seconds	Not clear if 30 or 60	8 weeks	Weekly clinic visit with nurse

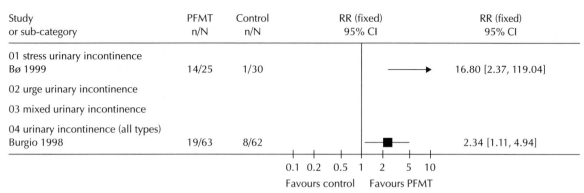

Study or sub-category	PFMT n/N	Control n/N	RR (fixed) 95% CI	RR (fixed) 95% CI
01 stress urinary incontinence				
Bø 1999	14/25	1/30		16.80 [2.37, 119.04]
02 urge urinary incontinence				
03 mixed urinary incontinence				
04 urinary incontinence (all types)				
Burgio 1998	19/63	8/62		2.34 [1.11, 4.94]

Figure 4.1   Patient-reported cure.

two trials: PFMT women were about 17 times more likely to report cure than controls in Bø 1999, but only about two and a half times as likely in Burgio 1998. The confidence intervals in both trials were wide (Figure 4.1).

Four trials contributed data to the patient-perceived cure or improvement comparison: women reported that they were 'improved' (Ramsay 1990), had '75% or more perceived improvement' (Burgio 1998), were 'dry' or 'improved' (Lagro-Janssen 1991), or were 'continent' or 'almost continent' (Bø 1999). Visual inspection of the plot showed that the results of the trial by Ramsay & Thou (1990) differed from those of the other three studies (Figure 4.2). This trial might be confounded by the choice of sham PFMT, which consisted of strong isometric hip adductor contractions that may have facilitated synergistic contractions in the muscles of the pelvic floor with a PFMT effect. Adherence rates in both groups were also very low. Assuming that PFMT has an effect, if exercise levels are suboptimal, then a training effect might not be evident or the size of effect might be diminished to the point where it is not detected. It is possible that women in the PFMT group were doing insufficient training to demonstrate an effect on the pelvic floor muscles. In the three remaining trials, the two in women with urodynamic stress incontinence (Lagro-Janssen 1991, Bø 1999) suggested a higher likelihood of cure or improvement than the single study in women with detrusor overactivity with or without urodynamic stress incontinence (Burgio 1998).

Symptom and condition specific quality of life assessment

Two trials used psychometrically robust questionnaires for assessment of incontinence symptoms,

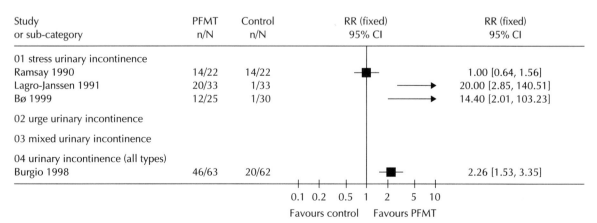

Study or sub-category	PFMT n/N	Control n/N	RR (fixed) 95% CI	RR (fixed) 95% CI
01 stress urinary incontinence				
Ramsay 1990	14/22	14/22		1.00 [0.64, 1.56]
Lagro-Janssen 1991	20/33	1/33		20.00 [2.85, 140.51]
Bø 1999	12/25	1/30		14.40 [2.01, 103.23]
02 urge urinary incontinence				
03 mixed urinary incontinence				
04 urinary incontinence (all types)				
Burgio 1998	46/63	20/62		2.26 [1.53, 3.35]

Figure 4.2   Patient-reported cure or improvement.

the impact of these symptoms on quality of life, or both. Bø 1999 used the Bristol Female Lower Urinary Tract Symptoms Questionnaire (B-FLUTS), which has established validity, reliability and responsiveness to change for evaluation of urinary incontinence symptoms in women (Donovan et al., 2005). Two parts of the questionnaire were reported: the lifestyle and sex life questions. Data were reported as frequencies, rather than mean scores. Fewer women in the PFMT group reported that urinary incontinence symptoms interfered with activity, or were problematic (Table 4.3). Schagen van Leeuwen 2004 reported mean change in the Quality of Life in people with Urinary Incontinence (I-QoL) score; I-QoL has established validity, reliability and responsiveness to change for assessing quality of life impact of urinary incontinence (Donovan et al. 2005). Although quality of life was better in the PFMT group, it was not clear if there were important differences between PFMT and control groups; the means were presented without a measure of dispersion.

Other outcomes of interest

Five studies used urinary diaries to count leakage episodes (Lagro-Janssen 1991, Burns 1993, Burgio 1998, Bø 1999), although Yoon 2003 did not report these data. To enable comparison between trials, the data were presented as number of leakage episodes in 24 hours (Figure 4.3). Visual inspection of the forest plot suggested that the effect size might be greater in the Lagro-Janssen 1991 trial, while the

effect size appeared similar in the three remaining trials (Burns 1993, Burgio 1998, Bø 1999). It seemed that PFMT women experienced about one less leakage episode per 24 hours compared to controls.

Five trials attempted to measure treatment adherence using exercise diaries (Ramsay 1990, Burns 1993, Bø 1999, Bidmead 2002) and self-report (Lagro-Janssen 1991). Bø 1999 reported the highest rate of adherence to PFMT (95%). Bidmead 2002 found that 75% of women allocated to PFMT had excellent (daily) or good (training more than three times a week) adherence to exercise. Women in the Lagro-Janssen 1991 study rated their adherence as excellent or good (62%), reasonable (20%), or poor or none (18%). Ramsay 1990 stated that adherence was poor, with PFMT occurring at '15% of the requested level', with similar rates of exercise between PFMT and sham PFMT groups. Burns 1993 did not present any data on this.

Discussion

Of the 13 trials that addressed the review hypothesis, only six reported data (suitable for analysis) for the primary outcomes of interest. Of these six studies, one was probably confounded by the choice of sham PFMT programme (Ramsay 1990). Statistically significant and clinical important heterogeneity was observed in each of the comparisons. The difficulties posed by variability in methodological quality of trials, heterogeneity, and outcome measurement and reporting are explored further

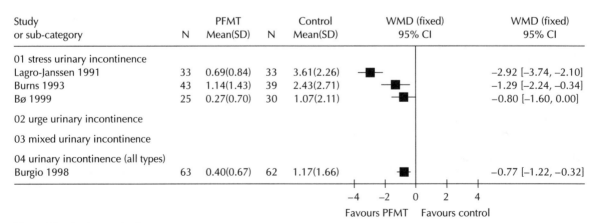

Study or sub-category	N	PFMT Mean(SD)	N	Control Mean(SD)	WMD (fixed) 95% CI	WMD (fixed) 95% CI
01 stress urinary incontinence						
Lagro-Janssen 1991	33	0.69(0.84)	33	3.61(2.26)		−2.92 [−3.74, −2.10]
Burns 1993	43	1.14(1.43)	39	2.43(2.71)		−1.29 [−2.24, −0.34]
Bø 1999	25	0.27(0.70)	30	1.07(2.11)		−0.80 [−1.60, 0.00]
02 urge urinary incontinence						
03 mixed urinary incontinence						
04 urinary incontinence (all types)						
Burgio 1998	63	0.40(0.67)	62	1.17(1.66)		−0.77 [−1.22, −0.32]

−4   −2   0   2   4
Favours PFMT   Favours control

Figure 4.3   Leakage episodes.

Table 4.3 Incontinence specific quality of life.

Study	Outcome	Measure	PFMT	Control	Difference
Aksac 2003	Social Activity Index. Sum of visual analogue scale scores for perceived difficulty participating in 9 specified social situations. A lower score indicates more perceived problem	Median (standard deviation)	7.5 (1.2), n = 20	3.6 (0.6), I = 10	Not estimable
Bø 1999	Bristol Female Lower Urinary Tract Symptoms Questionnaire (BFLUTS). For analysis positive findings ('a little', 'somewhat' and 'a lot', or 'a bit of a problem', 'quite a problem' and 'a serious problem') were grouped together and reported as frequencies. Only the lifestyle questions (28–31, 33) and sex life questions (21–24) were reported	Number with positive findings	Avoiding places and situations: 7, n = 25. Interference with social life: 1, n = 25 Interference with physical activity: 11, n = 25. Overall interference with life: 14, n = 25 Unsatisfied if had to spend rest of life as now: 10, n = 25. Sex life spoilt by urinary symptoms: 3, n = 20. Problem with sex life being spoilt: 2, n = 20. Problem with painful intercourse, 2, n = 20. Urinary incontinence with intercourse: 2, n = 20	Avoiding places and situations: 10, n = 30. Interference with social life: 12, n = 30. Interference with physical activity: 24, n = 30. Overall interference with life: 25, n = 30. Unsatisfied if had to spend rest of life as now: 11, n = 30. Sex life spoilt by urinary symptoms: 13, n = 25. Problem with sex life being spoilt: 13, n = 25. Problem with painful intercourse: 10, n = 25. Urinary incontinence with intercourse: 10, n = 25	Avoiding places and situations: relative risk (RR) 0.84, 95% confidence interval (CI) 0.37 to 1.88 Interference with social life: RR 0.10, 95% CI 0.01 to 0.72 Interference with physical activity: RR 0.55, 95% CI 0.34 to 0.89 Overall interference with life: RR 0.67, 95% CI 0.46 to 0.99. Unsatisfied if had to spend rest of life as now: RR 0.11, 95% CI 0.02 to 0.79. Sex life spoilt by urinary symptoms: RR 0.29, 95% CI 0.10 to 0.87. Problem with sex life being spoilt: RR 0.19, 95% CI 0.05 to 0.76. Problem with painful intercourse: RR 0.25, 95% CI 0.06 to 1.01. Urinary incontinence with intercourse: RR 0.25, 95% CI 0.06 to 1.01
	Social Activity Index	Mean (standard deviation)	9.3 (1.0), n = 25	7.9 (2.2), n = 30	Mean difference (MD) 1.4, 95% CI 0.4 to 2.4
Schagen van Leeuwen 2004	Incontinence Quality of Life (I-QoL) score	Mean change (standard deviation)	7.8 (?), n = ?	4.8 (?), n = ?	4.8 (?), n = ?

in the section below on issues that arose when carrying out the review.

Patient-perceived cure was more likely after PFMT than control. The trial with the greater effect size included SUI women only; the other recruited women with detrusor overactivity with or without urodynamic stress incontinence. Of the two diagnoses, and based on a biological rationale, it is reasonable to expect that PFMT might have more effect on SUI than urge or mixed incontinence. However, other factors might also contribute to the difference between the two trials. For example, in the trial with the greater effect size, cure was defined as 'unproblematic' incontinence, whereas in the other trial women reported that they were 'dry'. These descriptors might measure different things. Cure was also more likely in the trial where women trained for longer (6 months versus 8 weeks), and were younger on average (mean age around 50 compared to 67 years).

Four studies grouped cure and improvement. The data from the Ramsay 1990 trial were presented (Figure 4.2), but were thought to be confounded. The other three studies all found statistically significant differences in favour of PFMT, although the estimated size of treatment effect varied considerably. The two trials in women with urodynamic stress incontinence observed similarly large treatment effects, while the suggested effect was much less in the single study in women with detrusor overactivity incontinence with or without urodynamic stress incontinence. As with patient-reported cure, the trials with larger effect sizes recruited noticeably younger women. Finally, although there was some similarity in the exercise content of the PFMT programmes, the two trials with greater effects had the longer treatment durations (3 and 6 months, versus 8 weeks).

Overall, the differences in likelihood of cure or improvement after PFMT compared to control suggested by the review are sufficient to be of interest to women. As discussed above, the proportion of women who are cured or improved might be greater if women have SUI rather than urge or mixed urinary incontinence and train for longer. When interpreting these data, it is worth noting that there is a relationship between age and diagnosis: younger women are more likely to have SUI, and older women urge or mixed incontinence (Hannestad et al., 2000). Without individual patient data analysis it was not possible to tell if diagnosis, age, or duration of training, or all these factors might be associated with greater treatment effect. The possible association between these factors and treatment outcome requires further testing.

Based on evidence from single trials, it seems that there might be improved incontinence-specific quality of life (lifestyle and sex life) in women treated with PFMT compared to controls, but there might be less or no effect on generic quality of life (Burgio 1998, Bø 1999). Incontinence-specific quality of life measures have only recently been developed. Some of the included trials predated the development of these instruments. It is interesting that, although generic measures of quality of life have been available for longer, they too are only recent additions in incontinence research.

It seemed that the difference in leakage episodes between PFMT and control treatments was about one fewer per day in the PFMT group. It is not clear how important this difference might be for women; this might well depend on how often they leak. If they are leaking often, then this difference might not seem so important. Leakage frequency was similar between two trials in urodynamic stress incontinent women and the single study in women with detrusor overactivity with or without urodynamic stress incontinence, although the likelihood of self-reported cure and improvement appeared quite different in these diagnostic groups. It is possible that the effect of treatment on leakage episodes is similar, but women with detrusor overactivity incontinence (with or without urodynamic stress incontinence) probably also experience urgency and frequency in addition to urge incontinence. PFMT might be less effective in addressing urgency and frequency than incontinence. If so, then women with urge urinary incontinence will be less likely to report that PFMT has cured or improved their condition, because two of their symptoms might still be bothersome.

Treatment adherence is likely to have an impact on the size and direction of treatment effect, because adherence affects the exercise 'dose'. Although adherence data might be useful in interpreting trial results, treatment adherence is difficult to measure. It is interesting to note that the two trials reporting good to excellent rates of training adherence were also the two that demonstrated the greatest treatment effects for cure and improvement. Because these two trials also recruited young, urodynamic stress incontinence women, there are other potential explanations for this observation. Nevertheless, it is possible that treatment adherence contributed.

Issues that arose when carrying out the review

Methodological heterogeneity

Assessment of methodological quality in systematic reviews is done to evaluate the risk of bias in each included study. If the constituent studies are at high risk of bias, we can be less sure about the validity of the review findings. Empirical work has shown that differences in methodological quality can lead to bias in meta-analysis (Schulz et al., 1995; Egger et al., 2002). We agreed, based on the assessment tool used, that the methodological quality of the included studies in the PFMT review was variable.

We had planned, but were not able to undertake because of the small number of trials, a sensitivity analysis (to investigate how sensitive the results were to differences in methodological quality). To do this we would have needed to rank the included studies in some way, based on our quality assessment (Detsky et al., 1992).

Many instruments have been developed to help with methodological quality assessment (Moher et al., 1995), many of which are scales that are scored and summed. One of the difficulties inherent in assessing methodological quality is that judgements are made using information from the trial report, which may not accurately represent what was done (Huwiler-Muntener et al., 2002; Soares et al., 2004). However, the biggest problem is that, although well intentioned, existing quality assessment instruments are unlikely to measure quality validly (Jüni et al., 1999; Herbison et al., 2006). Other ways of exploring the impact of study quality are needed (Greenland & O'Rourke, 2001; Verhagen et al., 2001).

We do not know to what extent the variable methodological quality of the trials has affected the findings of the review. It was interesting to note that, of all the studies that contributed data to the review, the largest treatment effect (for cure and improvement, and leakage episodes) was observed

in the trial by Lagro-Janssen 1991. In this trial treatment allocation was by alternation, and this might be the trial at greatest risk of bias in the review (Egger et al., 2002).

Other sources of heterogeneity

None of the three plots (Figures 4.1, 4.2 and 4.3) reproduced in this chapter give a summary statistic because visual inspection, and the statistical tests for heterogeneity, suggested important differences between the studies. Although we thought that some of the heterogeneity might be related to methodological quality, we could also find reasonable clinical explanations for the differences.

Review authors face the conundrum of how much difference between primary studies is useful and how much is too much. It has been said that too much disparity between the included studies leads to comparison of apples and oranges (Sharpe, 1997). However, meta-analysis offers the opportunity to assess the direction and size of treatment effect across a variety of studies. Consistency of effect across a number of primary studies suggests 'robustness' of the findings, and the ability to generalise to a wider range of patients.

While homogeneity can be examined statistically, the test is underpowered and there may be considerable heterogeneity before this becomes statistically significant (Herbison, 1999). Furthermore, statistically significant heterogeneity might exist in the absence of clear clinical differences in the primary studies, but clinical differences in the studies might be important despite a lack of statistically significant heterogeneity (Flather et al., 1997). In fact, some would argue that statistical testing of heterogeneity is essentially irrelevant. Because some clinical heterogeneity will always exist, it is probably more useful to assess the importance of the differences between the studies than to rely on a test of the difference (Thompson, 2001).

Various methods of assessing and adjusting for heterogeneity have been proposed. The recommended approach varies depending on the degree of difference. Some variability might be adequately incorporated using a random effect model (Deeks et al., 2001). Other methods are recommended for substantial heterogeneity (Sterne et al., 2001). Subgroup analysis (i.e. grouping trial by a particular feature or characteristic, as we did with diagnosis) can give insight (Lau et al., 1997). However, meaningful investigation of heterogeneity by subgroup analysis often requires access to individual patient data (Davey Smith & Egger, 2001; Thompson, 2001), but this relies on the researchers having kept the data and being prepared to share it. Meta-regression, the investigation of significant associations between the treatment effect and other covariates (e.g. age), is another appropriate statistical method for assessing heterogeneity (Thompson, 2001); however, this probably requires at least 20 studies per comparison.

In summary, the question of how much heterogeneity is too much continues to be problematic. It seems reasonable to examine the primary studies for important clinical and methodological differences and discuss the legitimacy of combining the studies in meta-analysis. If meta-analysis is attempted, any observed heterogeneity should be investigated and an explanation offered.

Choice and reporting of outcome measures

The review yielded few data for any of the pre-specified outcomes of interest. We knew we were unlikely to find many trials that had measured incontinence-specific quality of life, which was one of two primary outcomes of interest, because of the lag time between development of these measures and the publication of research that has used them. Nevertheless, we chose our outcome measures to reflect what was likely to matter most to women, not what we thought most studies had measured. Just as it is recommended that trials avoid surrogate primary measures of outcome (e.g. urodynamic measure of bladder capacity rather than the bother associated with frequency, urgency or leakage), the same is true for reviews. Another important contributor to the lack of review data was that the original trial data were poorly reported (e.g. measure of central tendency but no measure of dispersion). It was also difficult to compare data when different measures had been used for the same outcome (e.g. perineometry and electromyography for muscle function).

The pad or paper towel test, used in 9 of the 13 included studies in this review, is a good illustration of the problem faced by reviewers and researchers when choosing, reporting and interpreting outcome. Although quantification of urine loss is one measurement domain recommended by the Outcome Research in Women Subcommittee of the Standardisation Committee of the International Continence Society (Lose et al., 1998), the pad test was not a pre-specified outcome in this review because each of the included studies used a different test. There are many tests: short and long, office- and home-based. The activities within the tests vary, and the test may begin with a standardised bladder volume or not. Pad test data can be presented in many different ways, including number cured (although the cut-off for cure varies), amount of leakage (as a mean or median, with measure of dispersion), or a measure of change from baseline (either percentage change or amount of change in millilitres or grams). Further, we need to know what matters most to women (i.e. whether it is the amount leaked, reduction in amount leaked, percent reduction, no leakage at all, number of times leakage occurred or something else), so that pad test data can be presented in a meaningful way and usefully interpreted.

It is very frustrating (for both reviewers and readers) that so many systematic reviews end with a similar statement along the lines of more research being needed before we can be sure about the effect of the treatment being reviewed. We have said it ourselves in the conclusions of this review! Contributing factors in our review were the lack of consistency in choice of outcomes and measurement instruments, and often poor data reporting in the included studies, which limited the possibilities for combining results from individual studies. In the conclusions of our review (see below) we have made specific suggestions about further research. What can be reported in reviews depends on the decisions that researchers (and journals publishing research) have made, and so one useful thing that reviews can do is highlight areas where consensus is needed in the methods and reporting of clinical trials.

Conclusion

Implications for practice

Based on the few data available, it seems that PFMT is better than no treatment, placebo drug, or inactive control treatments for women with stress, urge or mixed incontinence. Women treated with PFMT were more likely to report cure or improvement, and have fewer leakage episodes per day than controls. Condition-specific quality of life might also be better after PFMT, but this finding needs confirmation from further studies. The trials suggested that the treatment effect might be greater in women with stress urinary incontinence only, who tended to be younger (in their 40s and 50s), and from participating in a supervised PFMT programme for at least 3 months. These are hypotheses that need further testing. It seems likely that treatment effect will be enhanced if the PFMT programme is based on sound physiological principles, a correct contraction is confirmed prior to training, and women are supported to maintain treatment adherence. Overall, there is some support for the widespread recommendation that PFMT be included in first-line conservative management programmes for women with stress, urge or mixed urinary incontinence.

Implications for research

The outcomes of incontinence research would be much more useful if trialists selected a primary outcome measure that mattered to women, chose secondary measures to cover a range of domains, and opted for tools with established validity, reliability and responsiveness. Domains that require particular attention in future are quality of life (condition-specific and generic) and socio-economics, as these have been poorly addressed to date. Researchers might reconsider the past emphasis on self-reported cure or improvement as the principal means to collect data in the domain of women's observations. Two recent trials included in the review asked women if they wanted further treatment and/or were satisfied with treatment outcome, or both. Questions such as these have potential merit; asking women if they are cured or better with treatment may not differentiate those who are better and do not want any further intervention from those who are better but not sufficiently so to be satisfied with the treatment outcome. As PFMT often precedes other more invasive treatment options, such as surgery, the proportion of women satisfied with outcome of PFMT

(and for how long they remain so) might be important information for women, clinicians and service planners. There is also scope for the use of validated questionnaires that evaluate the bother or distress associated with symptoms (for example, the Urogenital Distress Inventory).

The reporting of methods and data could be much improved. Some included studies collected data for outcomes of interest, but did not report it at all or not in a useful manner (for example, point estimates without a measure of dispersion). It was also difficult to assess one of the primary ways to minimise risk of bias – allocation concealment – because the methods of randomisation were usually poorly described. Trialists should refer to the CONsolidated Standards Of Reporting Trials (CONSORT) statements for appropriate standards of trial reporting (Begg et al., 1996; Moher et al., 2001).

In essence, there is a need for at least one large, pragmatic, well-conducted and explicitly reported trial comparing PFMT with control to investigate the longer-term clinical effectiveness of PFMT. Such a trial would recruit women with symptoms of stress, urge or mixed urinary incontinence based on clinical history and physical examination. This trial would also have a sample size based on a clinically important difference in condition-specific quality of life, and large enough for subgroup analysis on the basis of diagnosis and age. Random allocation to groups should be hidden, and stratification or minimisation procedures would ensure an even distribution of women with different diagnoses across both arms of the trial. One arm of the study would comprise a supervised PFMT programme derived from sound exercise science, include confirmation of a correct voluntary pelvic floor muscle contraction, and incorporate appropriate adherence measures. The choice of programme would have to be set against the resource implications of intensively supervised individual programmes and the opportunity cost this represents. Careful clinical judgement is needed about what sort of programme could actually be applied in everyday practice and in different countries, with their different healthcare delivery systems. The other arm of the trial would be a control treatment, for example explanation of anatomy and physiology of the bladder and pelvic floor and advice on good bladder habits, with the same explanation and advice given in both arms. The outcome should be measured at an appropriate time, and should also be measured some time after the treatment has stopped. Such a trial would require substantial funding and multiple recruitment centres.

References

Aksac, B., Aki, S., Karan, A., Yalcin, O., Isikoglu, M. & Eskiyurt, N. (2003) Biofeedback and pelvic floor exercises for the rehabilitation of urinary stress incontinence. *Gynecologic and Obstetric Investigation*, 56 (1), 23–7.

Begg, C., Cho, M., Eastwood, S. et al. (1996) Improving the quality of reporting of randomized controlled trials. The consort statement. *Journal of the American Medical Association*, 276 (8), 637–9.

Bidmead, J., Mantle, J., Cardozo, L., Hextall, A. & Boos, K. (2002) Home electrical stimulation in addition to conventional pelvic floor exercises: a useful adjunct or expensive distraction? (abstract 68). *Neurourology and Urodynamics*, 21 (4), 372–3.

Bø, K., Talseth, T. & Holme, I. (1999) Single blind, randomised controlled trial of pelvic floor exercises, electrical stimulation, vaginal cones, and no treatment in management of genuine stress incontinence in women. *British Medical Journal*, 318 (7182), 487–93.

Burgio, K.L., Locher, J.L., Goode, P.S. et al. (1998) Behavioral vs drug treatment for urge urinary incontinence in older women: A randomized controlled trial. *Journal of the American Medical Association*, 280 (23), 1995–2000.

Burns, P.A., Pranikoff, K., Nochajski, T.H., Hadley, E.C., Levy, K.J. & Ory, M.G. (1993) A comparison of effectiveness of biofeedback and pelvic muscle exercise treatment of stress incontinence in older community dwelling women. *Journal of Gerontology*, 48 (4), M167–M174.

Davey Smith, G. & Egger, M. (2001) Going beyond the grand mean: Subgroup analysis in meta-analysis of randomised trials. In: *Systematic Reviews in Health Care: Meta-analysis in Context* (Egger, M., Davey Smith, G. & Altman, D., eds), pp. 143–56. BMJ Publishing, London.

Deeks, J.J., Altman, D.G. & Bradburn, M.J. (2001) Statistical methods for examining heterogeneity and combining results from several studies in meta-analysis. In: *Systematic Reviews in Health Care: Meta-analysis in Context* (Egger, M., Davey Smith, G. & Altman, D.G., eds), pp. 285–312. BMJ Publishing, London.

Detsky, A., David, N., O'Rourke, K., McGeer, A. & L'Abbé, K. (1992) Incorporating variations in the quality of individual randomized trials into meta-analysis. *Journal of Clinical Epidemiology*, 45, 255–65.

Donovan, J., Bosch, R., Gotoh, M. et al. (2005) Symptom and quality of life assessment. In: *Incontinence. Vol. 1 Basics and Evaluation* (Abrams, P., Cardozo, L., Khoury, S. & Wein, A. eds). Health Publication Ltd., Plymouth, UK.

Egger, M., Ebrahim, S. & Davey Smith, G. (2002) Where now for meta-analysis? *International Journal of Epidemiology*, 31 (1), 1–5.

Flather, M.D., Farkouh, M.E., Pogue, J.M. & Yusuf, S. (1997) Strengths and limitations of meta-analysis: Larger studies may be more reliable. *Controlled clinical trials*, 18 (6), 568–79.

Godec, C., Cass, A.S. & Ayala, G.F. (1975) Bladder inhibition with functional electrical stimulation. *Urology*, 6, 6630–66.

Greenland, S. & O'Rourke, K. (2001) On the bias produced by quality scores in meta-analysis, and a hierarchical view of proposed solutions. *Biostatistics*, 2, 463–71.

Hannestad, Y.S., Rortveit, G., Sandvik, H. & Hunskaar, S. (2000) A community-based epidemiological survey of female urinary incontinence: The Norwegian Epincont study. Epidemiology of incontinence in the county of Nord-Trondelag. *Journal of Clinical Epidemiology*, 53 (11), 1150–7.

Hay-Smith, E.J.C. & Dumoulin, C. (2006) *Pelvic Floor Muscle Training Versus No Treatment, or Inactive Control Treatments, for Urinary Incontinence in Women.* The Cochrane Database of Systematic Reviews Issue 1, Art. No.: CD005654. John Wiley & Sons, Chichester.

Henalla, S., Millar, D. & Wallace, K. (1990) Surgical versus conservative management for post-menopausal genuine stress incontinence of urine (abstract 87). *Neurourology and Urodynamics*, 9 (4), 436–7.

Henalla, S.M., Hutchins, C.J., Robinson, P. & MacVicar, J. (1989) Non-operative methods in the treatment of female genuine stress incontinence. *Journal of Obstetrics and Gynaecology*, 9, 222–5.

Herbison, P. (1999) Problems with meta-analysis. *The New Zealand Medical Journal*, 112 (1081), 38–41.

Herbison, P., Hay-Smith, J. & Gillespie, W.J. (2006) Adjustment of meta-analyses on the basis of quality scores should be abandoned. *Journal of Clinical Epidemiology*, 59, 1249–56.

Higgins, J. & Green, S. (eds) (2005) Cochrane Handbook for Systematic Reviews of Interventions 4.2.5 (updated May 2005) http://www.cochrane.org/resources/handbook/hbook.htm (accessed 31 October 2005).

Hofbauer, V.J., Preisinger, F. & Nurnberger, N. (1990) Der stellenwert der physikotherapie bei der weiblichen genuinen streß-inkontinenz. *Zeitschrift fur Urologie und Nephrologie*, 83, 249–54.

Hunskaar, S., Burgio, K., Diokno, A.C., Herzog, A.R., Hjälmås, K. & Lapitan, M.C. (2002) Epidemiology and natural history of urinary incontinence (UI). In: *Incontinence* (Abrams, P., Cardozo, L., Khoury, S. & Wein, A., eds). Health Publication Ltd, Plymouth, UK.

Huwiler-Muntener, K., Juni, P., Junker, C. & Egger, M. (2002) Quality of reporting of randomized trials as a measure of methodologic quality. *Journal of the American Medical Association*, 287 (21), 2801–4.

Jüni, P., Witschi, A., Bloch, R. & Egger, M. (1999) The hazards of scoring the quality of clinical trials for meta-analysis. *Journal of the American Medical Association*, 282 (11), 1054–60.

Lagro-Janssen, T.L.M., Debruyne, F.M.J., Smits, A.J.A. & Van Weel, C. (1991) Controlled trial of pelvic floor exercises in the treatment of urinary stress incontinence in general practice. *British Journal of General Practice*, 41, 445–9.

Lau, J., Ioannidis, J.P. & Schmid, C.H. (1997) Quantitative synthesis in systematic reviews. *Annals of Internal Medicine*, 127 (9), 820–6.

Lose, G., Fantl, J.A., Victor, A. et al. (1998) Outcome measures for research in adult women with symptoms of lower urinary tract dysfunction. *Neurourology and Urodynamics*, 17 (3), 255–62.

Miller, J.M., Ashton-Miller, J.A. & DeLancey, J.O.L. (1998) A pelvic muscle precontraction can reduce cough-related urine loss in selected women with mild SUI. *Journal of the American Geriatrics Society*, 46 (7), 870–4.

Moher, D., Jadad, A.R., Nichol, G., Penman, M., Tugwell, P. & Walsh, S. (1995) Assessing the quality of randomized controlled trials: An annotated bibliography of scales and checklists. *Controlled clinical trials*, 16 (1), 62–73.

Moher, D., Schulz, K.F., Altman, D.G., The Consort Group (2001) The consort statement: Revised recommendations for improving the quality of reports of parallel-group randomized trials. *Journal of the American Medical Association*, 285 (15), 1987–91.

Polden, M. & Mantle, J. (1990) *Physiotherapy in Obstetrics and Gynaecology*. Butterworth Heinemann, Oxford.

Ramsay, I.N. & Thou, M. (1990) A randomised, double blind, placebo controlled trial of pelvic floor exercises in the treatment of genuine stress incontinence (abstract 59). *Neurourology and Urodynamics*, 9 (4), 398–9.

Schagen van Leeuwen, J., Elser, D., Freeman, R. et al. (2004) Controlled trial of duloxetine alone, pelvic floor muscle training alone, combined treatment in women with stress urinary incontinence (SUI) (abstract). *European Urology Supplements*, 3 (2), 52.

Schulz, K.F., Chalmers, I., Hayes, R.J. & Altman, D.G. (1995) Empirical evidence of bias. Dimensions of methodological quality associated with estimates of treatment effects in controlled trials. *Journal of the American Medical Association*, 273 (5), 408–12.

Sharpe, D. (1997) Of apples and oranges, file drawers and garbage: Why validity issues in meta-analysis will not go away. *Clinical Psychology Review*, 17 (8), 881–901.

Soares, H.P., Daniels, S., Kumar, A. et al., Radiation Therapy Oncology Group (2004) Bad reporting does not mean bad methods for randomised trials: Observational study of randomised controlled trials performed by the Radiation Therapy Oncology Group. *British Medical Journal*, 328 (7430), 22–4.

Sterne, J.A., Egger, M. & Davey Smith, G. (2001) Systematic reviews in health care: investigating and dealing with publication and other biases in meta-analysis. *British Medical Journal*, 323 (7304), 101–5.

Thompson, S.G. (2001) Why and how sources of heterogeneity should be investigated. In: *Systematic Reviews in Health Care: Meta-analysis in Context* (Egger, M., Davey Smith, G. & Altman, D.G. eds), pp. 157–75. BMJ Publishing, London.

Verhagen, A.P., de Vet, H.C., de Bie, R.A., Boers, M. & van den Brandt, P.A. (2001) The art of quality assessment of RCTs included in systematic reviews. *Journal of Clinical Epidemiology*, 54 (7), 651–4.

Yoon, H.S., Song, H.H. & Ro, Y.J. (2003) A comparison of effectiveness of bladder training and pelvic muscle exercise on female urinary incontinence. *International Journal of Nursing Studies*, 40 (1), 45–50.

5 Biofeedback and Anal Sphincter Exercises for Faecal Incontinence in Adults

Christine Norton

Introduction

This chapter will describe a Cochrane review of conservative interventions for adults with faecal incontinence (Norton et al., 2006). The methods and findings of the review will be described and issues and problems arising will be discussed.

Background

The problem of faecal incontinence

Faecal incontinence (FI) has been defined as 'involuntary loss of stool that is a social or hygienic problem' (Norton et al., 2005). This has been a neglected topic in health care. Taboos and general distaste surrounding bowel function have contributed to under-recognition of the scale of the problem and a lack of research on investigation and treatment options (Lawler, 1997; Norton, 2004). The best epidemiological data available suggest that about 5% of community-dwelling adults have some degree of FI (Macmillan et al., 2004), with about 1% of the population having a problem severe enough to limit their lifestyle (Perry et al., 2002). This rises to much higher levels among specific patient groups, such as those with neurological disorders or chronic diarrhoea, and may be over 50% in frail residents of nursing homes (Potter et al., 2002). In most large studies the proportion of men and women with symptoms is roughly equal.

There can be little doubt that FI is an unpleasant and distressing condition, both for the patient and any carers involved. However, there have been few studies formally investigating the impact. It is thought that the vast majority of those with symptoms never seek help from healthcare professionals (Johanson & Lafferty, 1996). Those who do ask for treatment may encounter negative attitudes or therapeutic pessimism.

Nurses have traditionally taken little interest in the topic of FI, managing symptoms rather than addressing the possibility of improving symptoms. Even amongst continence specialists this has remained a neglected area, and the body of nursing knowledge on the topic is very limited. Nurses are well placed to help such patients, often being able to discuss such taboo topics openly (Norton, 2004), but it is only recently that information to assist in this has been easily available (Norton & Chelvanayagam, 2004).

FI is a symptom, not a diagnosis. A variety of possible causes and contributing factors may underlie the symptom (Norton & Chelvanayagam, 2004). Treatment options investigated to date are limited in their scope and in their success rates (Madoff et al., 2005; Norton et al., 2005).

Biofeedback and exercises

Biofeedback is the use of direct information about normally subconscious or involuntary bodily functions to enable the individual to attempt to modify those functions. Visual or auditory feedback (most commonly using computer technology) has been used to enable the patient to improve rectal sensitivity to stool presence, enhance voluntary anal sphincter performance via exercise training and/or to improve coordination between reflex and voluntary anorectal function.

Biofeedback is the most widely reported treatment option for faecal incontinence in adults, with over 60 papers published in English. Only one published paper has reported that biofeedback does not work (van Tets et al., 1996). However, most papers are case series, with all the bias and confounding variables that are inherent in that methodology, in addition to a publication bias in favour of positive studies that is well recognised in all areas of health care.

Pelvic floor muscle training (PFMT) attempts to improve anal sphincter strength and function by using a structured programme of voluntary exercises (squeezes). It has been shown in randomised studies to be effective for the treatment of some types of urinary incontinence, and there has been an assumption that the same intervention would be effective for faecal incontinence; however, very few studies have investigated the use of PFMT alone for this symptom.

Both of these interventions inevitably involve a complex combination of patient education and interaction with a therapist, incidental information on other aspects of care (such as advice on diet and practical management), and an element of emotional support and imparting therapeutic optimism. Given that both biofeedback and PFMT are costly financially and in terms of professional and patient time, it is important to know whether these treatments genuinely make a difference to patient symptoms or quality of life, and, if they are effective, which is the most important element of the complex mix? Alternative treatments for FI, such as surgery or irrigation, are usually more invasive than either biofeedback or PFMT, and carry higher costs and risks of morbidity, but would be justified if the latter options are ineffective.

The Cochrane Incontinence Group

The Cochrane Incontinence Group (www.cure. otago.ac.nz) was established in 1996 with the aim of reviewing the evidence base for interventions for urinary and faecal incontinence. In line with all other Cochrane groups, evidence from randomised controlled trials (RCTs) is taken as the gold standard for deciding whether an intervention gives health gain. Evidence from non-randomised studies are considered too prone to various sources of bias to allow definitive conclusions.

Two or more reviewers collaborate on each review. Before starting the review, a protocol is written and peer-reviewed. This pre-specifies the topics of interest, literature search strategy, comparisons between treatments that are considered most relevant and outcome measures that will be assessed. This process is designed to ensure that the review is a formal secondary research study, and not just an *ad hoc* dredging of studies to see what emerges. Detailed guidance is given by the Cochrane Collaboration on conducting all stages of the review, in a detailed online handbook (www. cochrane.org/resources/handbook). The Incontinence Group already keeps a detailed register of all known RCTs that might be of relevance to reviews on incontinence, gathered as a result of electronic and hand searching. The editorial base offers support to reviewers in the technicalities of searching and the practicalities of article retrieval.

Overview of the review

Aim

The aim of the review presented here was to search systematically for and combine evidence from all relevant RCTs on the effects of biofeedback and/or sphincter exercises for the treatment of FI in adults, in order to provide the best evidence currently available on which to base recommendations for clinical practice.

Objectives and hypotheses

The objective of the review was to determine the effectiveness of biofeedback and/or anal sphincter

---

Box 5.1   Hypotheses of the review.

(1) Anal sphincter exercises/pelvic floor muscle training alone are more effective than no treatment in alleviating faecal incontinence.
(2) Anal sphincter exercises/pelvic floor muscle training alone are more effective than any other treatment in alleviating faecal incontinence.
(3) Biofeedback alone is more effective than no treatment in alleviating faecal incontinence.
(4) Biofeedback alone is more effective than any other treatment in alleviating faecal incontinence.
(5) Anal sphincter exercises/pelvic floor muscle training in combination with biofeedback is more effective than either treatment alone, or than no treatment or any other treatment in alleviating faecal incontinence.
(6) One modality of anal sphincter exercises/pelvic floor muscle training and/or biofeedback is more effective than any other.

---

exercises/pelvic floor muscle training in the treatment of the symptom of faecal incontinence in adults. The hypotheses considered are shown in Box 5.1.

Methods

Trials selection

Two reviewers examined all the citations and abstracts derived from the electronic search strategy. Reports of potentially relevant trials were retrieved in full, and both reviewers applied the selection criteria to trial reports independently. Reviewers were not blind to the names of trial authors, institutions or journals.

Quality assessment

The methodological quality of identified trials was assessed independently by two reviewers, taking into account the quality of random alloca-

tion concealment, description of dropouts and withdrawals, whether data were analysed on an intention to treat basis, and whether therapists, participants or outcome assessors were blind to the treatments provided. Since it has been demonstrated that the quality of allocation concealment can affect the results of studies, each of the two reviewers rated the quality of allocation in three grades (Box 5.2). Studies were excluded if they were not randomised or quasi-randomised controlled trials in adults.

Outcome measures

There is no universally accepted single outcome measure for FI symptoms, and very little work has been done on what is most important to patients. It was decided to focus on measures of patient symptoms (questionnaires or diaries), satisfaction with status/outcome, proxy measures such as anal pressure, generic measures of health status (e.g. quality of life, activities of daily living or anxiety and depression) and costs.

Box 5.2   Grading used for quality of allocation concealment.

A, clearly adequate (e.g. central randomisation by telephone, numbered or coded identical containers administered sequentially, randomisation scheme controlled externally, etc.).
B, possibly adequate (e.g. sealed envelopes but not sequentially numbered or opaque, closed list of random numbers).
C, clearly inadequate (e.g. open list of random numbers, alternation, date of birth, day of week, case record number).

Data extraction and analysis

Data of interest were any quantitative data related to the pre-specified outcome measures. Data extraction from the included studies was undertaken independently by two reviewers. Missing information was sought from trial authors if necessary. Data were analysed using the Meta View statistical programme in Review Manager (RevMan).

Results

Thirty-five possible studies were identified by the search. Of these, some included children only, while others were not RCTs or did not include the target interventions. Two were abstract reports of subsequently published full papers. This left 11 studies to be included: 10 full papers (Latimer et al., 1984; Whitehead et al., 1985; Miner et al., 1990; Fynes et al., 1999; Heymen et al., 2000; Norton et al., 2003; Solomon et al., 2003; Davis et al., 2004; Mahony et al., 2004; Ilnyckyj et al., 2005) and one reported in abstract form (McHugh et al., 1986). The total number of participants randomised between these 11 studies was 564 (range 8–171 in different studies). All were hospital based in English-speaking countries.

Results from a single trial in this review suggest that anal biofeedback is superior to vaginal, and that electrical stimulation might enhance the results of exercises (Fynes et al., 1999). However, the trial focused on the use of electrical stimulation as an adjunct to biofeedback and compared two very different types of interventions (vaginal pelvic floor manometric pressure biofeedback and home exercise with anal electromyography (EMG) biofeedback, and home exercises in combination with anal electrical stimulation) rather than singling out the effects of electrical stimulation or biofeedback. Moreover, it is difficult to know how much of this improvement is a consequence of the natural history of faecal incontinence following childbirth, as a no-treatment group was not included. Another study found that adding electrical stimulation to exercise alone did not enhance the effectiveness of the exercises (Mahony et al., 2004).

Several studies compared exercises, with or without different methods of delivering biofeedback. All found no difference between groups (Heymen et al., 2000; Norton et al., 2003; Solomon et al., 2003),

whether EMG, pressure, ultrasound or home biofeedback was used, and no adjunctive effect to exercises alone. One study found that adding biofeedback and exercises after surgery to repair the anal sphincter produced no better results than surgery alone (Davis et al., 2004). Another study compared exercises, with or without biofeedback, and an arm of patients who received only education and support (no biofeedback or exercises): it was found that there was no additional benefit from the exercises or biofeedback over and above nurse-led patient teaching (Norton et al., 2003).

It also appears that training to enhance rectal discrimination of sensation may be helpful in reducing faecal incontinence, at least in the short term (Miner et al., 1990). It may be that adding this technique to the more commonly available pelvic floor muscle training would enhance results, but this cannot be a strong recommendation in view of the small numbers and lack of follow-up data.

It should be noted that pressure/EMG measurements may not be comparable between different studies because of equipment and technique variations. Within-study changes should be more reliable. There are no direct 'objective' measures of faecal incontinence. Changes in anorectal physiology measurements are proxy outcome measures and do not necessarily indicate changes in the patient's symptoms, which should be seen as the primary endpoint.

Conclusions of the review

There have been over 60 uncontrolled trial reports in the literature on the use of biofeedback for the management of faecal incontinence in adults (Norton et al., 2005). Some authors maintain that biofeedback is the treatment of choice for faecal incontinence on the basis of the findings of these observational studies. However, the results of this review show that there is not enough evidence from RCTs to support the effectiveness of sphincter exercises and/or biofeedback therapy for the management of people with faecal incontinence. While all studies reviewed showed improved symptoms in all groups, no major between-group differences were found in any study.

We found no evidence that one method of biofeedback or exercises gives any benefit over any other method, nor that either exercises or biofeedback offer an advantage over other forms of conservative management. Addition of biofeedback to surgical sphincter repair does not appear to improve outcome (Davis et al., 2004). It is not possible to draw strong conclusions for practice from the data analysed in this review. In particular, there is not enough evidence on which to select patients suitable for anal sphincter exercises and/or biofeedback, nor to know which modality of biofeedback or exercises is optimal. Reducing the threshold of discrimination of rectal sensation does seem to be clinically useful (Miner et al., 1990). Electrical stimulation and/or anal biofeedback may be superior to vaginal biofeedback in women with symptoms after childbirth (Fynes et al., 1999). However, based on the available evidence, these conclusions can only be tentative. No study reported any adverse events or deterioration in symptoms, and it seems likely that these treatments are relatively unlikely to do any harm.

Issues that arose from carrying out the review

Randomised versus non-randomised evidence

Randomised controlled trials are thought to provide sound evidence on the effects of healthcare interventions, mainly because they can eliminate selection bias. Methodological weaknesses in all trials but three (Norton et al., 2003; Solomon et al., 2003; Mahony et al., 2004) included in this review are likely to have compromised this assumption. There was wide variation among trial reports in the type of participants, type of interventions, use of outcome measures, duration of treatment and length of follow-up. Most trials were small and probably of insufficient power to detect any differences between intervention groups. The outcome measures used were often insufficiently reported to enable further statistical analyses. Length of follow-up was not clearly reported or was inadequate in many of the trials. The way in which data were reported in many of the trials (by not reporting measures of variance) made a quantitative synthesis of results (meta-analysis) impossible.

The low number of studies and participants mean that many possible treatment options have yet to be properly explored. Because the Cochrane Collaboration only considers RCTs, this can bias review conclusions towards those areas where there is some randomised evidence, at the expense of treatments that have yet to be the subject of RCTs. One small RCT (possibly underpowered) can discount the reports of case series with many more participants.

However, reviewers are obviously very conscious of this tendency. As experts in their clinical field, they will be aware of other non-RCT evidence and must make a judgement as to whether they should discuss such evidence and use it in reaching their conclusions.

The power of RCT evidence is that it can overturn accepted wisdom on clinical effectiveness. With bowel function disorders, as with many other areas of chronic disease management, there is a large and recognised effect of intervening *per se* (Whitehead et al., 1999). This is often termed the placebo response in trials of pharmacological agents, but is probably more usefully considered as a non-specific effect of treatment which should not so much be excluded as harnessed and maximised for patient benefit (Chaput de Saintonge & Herxheimer, 1994). Without an RCT, it would be easy to assume that these non-specific effects are attributable to the target intervention (e.g. biofeedback or exercises), without recognising that patient contact, time, information, support and education are factors in the change. It might then be assumed that expensive and complex computer or ultrasound equipment is needed to treat these patients. The RCT evidence suggests that it does not matter what equipment is used, or none at all, since patients improve at similar rates whatever intervention is used. This then challenges the accepted wisdom that 'biofeedback works for FI'. It is not even known if repeated patient contact is needed for improvement. One cohort study has suggested that telephone follow-up is as effective as face-to-face contact (Byrne et al., 2005), and this now needs testing in an RCT.

Those areas that have not yet been subject to RCT evaluation cannot be discounted. Absence of evidence of effect is not the same as evidence of absence of effect, and it is important that the review does not give the impression that treatments not yet subjected to an RCT do not work.

Outcome measures

There has been very limited work on developing or validating outcome measures for faecal incontinence. Almost all studies have reported researcher evaluation of outcome, or have used very simplistic and non-validated scores for symptoms. Little is known about what is important to patients with FI, with only two studies on this topic (Rockwood et al., 1999; Gardener et al., 2005).

The Cochrane Collaboration software for handling reviews is designed for ease of meta-analysis of data from large studies, usually with biological data (e.g. drug studies reporting quantitative measurements of continuous variables such as blood pressure or body weight). These data, if normally distributed, will often be presented as means and standard deviations or confidence intervals. If several studies have the same outcome measure, the software automatically summates them, taking account of different sample sizes, to give an estimate of overall effect. This can mean that several small, individually underpowered studies can together give meaningful results, or that the overall effect from several studies that gave conflicting results can be seen.

Few studies in FI have reported any outcome measures that can be entered into the Cochrane statistical package and, for the few that do, this may not be a valid thing to do. With a symptom such as faecal incontinence, there are few biological endpoints. In an attempt to substitute for this, various artificially constructed scores have been developed, but none has yet been subject to rigorous validation. There is a temptation to take such scores at face value as a continuous variable, but this could lead to spurious conclusions: it is by no means established that there is an equal distance between all data points, and values are possibly better treated as categorical data.

International relevance

This review was only able to assess studies published in the English language. A few non-English cohort studies are published (mainly in German or Spanish), the abstracts of which suggest that methods of biofeedback and exercise employed in other countries are probably quite similar to those in the included studies. However, little is know about what treatments (if any) are used with patients with FI in non-English-speaking parts of the world.

Translating the evidence into clinical recommendations

The clinical (as opposed to statistical) implications of the findings are difficult to draw. Logically, the evidence suggests that biofeedback, and perhaps even exercises, should be abandoned in favour of just talking to and educating patients. However, with small numbers of highly selected patients being included in studies, and all clinical series except one suggesting benefit, this may be a rash and premature conclusion. In an era when clinicians are being asked to base practice on good research evidence, there is a risk that publication of a review such as this could lead to decisions that biofeedback services should not be funded or that exercises are not worth doing. However much authors stress the paucity of the evidence, it tends to be the headlines that are noticed the most.

Relationship with other systematic reviews on the subject

There have been very few other reviews on this subject, and none of them were 'systematic'. Other Cochrane reviews have covered surgery, medication and neurological bowel management. None have found enough evidence for firm conclusions and recommendations. This leaves clinicians reliant on inferior evidence and expert opinion when making clinical management decisions.

Reflections on future reviews

Since the first Cochane review on biofeedback (1999), there has been a great increase in the quality of studies and the number of participants included. However, this evidence still only covers 11 studies and 500 patients. It must be debated whether exclusion of non-RCT evidence is sensible, given the paucity of RCT evidence on this topic. It would also be valuable to attempt to include any studies published in other languages.

Conclusion

Treatment options for faecal incontinence have not yet been investigated by means of well-designed trials. A Cochrane review of surgery for faecal incontinence (Bachoo et al., 2000) failed to draw conclusions about the effectiveness of different surgical interventions, mainly because of the dearth of controlled clinical trials concerning the most common operations (e.g. anterior overlapping anal sphincter repair), and the lack of trials comparing surgical methods with conservative treatments. A Cochrane review on drug treatments also failed to draw firm conclusions (Cheetham et al., 2003).

There is a need for well-designed RCTs with adequate sample sizes, validated outcome measures and long-term follow-up. In particular, studies should assess the effectiveness of different components of the package of care often called 'biofeedback', including exercises, feedback on sphincter function, rectal sensitivity training and coordination training, and the other advice and information that is often given to patients during the course of consultation (patient teaching, dietary advice, medication and bowel habit training). Very little attention seems to have been given to patients' perspectives on outcome in the studies reviewed, and there is no information on what patients view as a good or satisfactory outcome of treatment for faecal incontinence. Economic analyses should also be incorporated into future trials.

There is also a need for trials comparing exercises and/or biofeedback with other treatments, such as medication, dietary manipulation or surgery. In all future studies, there is a need to characterise participants in detail so that judgements can be made on which treatments are of benefit in which diagnostic categories.

References

Bachoo, P., Brazzelli, M. & Grant, A. (2000) Surgery for faecal incontinence in adults. *Cochrane Database of Systematic Reviews* 1999, Issue 3, Art. No. CD001757. John Wiley & Sons, Chichester.

Byrne, C.M., Solomon, M.J., Rex, J., Young, J.M., Heggie, D. & Merlino, C. (2005) Telephone vs face-to-face biofeedback for fecal incontinence: comparison of two techniques in 239 patients. *Diseases of the Colon and Rectum*, 48 (12), 2281–8.

Chaput de Saintonge, D.M. & Herxheimer, A. (1994) Harnessing placebo effects in health care. *Lancet*, 344, 995–8.

Cheetham, M., Brazzelli, M., Norton, C. & Glazener, C.M. (2003) Drug treatment for faecal incontinence in adults. *Cochrane Database of Systematic Reviews* 2002, Issue 3, Art. No. CD002116. John Wiley & Sons, Chichester.

Davis, K.J., Kumar, D. & Poloniecki, J. (2004) Adjuvant biofeedback following sphincter repair: a randomized study. *Alimentary Pharmacology and Therapeutics*, 20 (5), 539–49.

Fynes, M.M., Marshall, K., Cassidy, M., Behan, M., Walsh, D., O'Connell, P.R. & O'Herlihy, C. (1999) A prospective, randomized study comparing the effect of augmented biofeedback with sensory biofeedback alone on fecal incontinence after obstetric trauma. *Diseases of the Colon and Rectum*, 42 (6), 753–8.

Gardener, N., Avery, K., Abrams, P. & Norton, C. (2005) Methods of development of a symptom and quality of life assessment for bowel symptoms including anal incontinence – ICI-BS (Abstract 100, presented at the International Continence Society, Montreal). *Neurology and Urodynamics*, 24 (5/6), 558–9.

Heymen, S., Pikarsky, A.J., Weiss, E.G., Vickers, D., Nogueras, J.J. & Wexner, S. (2000) A prospective randomised trial comparing four biofeedback techniques for patients with faecal incontinence. *Colorectal Disease*, 2, 88–92.

Ilnyckyj, A., Fachnie, E. & Tougas, G. (2005) A randomized controlled trial comparing an educational intervention alone vs education and biofeedback techniques for patients with faecal incontinence. *Neurogastroenterology and Motility*, 17 (1), 58–63.

Johanson, J.F. & Lafferty, J. (1996) Epidemiology of fecal incontinence: the silent affliction. *American Journal of Gastroenterology*, 91 (1), 33–6.

Latimer, P.R., Campbell, D. & Kasperski, J. (1984) A components analysis of biofeedback in the treatment of faecal incontinence. *Biofeedback and Self-Regulation*, 9 (3), 311–24.

Lawler, J. (1997) *The Body in Nursing*. Churchill Livingstone, Melbourne.

Macmillan, A.K., Merrie, A.E.H., Marshall, R.J. & Parry, B.R. (2004) The prevalence of fecal incontinence in community-dwelling adults: a systematic review of the literature. *Diseases of the Colon and Rectum*, 47, 1341–9.

Madoff, R.D., Pemberton, J.H., Mimura, T. & Laurberg, S. (2005) Surgery for fecal incontinence. In: *Incontinence*, 3rd edn (Abrams, P. et al., eds), pp. 1565–88. Health Publications, Plymouth.

Mahony, R., Malone, P.A., Nalty, J., Behan, M., O'Connell, P.R. & O'Herlihy, C. (2004) Randomized clinical trial of intra-anal electromyographic biofeedback and intra-anal electromyographic biofeedback augmented with electrical stimulation of the anal sphincter in the early treatment of postpartum fecal incontinence. *American Journal of Obstetrics & Gynecology*, 191 (3), 885–90.

McHugh, S., Walma, K. & Diamant, N.E. (1986) Faecal incontinence: a controlled trial of biofeedback. *Gastroenterology*, 90, 1545.

Miner, P.B., Donnelly, T.C. & Read, N.W. (1990) Investigation of the mode of action of biofeedback in the treatment of faecal incontinence. *Digestive Diseases and Sciences*, 35 (10), 1291–8.

Norton, C. (2004) Nurses, bowel continence, stigma and taboos. *Journal of Wound Ostomy and Continence Nursing*, 31 (2), 85–94.

Norton, C. & Chelvanayagam, S. (2004) *Bowel Continence Nursing* Beaconsfield Publishers, Beaconsfield.

Norton, C., Chelvanayagam, S., Wilson-Barnett, J., Redfern, S. & Kamm, M.A. (2003) Randomized controlled trial of biofeedback for fecal incontinence. *Gastroenterology*, 125, 1320–9.

Norton, C., Whitehead, W.E., Bliss, D.Z., Metsola, P. & Tries, J. (2005) Conservative and pharmacological management of faecal incontinence in adults. In: *Incontinence* (Abrams, P. et al., eds), pp. 1521–63. Health Publications, Plymouth.

Norton, C., Cody, J. & Hosker, G. (2006) Effectiveness of biofeedback and/or sphincter exercises for the treatment of faecal incontinence in adults. *Cochrane Database of Systematic Reviews* 2006, Issue 3, Art. No. CD002111. John Wiley & Sons, Chichester.

Perry, S., Shaw, C., McGrother, C. et al. (2002) The prevalence of faecal incontinence in adults aged 40 years or more living in the community. *Gut*, 50, 480–4.

Potter, J., Norton, C. & Cottenden, A. (2002) *Bowel Care in Older People*. Royal College of Physicians, London.

Rockwood, T.H., Church, J.M., Fleshman, J.W. et al. (1999) Patient and surgeon ranking of the severity of symptoms associated with fecal incontinence: the fecal incontinence severity index. *Diseases of the Colon and Rectum*, 42, 1525–32.

Solomon, M.J., Pager, C.K., Rex, J., Roberts, R. & Manning, J. (2003) Randomised, controlled trial of biofeedback with anal manometry, transanal ultrasound, or pelvic floor retraining with digital guidance alone in the treatment of mild to moderate fecal incontinence. *Diseases of the Colon and Rectum*, 46 (6), 703–10.

van Tets, W.F., Kuijpers, J.H. & Bleijenberg, G. (1996) Biofeedback treatment is ineffective in neurogenic fecal incontinence. *Diseases of the Colon and Rectum*, 39 (9), 992–4.

Whitehead, W.E., Burgio, K.L. & Engel, B.T. (1985) Biofeedback treatment of faecal incontinence in geriatric patients. *Journal of the American Geriatrics Society*, 33, 320–24.

Part 2

Meta-synthesis and Meta-study of Qualitative Research

6 Overview of Methods

Myfanwy Lloyd Jones

Introduction

This chapter offers definitions of meta-study and meta-synthesis, and traces the development of those methodologies. It then discusses key methodological aspects that affect the process of undertaking a meta-study or meta-synthesis, including choice of topic, identification of relevant studies and choice of method used to synthesise study findings.

What are meta-study and meta-synthesis?

The recent dramatic increase in the volume of primary qualitative research (Lloyd Jones, 2004) has led to growing interest in the synthesis of such research. This can take two main forms:

- Descriptive synthesis, in which published studies are described using techniques such as narrative summary and tabulation, generally without seeking to reinterpret the findings
- Interpretive synthesis, in which data from published studies are synthesised and reinterpreted (Evans, 2005)

Meta-study and meta-synthesis together embrace the major approaches to interpretive synthesis. Meta-synthesis is a generic term that embraces a number of approaches to synthesising the findings from primary qualitative studies to produce new insights and understandings (Paterson & Thorne, 2003), while meta-study is a specific research approach in which the theory, methods and findings of qualitative research are analysed and synthesised to develop new ways of thinking about the topic of interest (Paterson & Thorne, 2003). Neither meta-study nor meta-synthesis involve the re-analysis of raw data from the primary qualitative studies.

Meta-study and meta-synthesis can be used to determine what is known and what is not known about a topic of interest, reflect on the processes and perspectives of the relevant body of research, explore the underlying methodological decisions and theoretical influences, and suggest future directions for researchers, theoreticians and clinicians (Paterson & Thorne, 2003), providing both a foundation for future research and a means of understanding and advancing a discipline (Thorne & Paterson, 1998).

Superficially, meta-synthesis may appear analogous to quantitative meta-analysis. However, its goal is different. Meta-analysis is an aggregative method of combining the findings of quantitative studies that address the same research question, in order to achieve increased statistical power and greater precision. In contrast, meta-synthesis uses interpretive methods to synthesise the findings of qualitative studies into a new conceptualisation in order to develop theory or theoretical description

(Schreiber et al., 1997). While meta-analysis combines the results of very similar studies, meta-synthesis can draw on studies which vary in important respects (for example, their populations or settings) to achieve a greater degree of conceptual development and insight than was possible in the original studies. Thus, a meta-synthesis is more than the sum of its parts: it offers a novel interpretation which is not contained in any one of the constituent studies but is derived from all of those studies together (Sandelowski, 2004).

Unlike a critical research review, meta-synthesis is an investigation of the results and processes of previous research that allows the researcher to go beyond understanding to explanations and predictions of patterns of human behaviour. It highlights which populations have been studied and which have not, and synthesises and interprets the results of previous studies to reflect the state of research in a specific area. New conceptualisations arise from the process of comprehending the meanings of the original studies, synthesising the merged data, and recontextualising them into a comprehensive meaning (Sherwood, 1999).

Schreiber et al. (1997) note that meta-synthesis can be used for three main purposes (although these may overlap):

- Theory building: drawing on a number of studies of related concepts to push the level of theory beyond that possible in a single study, as in Kearney's study of women's addiction recovery (Kearney, 1998b)
- Theory explication: fleshing out abstract concepts and reconceptualising the original studies, generally focusing on studies of a single concept. Thus, in her study of courage in people with chronic health problems, Finfgeld substantiates pre-existing concepts, reassesses their significance and clarifies their interrelationships, resulting in the generation of a new model and theories (Finfgeld, 1999)
- Theoretical description: synthesising the findings of studies which deal with the target phenomenon into a comprehensive, thickly descriptive product, as in Barroso & Powell-Cope's study of living with HIV (Barroso & Powell-Cope, 2000)

Meta-synthesis depends on the assumption that it is reasonable to generalise beyond individual qualitative studies. This assumption is not univer-sally accepted. Moreover, some researchers who accept the principle of generalisation nonetheless fear that meta-synthesis may downplay important differences between individual studies, thus losing qualitative research's emphasis on context and holism (Campbell et al., 2003). However, the prag-matic value of meta-synthesis transcends these concerns: it allows qualitative research to be dis-seminated more widely, in a form that enables healthcare providers and policy makers to make sense of the findings and use them as a founda-tion for evidence-based practice (Kearney, 1998b; Finfgeld, 2003; McCormick et al., 2003). For resear-chers, meta-study and meta-synthesis can portray the state of the art in their area of interest and give directions for further work by highlighting trends, problems and continuing issues (McCormick et al., 2003). Meanwhile, the findings of the original stud-ies remain unaltered and available for reference (Finfgeld, 2003). Indeed, although a meta-synthesis presents only one 'reading' of the evidence, other readings are possible and should be encouraged (Noblit & Hare, 1988).

A brief history

The first major landmark in the synthesis of qual-itative research was Glaser & Strauss's proposal that higher-level theory could be generated by applying the basic techniques of grounded theory to pre-existing substantive grounded theory reports, a process they termed 'grounded formal theory'. They used theoretical sampling to identify relevant studies, but did not suggest how to identify the sampling frame (Glaser & Strauss, 1967). Kearney (1998a) subsequently suggested that grounded for-mal theory could also draw on phenomenological reports and content analyses, although their role would be subsidiary to that of grounded theory studies or studies that adhered to essential ele-ments of the grounded theory approach. Her stud-ies of women's experiences of domestic violence included reports that, although not necessarily grounded theory studies, used constant comparison to develop theory grounded in data (Kearney, 2001). Finfgeld also successfully used grounded theory methods to synthesise studies conducted using any predetermined, explicit and widely accepted qual-itative method (Finfgeld, 1999).

Noblit & Hare (1988) subsequently proposed their 'meta-ethnography' method, which they claimed was suitable for synthesising all types of interpretive research, and not just ethnographic studies. Their major innovation was to specify that the primary researchers' interpretations of their data formed the material to be synthesised. A meta-ethnography was therefore an interpretation of interpretations, and was intended to encourage dialogue and critique (Noblit, 2004). Noblit & Hare (1988) noted that the synthesis could take one of three forms – reciprocal, refutational and line-of-argument – depending on whether the findings of the synthesised studies were similar or contradictory, or whether they related to different aspects of a phenomenon but could be arranged to create a coherent argument. They gave clearer procedural guidance than had hitherto been available but, like Glaser & Strauss, offered little advice on study selection. They implied that meta-ethnography would often be used to synthesise specific studies that were already known to the researchers; they suggested that, if this were not so, the search for relevant studies should be exhaustive, but did not advise how it should be undertaken. Moreover, they appeared to envisage the synthesis of only a small number of studies: none of the examples they presented involved more than six studies (Noblit & Hare, 1988).

By contrast, the third major development, the meta-study approach of Paterson et al., was influenced by systematic review methodology: it emphasised the importance of using explicit and reproducible criteria and methods to identify and appraise all research relevant to the focus of interest (Paterson et al., 2001) and recognised the consequent need for a method able to deal with large numbers of studies that might be theoretically and methodologically varied and might yield dissimilar kinds of knowledge (Thorne et al., 2002b). Sociologists had already developed the concept of meta-study, which involved three components: meta-theory, meta-method and meta-data-analysis (Zhao, 1991). Paterson et al. provided comprehensive guidance through these three analytic components, and added a fourth component, meta-synthesis, to complete the meta-study process (Paterson et al., 2001).

For Paterson et al. (2001), meta-theory involves a careful examination of the theoretical perspectives or frameworks underlying the relevant studies, with the aim of understanding why researchers with diverse disciplinary and theoretical perspectives may uncover different findings even if they have similar research questions and samples (Thorne et al., 2002b). Meta-method is used both to assess the methodological rigour of individual studies and to reveal insights about the effect of methodological trends on evolving knowledge in a given field (Paterson et al., 2001). Meta-data-analysis involves examining the findings of each study in the light of other relevant studies to identify similarities and differences between them. Finally, in meta-synthesis, study findings are integrated to develop new truths and understandings, using any systematic interpretive approach used in primary qualitative research (Paterson et al., 2001).

Paterson et al's meta-study approach encourages careful consideration of the context and related assumptions underlying the findings of each contributing study, and their effect on those findings. It has the dual benefit of increasing the caution and sensitivity with which generalisations are made (Kearney, 2004), while also permitting the inclusion of dissimilar studies. A meta-study may focus primarily on one of the four components: for instance, it may result in a critique or intellectual history rather than a synthesis or integration of study findings (Thorne et al., 2002a). However, Sandelowski (2004) has argued that a true meta-synthesis should result in a set of inferences, conclusions or generalisations that researchers are willing to advance and defend, and that should therefore have immediate utility for clinical practice.

Key methodological aspects

This section briefly discusses key methodological aspects which affect the nature and findings of meta-studies and meta-syntheses. Although they must inevitably be described sequentially, in practice these aspects represent processes that are likely to overlap: as Paterson et al. (2001:112) state, meta-study is 'a dynamic and iterative process of thinking, interpreting, creating, theorizing, and reflecting'.

Focus of study, inclusion and exclusion criteria, theoretical framework

The starting point for any meta-study or meta-synthesis is the identification of the focus of study

– a topic, issue, setting, or controversy suited to qualitative research and, in the words of Noblit & Hare (1988:27), 'worthy of the synthesis effort'. This focus may be broad, as in Sherwood's (1997) study of caring seen from the client's perspective, or narrow, as in the study by Britten et al. (2002) of the perceived meanings of medicines and their impact on medicine-taking and communication with healthcare professionals. However, as it is unusual to find clusters of qualitative research on the same topic, the focus will usually be broader than the questions addressed in the original studies (Morse, 1997).

In healthcare research, the focus should be broad enough to capture fully the phenomenon of interest, but specific enough for the findings to be meaningful to healthcare providers, policy makers and researchers (Finfgeld, 2003). It should be delineated sufficiently clearly to allow relevant studies to be identified using explicit inclusion and exclusion criteria (Sherwood, 1999). However, as studies are identified and read, the initial focus may change or be modified (Noblit & Hare, 1988), for instance, being broadened or narrowed in response to the volume of data found; the inclusion and exclusion criteria should then be modified appropriately.

Key inclusion and exclusion criteria relate to factors such as study samples, settings and themes. Some researchers also specify research methods in these criteria, as they feel that studies using different qualitative methods should not be combined (Estabrooks et al., 1994; Jensen & Allen, 1996; Morse, 1997). Others disagree (Paterson et al., 2001; Clemmens, 2003). Findings derived from different qualitative methods may be used to qualify rather than to disconfirm results, and may furnish explanations for anomalous findings (Barbour, 1998). In addition, there are pragmatic arguments for including any studies whose findings are relevant, regardless of methodology. Meta-studies that reject research on the basis of study design alone risk denying valuable insights that contribute to the interpretation of a phenomenon (Booth, 2001). Moreover, many publications lack adequate methodological information (Lemmer et al., 1999; Paterson et al., 2001), while others display discrepancies between the claimed research method and the actual approach used (Paterson et al., 2001; Sandelowski & Barroso, 2003a). However, the decision on whether to limit studies to those using specific qualitative methodo-

logies depends ultimately on the philosophical position of the researcher and the purpose of the meta-study (Schreiber et al., 1997).

Exclusion criteria based on the year or language of publication should not be adopted for convenience, but should be justified in terms of the focus of study. For example, Barroso and Powell-Cope (2000) limited their meta-synthesis of qualitative research on living with HIV infection to studies conducted in the USA because they considered that, for different reasons, the experience of HIV-positive individuals in other Western countries and in developing countries would not be comparable with the experience of those living in the USA.

Some researchers adopt a theoretical framework to help define relevant concepts and determine the basis for the interpretation of findings (Paterson et al., 2001). Indeed, Harding & Gantley (1997) have claimed that a theoretically informed approach is vital in order to progress beyond 'common sense' insights. However, researchers should not be constrained by a framework that, as the study progresses, turns out to be inappropriate (Paterson et al., 2001). Examples of meta-studies which use theoretical frameworks are Finfgeld's (2001) review of research on how childbearing and childrearing women try to resolve substance abuse problems, which uses the harm reduction framework and Transtheoretical Model of Change, Paterson et al.'s (1998) use of Curtin and Lubkin's model of chronic illness in their meta-synthesis of adapting to and managing diabetes, and Fredriksson's (1999) exploration of modes of relating in a caring conversation in relation to the elements of presence, touch and listening, which, in a previous qualitative study, he had found to be essential to a caring conversation.

Study identification

Meta-study and meta-synthesis techniques may be applied to any group of qualitative studies that is relevant to the focus of interest. However, the influence of systematic review methodology has led to a growing emphasis on exhaustive literature searching, guided by explicit inclusion and exclusion criteria, and designed to identify as many potentially relevant studies as possible in order to minimise the likelihood of excluding important information or views.

Most literature searches in nursing studies start with electronic databases such as the Cumulative Index of Nursing and Allied Health Literature (CINAHL). Because of the difficulty of finding appropriate keywords to identify qualitative studies (Evans, 2002; Lloyd Jones, 2004), and because of the need to identify negative or disconfirming cases, very broad search strategies may be required. However, even if very sensitive search strategies are used, electronic searching alone is not enough. Some qualitative journals are not indexed in the electronic databases (Barbour & Barbour, 2003), and many qualitative studies are published in book form: electronic searches occasionally identify complete books, but generally do not identify studies published as book chapters (Walsh & Downe, 2005). Electronic searches should therefore be supplemented with the other strategies from Bates's 'berrypicking' search technique (Bates, 1989):

- Footnote chasing ('citation snowballing'): following up appropriate citations from the reference lists of relevant studies (Booth, 2001)
- Citation searching, using an electronic citation search facility
- Systematic hand searching of runs of relevant journals
- Area scanning: browsing materials that are physically adjacent to materials located earlier in a search (Barroso et al., 2003)
- Author searching: searching electronic databases for other relevant work by the authors of relevant publications (Barroso et al., 2003)

In addition, subject experts and other researchers in the field may be asked to identify relevant studies (Hawker et al., 2002; Walsh & Downe, 2005).

Despite the recognised place of serendipity in identifying relevant studies, and the subsequent difficulty of recording an exact search trail (Hawker et al., 2002), researchers should be transparent about how their search strategies were initially determined, and how they evolved over time (Walsh & Downe, 2005). Ideally, in future, Booth's STARLITE standard for reporting literature searches will be generally adopted (Booth, 2006).

Study selection

Once researchers have identified the studies that satisfy their initial inclusion and exclusion criteria,

they must decide whether to include all of these, or only a sample. Unless all relevant studies are included, important information or views may be excluded (Sherwood, 1999), thus limiting understanding of the phenomenon and its context (Jensen & Allen, 1996). However, the feasibility of including all the relevant studies depends on both the number of studies and the researcher's theoretical position. Sandelowski et al. (1997) consider that the inclusion of more than ten topically similar studies in one meta-synthesis can impede deep analysis and threaten the interpretive validity of findings. They note that this may be overcome if what initially appears to be one large topic is divided into several separate meta-syntheses on related topics whose findings can then be combined to create an overall picture. On the other hand, Paterson et al. (2001) suggest that at least a dozen discrete studies are needed for meaningful meta-study, although working with more than 100 may be 'overly ambitious'.

If the number of studies is such that sampling is necessary, the danger of excluding relevant information will be reduced if the sampling strategy seeks to include a wide range of types of papers reflecting as many themes or schools of thought as possible (Booth, 2001). That strategy may be purposive, selecting studies to reflect diversity and promote generalisability (Barbour & Barbour, 2003; Finfgeld, 2003), or theoretical, aiming to achieving data saturation (Dingwall et al., 1998).

Some researchers recommend excluding studies that otherwise satisfy the inclusion and exclusion criteria if their methodological quality is poor (Estabrooks et al., 1994; Sherwood, 1999). Others consider that this is inappropriate in the absence of universal consensus as to what constitutes a good qualitative study (Sandelowski et al., 1997; Popay et al., 1998; Paterson et al., 2001). Finfgeld (2003) has proposed two fundamental quality criteria: that a study should appear to have been conducted using widely accepted qualitative methods, and that its findings should be well supported by the raw data. There is also a strong case for excluding studies in which the researcher's 'political' agenda is evident throughout (Paterson et al., 2001). If studies are to be excluded for reasons of quality, the criteria should be predefined and the studies excluded on this basis should be listed, together with the specific reasons for their exclusion.

Summary, analysis and synthesis of study findings

As noted earlier, Noblit & Hare (1988) established that in meta-synthesis the 'data' to be summarised, analysed and synthesised were the primary researchers' findings (their concepts, interpretations and explanations), not the raw data (quotations, incidents, etc.) underlying, and offered in support of, those findings. Sandelowski & Barroso (2002) differentiate further between study findings and the analytical procedures used to produce them (data displays, coding schemes, etc.). In their meta-synthesis on motherhood in HIV-positive women, they excluded reports that contained no findings but only raw data presented as if they were findings. They also excluded selected findings from the included studies if they discerned no data supporting those findings (Sandelowski & Barroso, 2003b). Estabrooks et al. (1994) support this approach, whereas Barbour & Barbour (2003) recommend seeking additional information from the original researchers.

Approaches that can be used to analyse and synthesise study findings include grounded formal theory (Glaser & Strauss, 1967), meta-ethnography (Noblit & Hare, 1988), and less structured approaches such as the interpretive descriptive method described by Thorne et al. (1997). The approach used should suit the research question and design (Paterson et al., 2001). Thus, grounded formal theory is appropriate if the objective is to develop theory in a target domain, and if the findings reported by studies in that domain are suited to theoretical transformation (Sandelowski & Barroso, 2003b). Kearney used grounded formal theory in a study whose aim was to construct a theory of women's experiences in violent relationships, by synthesising studies which used constant comparative techniques to develop concepts or theories from original data (Kearney, 2001). Meta-ethnography is appropriate if the objective is to explore the relationship between the findings of individual studies when these findings take the form of concepts or metaphors (Sandelowski & Barroso, 2003b), as in Beck's meta-synthesis of caring within nursing education (Beck, 2001). However, strict adherence to some methods may not always be possible. For example, grounded theory as described by Glaser & Strauss (1967) depends on the ongoing generation of new data until all categories are saturated. However, in meta-synthesis the primary data set is

finite, and may not permit data saturation; this may then result in a limited emerging theory (Paterson et al., 2001). Whatever method is used, it should be made transparent in the written report (Barbour, 2001).

There should be evidence that the researchers have made diligent efforts to look for uniqueness in the data and to develop fully the categories and subcategories they have identified (Finfgeld, 1999), developing and testing hypotheses by further data collection and analysis in the search for evidence to support or negate the emerging theory (Paterson et al., 2001). Divergent or deviant data should not be glossed over as they may contribute to the development of new perspectives (Walsh & Downe, 2005). Additional insights may be gained by grouping the studies for analysis in as many ways as possible (for example, in relation to their historical or sociocultural context, research design or theoretical orientation) and then comparing the groups with each other (Paterson et al., 2001).

Campbell et al. (2003) have suggested that, in meta-ethnography, the order in which studies are synthesised may affect the outcome of the synthesis. However, the use of constant comparison, which is implicit in Noblit & Hare's (1988) general account of meta-ethnography, and specified in relation to line-of-argument synthesis, should counter this tendency, as should grouping the studies for analysis in as many ways as possible, as recommended by Paterson et al. (2001).

Tabulation of relevant data aids transparency in data analysis and synthesis. For example, for each study included in their meta-synthesis, Britten et al. (2002) tabulate details of their methodology, key concepts (first-order constructs – the everyday understandings of ordinary people) and main explanations and theories (second-order constructs – the constructs of the social sciences). They then tabulate their synthesis of those key concepts and second-order interpretations, together with the third-order interpretations they develop from them, which they finally link in the text into a line of argument.

A meta-study that uses an existing organising construct or framework to give meaning to the disparate themes identified in the analysis runs the risk of introducing bias through selecting codes or categories that are more congruent with that interpretation of the phenomenon under study than with the primary researchers' intentions, or placing too much weight on limited data because they support that prior interpretation, or ignoring data that do not support that reasoning (Paterson et al., 2001). Paterson et al. (2001) have proposed a number of strategies to counteract these dangers. When published meta-studies include a tabulation of the summarised findings of the included studies in relation to the theoretical framework, as in Burke et al.'s (1998) study of family or parent stress with a child in a chronic condition, readers can assess the fit between their findings and the theoretical framework.

Paterson et al. (2001) recommend comparing a tabulation of the specific constructs studied in the included studies with a table of relevant concepts in the field, derived from a literature review, in order to identify whether the included studies omit some themes or participant groups. This exercise enables researchers to gain insights by exploring the reasons for the omissions, and can also reveal differences in the primary researchers' interpretations of the phenomenon under study.

Some researchers utilise one or more strategies to attempt to safeguard the validity of their findings. Britten et al. (2002) recommend consulting the primary researchers to test the validity of the third-order interpretations and the extent to which they are supported by the primary data. In their meta-synthesis of studies of the lay meanings of medicines, the first author undertook the data analysis and synthesis, and fed the results back to the other authors (who included the authors of two of the synthesised papers) to confirm the congruence of her third-order interpretations with their own data. Jensen & Allen (1994) sought to validate the findings of their meta-synthesis of research on wellness–illness both internally, with the quotes of the studies' participants, and externally, through comparisons with other theoretical literature. Other possible methods include comparing the findings with oral testimony from relevant participants or with randomly or theoretically selected case studies (Booth, 2001), or using key informants to assess the appropriateness of the meta-synthesis findings as a reflection of their own experience (Paterson, 2003).

Interpretation of results and dissemination of findings

Authors should interpret the results of their meta-study or meta-synthesis in such a way as to determine its meanings for its intended audience; those meanings may relate to understandings of phenomena, or may identify issues that need addressing (Noblit & Hare, 1988). They should place the studies synthesised in a wider context (Noblit & Hare, 1988) and convey explicitly how the final synthesis is greater than the sum of its constituent parts (Walsh & Downe, 2005).

The findings of most meta-studies and meta-syntheses will be disseminated in scientific publications – journals, books or reports. However, in principle, other forms of dissemination may be used, including fiction, poetry, dance, drama and visual art (Annells, 2005). The choice of form should depend on the intended audience (Noblit & Hare, 1988). Whatever form is chosen, the phenomenon of interest should be clearly defined, and the essential patterns and explanatory themes defined (Sherwood, 1999).

Assessing the quality of a meta-synthesis

The summary above touches on many elements of quality in meta-synthesis. However, three main factors have been identified that may be used as an index of quality:

Credibility   A meta-synthesis should be rooted in the original data, and should present such faithful descriptions or interpretations of a human experience that people having that experience would immediately recognise it as their own (Jensen & Allen, 1996). Credibility is enhanced if the inferences drawn in the meta-synthesis are supported by raw data in the form of quotations from the original studies (Finfgeld, 2003).

Fittingness   The findings should fit into contexts outside those of the specific studies included in the meta-synthesis. They should be grounded in the life experiences studied, and reflect their typical and atypical elements (Jensen & Allen, 1996). While a meta-synthesis may be externally validated by comparison with the theoretical literature (Jensen & Allen, 1994), it should be remembered that such literature is not itself infallible.

Auditability   The purpose of the meta-synthesis should be explicit, and the methods used should be described in sufficient detail to allow the study to be replicated (Paterson et al., 2001). However, because of the nature of interpretive research, it should be recognised that the synthesis is an interpretation (Noblit & Hare, 1988), and that replication would not necessarily result in identical findings.

Conclusion

Meta-study and meta-synthesis are exciting and rigorous methods of exploring and building upon existing qualitative research. Inevitably, they have some limitations as a consequence of their dependence on the existence of sufficient relevant primary research studies, and on the quality of those studies. Moreover, as Kearney (2001) has noted, they run the risk of synthesising data relating to experiences that are culturally or historically incomparable in ways that are not apparent from the published reports. Following involvement in a meta-study of the body of qualitative literature about the chronic illness experience, Thorne (2004:1357) suggested that 'metastudy tends to serve us far better as a method for rigorously and systematically deconstructing existing bodies of qualitative research findings than it does as a technique for synthesizing powerful new products'. This view may be coloured by the size of that meta-study, which included 292 studies (Paterson, 2001); as noted above, Sandelowski et al. (1997) would consider the inclusion of so many studies to be problematic. Despite their caveats, Paterson and Thorne's research group was able to use the meta-study approach to develop the Shifting Perspectives Model of chronic illness (Paterson, 2001).

Meta-study and meta-synthesis have been shown to be valuable tools for interpreting and comparing qualitative study findings across settings and populations. They can lend credibility to some conclusions, while exposing the gaps and weaknesses in others (Paterson & Thorne, 2003). Thus, for example, Kearney & O'Sullivan (2003) found that popular theories of lifestyle change largely failed to account for key aspects of identity shift and behaviour change. Meta-study and meta-synthesis can also reveal how the dominant perspectives and methodologies within a field of study may have shaped interpretations (Paterson & Thorne, 2003), as in Slade's (2002) identification of the distinct medical and patient perspectives

on outcome measurement in mental health care, and how those dominant perspectives may have changed over time, as in Thorne & Paterson's (1998) identification of a shift in the 1990s from a negative to a perhaps unduly positive view of chronic illness. Finally, they have a key role in disseminating qualitative research findings to relevant audiences.

References

Annells, M. (2005) A qualitative quandary: alternative representations and meta-synthesis. *Journal of Clinical Nursing*, 14 (5), 535–6.

Barbour, R.S. (1998) Mixing qualitative methods: quality assurance or qualitative quagmire? *Qualitative Health Research*, 8 (3), 352–61.

Barbour, R.S. (2001) Checklists for improving rigour in qualitative research: a case of the tail wagging the dog? *British Medical Journal*, 322, 1115–17.

Barbour, R.S. & Barbour, M. (2003) Evaluating and synthesizing qualitative research: the need to develop a distinctive approach. *Journal of Evaluation in Clinical Practice*, 9 (2), 179–86.

Barroso, J. & Powell-Cope, G.M. (2000) Metasynthesis of qualitative research on living with HIV infection. *Qualitative Health Research*, 10 (3), 340–53.

Barroso, J., Gollop, C.J., Sandelowski, M., Meynell, J., Pearce, P.F. & Collins, L.J. (2003) The challenges of searching for and retrieving qualitative studies. *Western Journal of Nursing Research*, 25 (2), 153–78.

Bates, M.J. (1989) The design of browsing and berry-picking techniques for online search interface. *Online Review*, 13, 407–24.

Beck, C.T. (2001) Caring within nursing education: a metasynthesis. *Journal of Nursing Education*, 40 (3), 101–9.

Booth, A. (2001) Cochrane or cock-eyed? How should we conduct systematic reviews of qualitative research? Paper presented at the Qualitative Evidence-based Practice Conference, Taking a Critical Stance, Coventry University, 14–16 May 2001.

Booth, A. (2006) Brimful of STARLITE: towards standards for reporting literature searches. *Journal of the Medical Library Association*, 94 (4), 421–9.

Britten, N., Campbell, R., Pope, C., Donovan, J., Morgan, M. & Pill, R. (2002) Using meta ethnography to synthesise qualitative research: a worked example. *Journal of Health Services & Research Policy*, 7 (4), 209–15.

Burke, S.O., Kauffman, E., Costello, E., Wiskin, N. & Harrison, M.B. (1998) Stressors in families with a child with a chronic condition: an analysis of qualitative studies and a framework. *Canadian Journal of Nursing Research*, 30 (1), 71–95.

Campbell, R., Pound, P., Pope, C., Britten, N., Pill, R., Morgan, M. & Donovan, J. (2003) Evaluating meta-ethnography: a synthesis of qualitative research on lay experiences of diabetes and diabetes care. *Social Science and Medicine*, 56 (4), 671–84.

Clemmens, D. (2003) Adolescent motherhood: a meta-synthesis of qualitative studies. *MCN, American Journal of Maternal Child Nursing*, 28 (2), 93–9.

Dingwall, R., Murphy, E., Watson, P., Greatbatch, D. & Parker, S. (1998) Catching goldfish: quality in qualitative research. *Journal of Health Services Research and Policy*, 3 (3), 167–72.

Estabrooks, C.A., Field, P.A. & Morse, J.M. (1994) Aggregating qualitative findings: an approach to theory development. *Qualitative Health Research*, 4 (4), 503–11.

Evans, D. (2002) Database searches for qualitative research. *Journal of the Medical Library Association*, 90 (3), 290–3.

Evans, D. (2005) Systematic reviews of interpretive research: interpretive data synthesis of processed data. *Australian Journal of Advanced Nursing*, 20 (2), 22–6.

Finfgeld, D.L. (1999) Courage as a process of pushing beyond the struggle. *Qualitative Health Research*, 9 (6), 803–14.

Finfgeld, D.L. (2001) Emergent drug abuse resolution models and their implications for childbearing and childrearing women. *Health Care for Women International*, 22, 723–33.

Finfgeld, D.L. (2003) Metasynthesis: the state of the art – so far. *Qualitative Health Research*, 13 (7), 893–904.

Fredriksson, L. (1999) Modes of relating in a caring conversation: a research synthesis on presence, touch and listening. *Journal of Advanced Nursing*, 30 (5), 1167–76.

Glaser, B.G. & Strauss, A.L. (1967) *The Discovery of Grounded Theory*. Aldine de Gruyter, New York.

Harding, G. & Gantley, M. (1997) Qualitative methods: beyond the cookbook. *Family Practice*, 15, 76–9.

Hawker, S., Payne, S., Kerr, C., Hardey, M. & Powell, J. (2002) Appraising the evidence: reviewing disparate data systematically. *Qualitative Health Research*, 12 (9), 1284–99.

Jensen, L.A. & Allen, M.N. (1994) A synthesis of qualitative research on wellness–illness. *Qualitative Health Research*, 4 (4), 349–69.

Jensen, L.A. & Allen, M.N. (1996) Meta-synthesis of qualitative findings. *Qualitative Health Research*, 6 (4), 553–60.

Kearney, M. (2004) Interpretive practice and theory building. *Qualitative Health Research*, 14 (10), 1351–5.

Kearney, M.H. (1998a) Ready-to-wear: discovering grounded formal theory. *Research in Nursing and Health*, 21 (2), 179–86.

Kearney, M.H. (1998b) Truthful self-nurturing: a grounded formal theory of women's addiction recovery. *Qualitative Health Research*, 8 (4), 495–512.

Kearney, M.H. (2001) Enduring love: a grounded formal theory of women's experience of domestic violence. *Research in Nursing and Health*, 24 (4), 270–82.

Kearney, M.H. & O'Sullivan, J. (2003) Identity shifts as turning points in health behavior change. *Western Journal of Nursing Research*, 25 (2), 134–52.

Lemmer, B., Grellier, R., and Steven, J. (1999) Systematic review of nonrandom and qualitative research literature: exploring and uncovering an evidence base for health visiting and decision making. *Qualitative Health Research*, 9 (3), 315–28.

Lloyd Jones, M. (2004) Application of systematic review methods to qualitative research: practical issues. *Journal of Advanced Nursing*, 48 (3), 271–8.

McCormick, J., Rodney, P. & Varcoe, C. (2003) Reinterpretations across studies: an approach to meta-analysis. *Qualitative Health Research*, 13 (7), 933–44.

Morse, J.M. (1997) Responding to threats to integrity of self. *Advances in Nursing Science*, 19 (4), 21–36.

Noblit, G. (2004) Insights from the metaethnographic tradition. *Qualitative Health Research*, 14 (10), 1347–51.

Noblit, G.W. & Hare, R.D. (1988) *Meta-ethnography: Synthesizing Qualitative Studies*. Sage, Newbury Park.

Paterson, B.L. (2001) The shifting perspectives model of chronic illness. *Journal of Nursing Scholarship*, 33 (1), 21–6.

Paterson, B.L. (2003) The koala has claws: applications of the shifting perspectives model in research of chronic illness. *Qualitative Health Research*, 13 (7), 987–94.

Paterson, B.L. & Thorne, S. (2003) The potential of meta-synthesis for nursing care effectiveness research. *Canadian Journal of Nursing Research*, 35 (3), 39–43.

Paterson, B.L., Thorne, S. & Dewis, M. (1998) Adapting to and managing diabetes. *Image – the Journal of Nursing Scholarship*, 30 (1), 57–62.

Paterson, B.L., Thorne, S.E., Canam, C. & Jillings, C. (2001) *Meta-study of Qualitative Health Research*. Sage Publications, Thousand Oaks, California.

Popay, J., Rogers, A. & Williams, G. (1998) Rationale and standards for the systematic review of qualitative literature in health services research. *Qualitative Health Research*, 8 (3), 341–51.

Sandelowski, M. (2004) Metasynthesis, metastudy, and metamadness. *Qualitative Health Research*, 14 (10), 1357–60.

Sandelowski, M. & Barroso, J. (2002) Finding the findings in qualitative studies. *Journal of Nursing Scholarship*, 34 (3), 213–19.

Sandelowski, M. & Barroso, J. (2003a) Creating meta-summaries of qualitative findings. *Nursing Research*, 52 (4), 226–33.

Sandelowski, M. & Barroso, J. (2003b) Toward a meta-synthesis of qualitative findings on motherhood in HIV-positive women. *Research in Nursing and Health*, 26 (2), 153–70.

Sandelowski, M., Docherty, S. & Emden, C. (1997) Qualitative metasynthesis: issues and techniques. *Research in Nursing & Health*, 20 (4), 365–71.

Schreiber, R., Crooks, D. & Stern, P.N. (1997) Qualitative meta-analysis. In: *Completing a Qualitative Project: Details and Dialogue* (Morse, J. M., ed.), pp. 311–326. Sage, Thousand Oaks, California.

Sherwood, G. (1999) Meta-synthesis: merging qualitative studies to develop nursing knowledge. *International Journal for Human Caring*, 3 (1), 37–42.

Sherwood, G.D. (1997) Meta-synthesis of qualitative analyses of caring: defining a therapeutic model of nursing. *Advanced Practice Nursing Quarterly*, 3 (1), 32–42.

Slade, M. (2002) What outcomes to measure in routine mental health services, and how to assess them: a systematic review. *Australian and New Zealand Journal of Psychiatry*, 36, 743–53.

Thorne, S. (2004) The metastudy perspective. *Qualitative Health Research*, 14 (10), 1355–7.

Thorne, S. & Paterson, B. (1998) Shifting images of chronic illness. *Image – the Journal of Nursing Scholarship*, 30 (2), 173–8.

Thorne, S., Kirkham, S.R., & MacDonald-Emes, J. (1997) Focus on qualitative methods. Interpretive description: a noncategorical qualitative alternative for developing nursing knowledge. *Research in Nursing and Health*, 20 (2), 169–77.

Thorne, S., Joachim, G., Paterson, B. & Canam, C. (2002a) Influence of the research frame on qualitatively derived health science knowledge. *International Journal of Qualitative Methods*, 1 (1). http://www.ualberta.ca/~ijqm/

Thorne, S., Paterson, B., Acorn, S., Canam, C., Joachim, G. & Jillings, C. (2002b) Chronic illness experience: insights from a metastudy. *Qualitative Health Research*, 12 (4), 437–52.

Walsh, D. & Downe, S. (2005) Meta-synthesis method for qualitative research: a literature review. *Journal of Advanced Nursing*, 50 (2), 204–11.

Zhao, S.Y. (1991) Metatheory, metamethod, meta-data-analysis – what, why and how. *Sociological Perspectives*, 34 (3), 377–90.

7

Coming Out as Ill: Understanding Self-disclosure in Chronic Illness from a Meta-synthesis of Qualitative Research

Barbara L. Paterson

Introduction

In many research studies, both researchers and the people who participate in the research use the metaphor of 'coming out' to describe self-disclosure, or revealing of the authentic self to others (Antaki et al., 2005), in chronic illness. For example, one woman writes, 'I frequently found myself faced with the decision of whether to "come out" about my disease – when, to whom, under what circumstances, to what extent and in what manner' (Myers, 2004:256).

In this chapter, I illustrate the processes and procedures of meta-study, a particular approach to meta-synthesis of qualitative research, that I took to conduct a meta-study of 33 qualitative research reports about the 'coming out' experience, or self-disclosure, of people as HIV positive. Meta-study represents an attempt not only to compile and analyse the findings of various research reports, but also to reflect on the processes and perspectives of research in a way that acknowledges that researchers' decisions about the research design and their interpretations of the data occur within a broader sociocultural, disciplinary and historical context that shapes and is shaped by those decisions. The derivations of meta-study are located in both anthropological and sociological traditions of meta-theory, in which scholars have worked to synthesise diverse theoretical perspectives about particular phenomena to form a grand theory.

It is important to understand that the synthesis that occurs in meta-study is as much a social construction as the meta-synthesist's interpretations of individual research studies. Meta-study can provide fascinating insights about the prevailing ideas, methods and conclusions of research conducted within particular fields of study over time, but it also raises many questions with few definitive answers. The procedures of meta-study are detailed in our book about the method (Paterson et al., 2001) and elsewhere (Thorne & Paterson, 1998; Paterson, 2001, 2003a, b; Thorne et al., 2002a, b; Paterson et al., 2003).

The meta-study project

The primary research

For the project discussed in this chapter, I selected primary research reports (that is, qualitative research that formed the sample of the meta-study project) focusing on HIV-positive adults' self-disclosure of their serostatus to others. The details of the 33 studies are given in Appendix 7.1. These primary research reports were selected from published literature in the health and social sciences and unpublished doctoral theses reported from January 1990 to January 2006. Available research reports were identified by means of a search in

Table 7.1   Overview of primary research studies included in the meta-study.

Focus of study	Stated research methods	Theoretical framework[a]	Sample profile	Data collection
Effect of treatment on and by disclosure ($n = 1$)	Qualitative descriptive ($n = 25$)	Not identified ($n = 25$)	All women ($n = 13$)	Single individual interviews ($n = 29$)
Disclosure experience ($n = 17$)	Grounded theory ($n = 4$)	Stigma ($n = 5$)	All men ($n = 14$)	Multiple individual interviews ($n = 4$)
Decision making *re* disclosure ($n = 5$)	Phenomenology ($n = 2$)	Social support ($n = 1$)	Receiving antiretroviral treatment ($n = 1$)	
Disclosure in workplace ($n = 1$)	Case study ($n = 1$)	Decision making ($n = 1$)	No restriction other than person is HIV positive ($n = 5$)	
Disclosure in health care settings ($n = 1$)	Narrative analysis ($n = 1$)	Social action ($n = 1$)		
Impact of disclosure ($n = 3$)		Social cognitive learning ($n = 1$)		
Factors that influence intention to disclose ($n = 3$)		Communication privacy management ($n = 1$)		
Methods of disclosure ($n = 1$)				
Non-disclosure ($n = 1$)				

[a]Note: three studies had more than one theory as a framework.

computerised databases (e.g. the Cumulative Index of Nursing and Allied Health Literature (CINAHL), Sociological Abstracts, Digital Dissertations), as well as the reference lists of relevant studies. Selected primary research reports met the following criteria:

(1)   the researcher investigated self-disclosure of HIV from the perspective of the discloser as a person with HIV;
(2)   participants were adults (18 years and older);
(3)   the research approach was qualitative and interpretive;
(4)   the researcher(s) included clear details about the research design and the findings; and
(5)   the findings were presented as detailed, descriptive textual or narrative accounts of the phenomenon under study.

Over 100 research reports were reviewed. Of these, 33 qualitative research reports met the selection criteria and were selected for the meta-study.

Sample characteristics

An overview of the primary research reports is given in Table 7.1. Most of the primary research reports occurred in the years 2000–2006 ($n = 27$); the remaining six studies were in the years 1992–1999. One of the research studies was quantitative with a smaller but distinct qualitative component; two were qualitative with a minor quantitative segment. A variety of research approaches were represented in the body of primary research, including phenomenology ($n = 2$), grounded theory ($n = 4$), case method ($n = 1$), narrative analysis ($n = 1$), and generic or unspecified qualitative approaches that are descriptive in nature ($n = 25$). Interviewing was the data collection strategy used in all studies, although one researcher (Strawn, 1997) asked participants to identify their social support network and the closeness of their relationship by indicating this on a Personal Network Map. Single individual interviews were the data collection strategy used in all but four of the studies. The focus of the majority of the studies ($n = 17$) was the general experience of self-disclosure. Others investigated specific aspects of self-disclosure, such as the influence of HIV treatment on disclosure decisions, or self-disclosure in specific settings, such as the workplace.

Participants in this body of research had a wide range of ages, educational levels and ethnicity. The reported annual household income of participants was generally low (below US$25 000), largely because several of the primary research studies included only people in socially marginalised groups (e.g. injection drug users) and those who were symptomatic and unlikely to be fully employed. All of the primary researchers recruited participants from AIDS-specific clinics or AIDS-related organisations; however, researchers in seven studies included other means of recruitment, such as the snowball technique or advertisements in gay magazines.

Preparing for the meta-study

The quality of the preparation efforts that provide the foundation for meta-study research is crucial to the effectiveness and credibility of this work. In preparation for the meta-study research project about self-disclosure in HIV, I read 15 qualitative research reports about self-disclosure of HIV positive serostatus that had been conducted since 1980. This enabled me to narrow my research questions (i.e. What is the nature of the self-disclosure experience in HIV infection and what are the contexts that facilitate or constrain self-disclosure?), as well as to identify the selection criteria I would need to apply to locate relevant primary research for the meta-study. For example, I determined that I would include research that had been conducted about self-disclosure of HIV-positive serostatus since 1990, because 1990 marked the beginning of a shift away from sole focus on gay men in research about self-disclosure of HIV-positive serostatus (Noone, 2000), and because within the past 15 years treatment for HIV has been revolutionised by the developments in antiretroviral therapy.

I developed an appraisal tool to provide a systematic means of coding the data and an audit trail of data analysis decisions in the meta-study (see Appendix 7.2). This tool was refined as I located

new literature and asked different questions about the data that were needed to answer the research questions. For example, initially I did not think it was important to include details about how the authors of the various reports attended to ethical considerations of their studies. I thought that it would be interesting to note if the primary researchers draw attention in their discussion of the findings to the ethics of conducting such research, or in other words, the paradox of asking people to acknowledge that they do not always disclose their serostatus to others in a climate where non-disclosure is illegal. I included a section in the appraisal tool to identify researchers' discussions on the ethical implications of the research. The findings led me to ask why so few of them appeared to have considered the ethical conundrums of such research.

In group efforts in meta-study research, each primary research report is analysed by more than one research team member independently, and then discussed among the team to arrive at a consensual decision about the research (Paterson et al., 2001). As a sole researcher, I addressed the criteria of rigour as truth value, applicability, consistency and neutrality (Lincoln & Guba, 1985) by reading each primary research report at least five times, and by documenting my appraisal of the primary research reports, as well as my methodological procedures and decisions, such as how I determined which reports met the selection criteria of an adequate demographic profile of the participants and which did not. In addition, I checked all my interpretations of the findings with five experts in the field, including two people who are HIV positive, two researchers in the field, and an executive officer of an AIDS organisation.

The analytic components of meta-study

In meta-study research, the theory, research methods and findings of individual research reports are considered as data. The meta-study researcher analyses these data to identify the similarities, differences and patterns that exist. These are then synthesised to generate new or expanded theory about the phenomenon under study. The analysis in meta-study occurs in three phases: meta-data-analysis, meta-method and meta-theory. These can occur simultaneously as the primary research reports are reviewed. For example, in the meta-data-analysis component, I looked for findings that appeared to contradict one another or were contrary to my own experience. Then I searched for further data to support why this contradiction existed, including evidence that the choice of the research design (meta-method) or the theoretical framework (meta-theory) had influenced this occurrence.

Meta-data-analysis

Meta-data-analysis is the analysis of the findings reported by primary researchers in reports of their research (Paterson et al., 2001). In meta-data-analysis, the meta-study researcher compares the findings of individual research studies with those found in all primary research reports and in a sample (e.g. those with a similar sample profile) of the primary research that has been selected for review (Noblit & Hare, 1988). Meta-data-analysis is essentially an 'analysis of the analysis' of data provided by primary researchers.

I used the procedures advocated by Noblit & Hare (1988), pioneers of meta-ethnography, to conduct the meta-data-analysis of primary research about self-disclosure in HIV. This entailed identifying, comparing and contrasting the key metaphors evident in the findings presented in primary research reports and hypothesising about the relationships between various findings. Key metaphors are words, phrases, ideas, concepts or categories that encapsulate research findings.

The key metaphor that I located within this body of research was 'calculus'. The expressions of the calculus metaphor in the body of primary research are represented in Table 7.2. One pair of researchers (Black & Miles, 2002:692) refer to the calculus of self-disclosure in HIV as a 'careful, reasoned, evaluative process' that is 'used to weigh the risks of disclosing against the costs'. As well as anticipating the possible outcomes of the disclosure, calculus entails considering personal goals, the needs of others, moral and social obligations, and the context (e.g. the nature of the relationship with the other, timing, setting) before deciding to fully or partially disclose or to withhold disclosure of the serostatus. Another consideration in such a calculus is whether the serostatus will become known to the other person in another way (Friedman, 2004).

Although the person may wish to choose when and to whom disclosure occurs, visible symptoms (e.g. Kaposi's sarcoma) or other circumstances, such as others' lack of confidentiality, can result in the ill person being 'outed' as HIV positive. In general, primary researchers described planned, controlled self-disclosure as eliciting positive outcomes, and spontaneous self-disclosure as costly.

A critical step in meta-data-analysis is hypothesising about relationships between data and then testing those hypotheses by returning to the texts of primary research reports to determine if there is sufficient evidence to support the hypotheses. In much of the primary research, self-disclosure is depicted as enabling the person to embrace a new identity that incorporates the illness and/or to sustain an identity as a 'good' person, despite the stigmatising judgements of others. Non-disclosure, on the other hand, is represented as internalised stigma (believing the stigmatising attitudes of others to be appropriate and true), cowardice, irresponsibility and/or immorality.

I hypothesised that the focus on disclosure as 'good' and the emphasis on non-disclosure as evidence of personal inadequacy would vary according to the recipient of the disclosure (i.e. sexual partners, employers, children). I re-read all the reports, listing the phrases and terms that suggested that disclosure was moral and non-disclosure immoral. I concluded that there were indeed differences in the implication of morality among studies that focused on the experience of gay men with sexual partners and those of mothers who were deciding whether to disclose to their children. Mothers were portrayed as protective and strategic when they concluded that their children were too young or vulnerable to receive the news about the serostatus. Gay men, however, were represented as cowardly, irresponsible, in denial and/or immoral when they chose not to disclose their serostatus to sexual partners.

Meta-method

Meta-method involves the analysis of research methods used in the primary research to establish how researchers have attended to the rigour and epistemological integrity of their use of particular qualitative methods. It also includes determining how researchers' interpretations of qualitative

Table 7.2   Expressions of the calculus metaphor.

Metaphor	Source
'It may help me to accomplish my goals and/or to achieve what I need' and 'It may mean that my goals and/or needs will not be met'	Friedman, 2004; Schrimshaw & Siegel, 2002; Klitzman et al., 2004; de Ritter, 2001; Maman et al., 2001; Larkins et al., 2005; Farmer, 2004; Holt et al., 1998; Stirratt, 2004; Sauka & Lie, 2000; Sowell et al., 2003; Barnes, 1992; Black & Miles, 2002; Dane, 2002; Fesko, 2001; Gielen et al., 1997, 2000; Klitzman, 1999; Klitzman et al., 2004; Larkins et al., 2005; Nelson & Harvey, 1998; Ortiz, 2005; Parsons et al., 2004; Sheon & Crosby, 2004; Siegel et al., 2005; Strawn, 1997; Walsh, 2000; Yoshioka & Schustack, 2002
'It will cause the other to see me as a person' and 'It will cause the other to pay undue attention to my disease'	Paxton, 2004; Sauka & Lie, 2000; Schrimshaw & Siegel, 2002; Serovich et al., 2005; Stirratt, 2004; Vallerhard et al., 2005
'It will help our relationship' and 'It will damage our relationship'	Barnes, 1992; Black & Miles, 2002; Schrimshaw & Siegel, 2002; Bor et al., 2004; Dane, 2002; de Ritter, 2001; Farmer, 2004; Fesko, 2001; Friedman, 2004; Gielen et al., 1997, 2000; Holt et al., 1998; Klitzman, 1999; Larkins et al., 2005; Maman et al., 2001; Murphy et al., 2003; Nelson & Harvey, 1998; Noone, 2000; Ortiz, 2005; Parsons et al., 2004; Sauka & Lie, 2000; Siegel et al., 2005; Sowell et al., 2003; Strawn, 1997; Walsh, 2000; Yoshioka & Schustack, 2001
'I can decide where, when, to whom, and if I disclose' and 'It's only a matter of time before the other person knows'	de Ritter, 2001; Fesko, 2001; Friedman, 2004; Klitzman et al., 2004; Larkins et al., 2005; Sauka & Lie, 2000; Schrimshaw & Siegel, 2002; Sheon & Crosby, 2004; Siegel et al., 2005; Sowell et al., 2003; Strawn, 1997; Stirratt, 2004
'My needs are the priority' and 'Their need is greater than mine'	Black & Miles, 2002; Dane, 2002; Schrimshaw & Siegel, 2002; Larkins et al., 2005; Paxton, 2004; Stirratt, 2004; Vallerhard et al., 2005
'I am unskilled at disclosure' and 'I have learned the best way of doing this'	Chandra et al., 2003; Holt et al., 1998; Kimberly et al., 1995; Klitzman, 1999
'I have an obligation to disclose' and 'I need to protect myself by not disclosing'	Barnes, 1992; Black & Miles, 2002; Schrimshaw & Siegel, 2002; Bor et al., 2004; Dane, 2002; de Ritter, 2001; Farmer, 2004; Fesko, 2001; Friedman, 2004; Gielen et al., 1997, 2000; Holt et al., 1998; Klitzman, 1999; Larkins et al., 2005; Maman et al., 2001; Murphy et al., 2003; Nelson & Harvey, 1998; Noone, 2000; Ortiz, 2005; Parsons et al., 2004; Sauka & Lie, 2000; Siegel et al., 2005; Sowell et al., 2003; Stirratt, 2004; Strawn, 1997; Walsh, 2000; Yoshioka & Schustack, 2001
'It feels right to disclose now/in this setting/to this person' and 'It would be inappropriate/risky to disclose now/in this setting/to this person'	Black & Miles, 2002; de Ritter, 2001; Schrimshaw & Siegel, 2002; Farmerm 2004; Feskom 2001; Friedman, 2004; Gielen et al., 1997; Holt et al., 1998; Kimberly et al., 1995; Klitzman, 1999; Klitzman et al., 2004; Larkins et al., 2005; Nelson & Harvey, 1998; Ortiz, 2005; Paxton, 2004; Sheon & Crosby, 2004; Siegel et al., 2005; Sowell et al., 2003; Strawn, 1997; Stirratt, 2004; Vallerhard et al., 2005; Walsh, 2000
'It is liberating and empowering to me to disclose' and 'It will be a burden for the other to bear'	Schrimshaw & Siegel, 2002; Bor et al., 2004; de Ritter, 2001; Friedman, 2004; Gielen et al., 1997; Kimberly et al., 1995; Klitzman, 1999; Larkins et al., 2005; Noone, 2000; Paxton, 2004; Strawn, 1997; Stirratt, 2004; Vallerhard et al., 2005
'It is stressful to keep a secret about HIV serostatus' and 'Non-disclosure is a way to deal with the stress of living with HIV'	Black & Miles, 2002; de Ritter, 2001; Schrimshaw & Siegel, 2002; Farmer, 2004; Fesko, 2001; Friedman, 2004; Gielen et al., 1997; Holt et al., 1998; Kimberly et al., 1995; Klitzman, 1999; Klitzman et al., 2004; Larkins et al., 2005; Nelson & Harvey, 1998; Ortiz, 2005; Paxton, 2004; Sheon & Crosby, 2004; Siegel et al., 2005; Sowell et al., 2003; Strawn, 1997; Vallerhard et al., 2005; Walsh, 2000

methods have framed the design of the research and the nature of the findings that are generated in the research (Paterson et al., 2001; Thorne et al., 2002a, b). I conducted meta-method by performing an initial appraisal of the research question(s), the role of the researcher(s), and sampling, data collection and data analysis procedures in the individual studies (see Appendix 7.2). This revealed insights about the underlying assumptions, patterns and themes that were shared by primary researchers about the research methodologies they used. This was followed by an overall appraisal of the selected studies to determine how the methodology impacted and shaped the creation of knowledge about self-disclosure within the field.

One of the insights derived in meta-method was that there is minimal discussion by primary researchers about the participants' self-disclosure experiences that are not HIV related and how these may have affected their self-disclosure experience about their HIV-positive serostatus. We do not know, for example, how previous illness experiences, such as having type 1 diabetes as a young-ster, affect the decision to self-disclose HIV-positive serostatus. Neither do we know how the 'coming out' experience as a gay person influences self-disclosure decisions about HIV-positive serostatus. Few researchers explored participants' general disclosure preferences and how these were enacted or revised in the self-disclosure of HIV-positive serostatus. It would make sense that someone who is open with most people in most situations would maintain the same openness when they become HIV positive. Conversely, people who sustain tightly closed boundaries regarding personal information are unlikely to disclose their serostatus.

One of the procedures of meta-method is determining what has not been studied and what is missing in the researchers' investigation of the phenomenon under study. For example, although seven of the studies considered the cultural influences on disclosure decisions, including the culture of particular ethnic groups and the culture of gay men, there were no studies that specifically investigated the influence of culture in disclosure decisions that occurred in rural or religious communities. There was also a general focus on disclosure as oral in this body of research. The use of online support groups, net forums and chatting on the internet to facilitate disclosure was not widely explored.

Meta-theory

Meta-theory involves determining how the choice of theoretical frameworks is linked to conclusions made by primary researchers, as well as the implications of this linkage to how scholars and clinicians now understand the phenomenon under study (Paterson et al., 2001; Paterson, 2003a). I determined the theoretical frames for the research studies based on what the researchers identified as the theoretical framework and/or their use of particular theoretical stances to design the research (e.g. the interview questions) and to interpret the findings. I asked myself, 'How have these theoretical frames influenced how the researchers have made sense of their findings and what are the implications of this to how we now understand self-disclosure in HIV?'

In meta-theory, I recognised that few primary researchers stipulated a theoretical framework; however, several implied that they had been strongly influenced by stigma theory (Goffman, 1963), particularly as Goffman's original theory of stigma was expanded upon by others. Most often, the researchers discussed stigma as a significant deterrent to self-disclosure but did not conceptualise it. The contributions of stigma theory in understanding the data and generating new insights about self-disclosure are limited as a result.

Meta-synthesis

The synthesis phase of meta-study follows the analytical phases. It can best be described as digging deep to generate new knowledge about the phenomenon under study (Paterson et al., 2001). Meta-synthesis extends the comparisons of data across and between primary research studies that occurred in the analytical phases, to challenge common understandings of the phenomenon under study and the way in which it should be studied. One of the significant steps in meta-synthesis is to consider how the sociocultural, historical and disciplinary context have shaped the way primary researchers have understood and presented the phenomenon under study.

In the meta-synthesis component of the meta-study, I read widely in related fields, such as self-disclosure in psychotherapy, coming out as a gay or lesbian person, and in chronic physical and mental illness. I also read extensively in topic areas that were referenced by researchers in the self-disclosure field, such as privacy, decision making and stigma theory. Such reading gave insights about alternate perspectives regarding the phenomenon under study, leading to new insights about why and how primary researchers and participants constructed self-disclosure in the way they did. It also revealed aspects of the disciplinary, sociocultural and historical contexts that assisted me to synthesise the analytical findings.

The goal of meta-synthesis is to deconstruct current understandings of the phenomenon under study in order to contribute new insights to the field of scholarship. In the meta-synthesis component of the meta-study, I determined that the theoretical perspectives that predominate in this body of research (i.e. disease progression or risk–benefit calculus) are limited in their ability to explicate self-disclosure of HIV-positive serostatus, particularly as enacted beyond the individual in a sociocultural context. For example, they do not explain why people who fully accept their diagnosis, have lived with the diagnosis of HIV for several years, and believe that the risks of disclosure to be few may still be reluctant to self-disclose in certain settings or situations. Gay men in bath houses may not reveal their positive serostatus although they are 'out' about their disease, not because they think there are too many risks but because the social norms of bath houses dictate that people do not talk (Larkins et al., 2005).

The meta-synthesis revealed an understanding of the self-disclosure experience of people who are HIV positive that challenges previous interpretations of the phenomenon. Antaki et al. (2005:195) describe self-disclosure 'as a performed and situated social action'. Likewise, the meta-synthesis pointed to self-disclosure as social theatre in which the person negotiates an identity as an individual who is HIV positive in the context of their immediate and broader sociocultural environment. Although primary researchers have pointed to self-disclosure of HIV-positive serostatus as an outcome of the disease trajectory and/or as a calculated response, the notion of self-disclosure as social theatre implies that people enact self-disclosure as a social performance to address their personal needs and goals and/or those of others, as well as the often competing norms, values and ethical paradigms that exist

about self-disclosure within their family unit, community, cultural group and society. Rather than being a deliberate and rational decision making by the individual, this notion of self-disclosure is one of responsiveness that is interactional and relational. It may be calculated or spontaneous, as well as cognitive and/or affective in nature, depending on how the individual interprets and performs their personal and sociocultural scripts in particular settings and with particular people. Understanding self-disclosure in this way will lead researchers to creative and relevant research approaches that:

(1) capture the multiple and often conflicting goals and expectations of both the discloser and the receiver of the information;
(2) consider how the self-discloser has been framed or represented by not only the person who is HIV positive and the recipient, but by their family unit, cultural group, community and society; and
(3) account for the influence and interactivity of micro-, meso- and macro-level factors that contribute to the social construction of self-disclosure of serostatus as ideal.

Challenges in the meta-study project

Meta-study is a complex research method that is relatively early in its development. As such, it presents challenges that do not have immediate solutions. This meta-study project entailed several such challenges. The two that I will highlight relate to conducting meta-study as a sole researcher and selecting primary research.

Conducting meta-study alone

This was the first time that I attempted to conduct a meta-study by myself. If you are aware of meta-study as an approach, you will also be aware that in our book about the method (Paterson et al., 2001), we strongly advise researchers to avoid trying to conduct a meta-study on their own. We stress that to conduct a meta-synthesis requires a diverse set of experience, knowledge and perspectives. This chapter is a case of 'Do not what I do, but do what I say', as I was the sole researcher in this project.

I am often asked if it possible to conduct meta-study research on one's own. After this experience, I would say with considerable passion, 'It can be done, but it's not the best way.' Graduate students could conduct a meta-study because they have the benefit of receiving insights from their supervisors, but I strongly advise researchers to consider conducting meta-study as a research team and not as a solitary activity. As I discovered in a new way in this project, solitary meta-study is fraught with challenges. Not only did the project take much longer than I expected, but I greatly missed the benefits of discussing what I interpreted in the primary research with colleagues who had different perspectives and experiences from mine. I would have benefited greatly from input about how the discipline of psychology has framed self-disclosure in therapy and the influence of that in the primary research conducted by researchers in this field who cited psychological research as background to their investigations.

Because I am representing the work of primary researchers in my synthesis, I owe it to them to be as reflective and as informed as possible about their work and the implications of their research designs and findings. I find myself, at the conclusion of this meta-study project, worried that I may not have synthesised the primary research well or missed a crucial aspect of the analysis or synthesis because of the limitations of my personal understandings and experience. It is possible that I selected primary research studies and interpreted the data they held without knowledge of the major conceptual, theoretical or methodological debates within the field. Perhaps self-disclosure is a construct that includes other terms that I do not know; therefore, I may have missed critical primary research by overlooking research reports that did not refer to self-disclosure but used other terminology. Although I shared the analysis and synthesis with five experts in the field, they did not have time to read all the primary research reports or to engage with me in discussions about the primary research throughout the meta-study. They gave feedback only about the end-product of the meta-study. Including researchers who are familiar with aspects of the phenomenon under study, research methods and/or relevant theories that I do not know might have provided alternative depictions of self-disclosure in this synthesis.

Selecting primary research

When I speak about meta-study, people always ask me how I know that I have all the qualitative research reports that are relevant to the meta-study. I have answered this in various ways over the years, such as, 'You can only do your best. You need to make it clear what studies you have used. In this era of knowledge explosion and multiple sources of research reports, it is impossible to guarantee that you have every relevant primary research report that exists.' I was struck by how, after months of searching through databases and the reference lists in reports, I did not identify any relevant primary research about self-disclosure in any other language than English. It would be foolish to assume that all the research in this field was conducted in English. Rather, it points to the limitations of our traditional search methods in locating research conducted in non-English-speaking countries.

In this project, I learned that it is not only the comprehensiveness of the primary research that should be addressed, but also the inclusion criteria that are applied in a meta-study. For example, I need to acknowledge that my decision to include only research that specifically addressed self-disclosure has implications for what was revealed about the phenomenon under study. Because it is possible that asking people to discuss their experience of living with the illness may reveal different data from asking them directly about disclosure (MacLeod & Austin, 2003), the inclusion of primary research reports that discussed disclosure as a significant theme but not the sole focus of the research would have offered an opportunity to make cross-comparisons between the data in both bodies of research.

An aspect of selecting primary research that presented a challenge in the meta-study was determining which studies should be excluded because of a lack of rigour in the research or 'How bad is too bad to be included in the meta-study?' In my initial writing about meta-study (Paterson et al., 2001), I stated that it was necessary to exclude studies where the researchers' political agenda determined how data were collected and interpreted. I also stated that primary research studies should be excluded when it appeared that the data the researchers provided were too limited or unclear to justify the researchers' interpretations. I have changed my mind about these things.

Several meta-synthesis researchers (Eastabrooks et al., 1994; Barroso & Powell-Cope, 2000; Walsh & Downe, 2005) have detailed how they rate qualitative research reports according to criteria of relevance, congruence and methodological rigour; typically, they exclude those that receive 'unfavourable ratings' (Barroso & Powell-Cope, 2000:340). Although in the first meta-study, this was a significant issue in deciding what research should be excluded, I have come to understand primary research reports in a similar way as I view participants in qualitative research studies: some are more articulate and revealing than others, but I do not disqualify them on that basis.

In a study of people with traumatic brain injury, for example, I encountered participants who experienced some significant short-term memory deficits. If I had simply excluded them on the basis of their limitations in responding to interview questions, I would have missed the opportunity to explore with them the meaning of such deficits in their experience as an injury survivor. Further, these participants were helpful in articulating why clinicians who interviewed them had often found that they gave contradictory responses. Similarly, in meta-study research, primary research reports that seem on first reading to be missing vital components of what we now consider to be standard components of a qualitative research report (e.g. demographic details of the sample) include research findings that are, in fact, extremely revealing for the meta-study.

The only research reports that I did not include were surveys requiring some open-ended answers to a structured interview; typically, such research reports presented the data as a list of words or short phrases such as 'I don't ever tell', and the responses were categorised by percentages or numbers of respondents who answered in this way. Using criteria espoused by Sandelowski et al. (2004), I did not consider such reports to be qualitative research.

The perspective that all qualitative research reports that meet the inclusion criteria should be included in a meta-synthesis is mirrored by others (Jensen & Allen, 1996). My views have changed about this matter over the years because I learned in previous meta-study projects that what appear

to be methodological flaws in published qualitative research can often be the outcome of editorial decisions about what aspects of the research deserve reporting. Despite the fact that some primary research in this meta-study project contained few details about the research approach, the findings contribute significantly to an understanding of how self-disclosure has been constructed in this body of research. I maintain that research reports that meet my criteria of being qualitative (e.g. findings are presented as narrative or textual accounts) contribute to the depth and breadth of meta-study research.

Conclusion

This chapter has offered readers a glimpse of the processes and phases of meta-study, a research approach to synthesise qualitative research. This synthesis has revealed the body of primary research as limited in its capacity to address the complexity and contextual bases of self-disclosure of HIV serostatus. Meta-study demands that researchers engage in analytical and synthesis processes to articulate how the parts inform the whole of the phenomenon under study, as well as the historical and sociocultural situatedness of the body of research (Zimmer, 2006). Although I have not had the space to describe each step and decision in the meta-study project, I trust that I have offered sufficient detail to demonstrate that meta-study, although complex, offers significant contributions to understanding the history of the research in a particular field of study, as well as to understanding the directions for future research.

References

Antaki, C., Branes, R. & Leudar, I. (2005) Self-disclosure as a situated interactional practice. *British Journal of Social Psychology*, 44, 181–99.

Barnes, D.B. (1992) The disclosure of HIV status in health care settings: processes, patterns and consequences. Unpublished doctoral dissertation, University of California, San Francisco.

Barroso, J. & Powell-Cope, G.M. (2000) Metasynthesis of qualitative research on living with HIV infection. *Qualitative Health Research*, 10 (3), 340–53.

Black, B.P. & Miles, M.S. (2002) Calculating the risks and benefits of disclosure in African American women who have HIV. *Journal of Obstetric, Gynecologic and Neonatal Nursing*, 31 (6), 688–97.

Bor, R., Du Plessis, P. & Russell, M. (2004) The impact of disclosure on the index patient's self-defined family. *Journal of Family Therapy*, 26, 167–92.

Chandra, P.S., Deepithivarma, S. & Manjula, V. (2003) Disclosure of HIV infection in South India. *AIDS Care*, 15 (2), 207–15.

Dane, B. (2002) Disclosure. The voices of Thai women living with HIV/AIDS. *International Social Work*, 45 (2), 185–205.

de Ritter, N.F. (2001) Perspectives of disclosure and permanency planning of HIV-symptomatic mothers with dependent children (Immune deficiency). Unpublished doctoral dissertation, New York University, New York.

Eastabrooks, C., Field, P.A. & Morse, J.M. (1994) Aggregating qualitative findings: An approach to theory development. *Qualitative Health Research*, 4, 503–11.

Farmer, S.P. (2004) A phenomenological study of HIV disclosure to family among gay Mexican–American men. Unpublished doctoral dissertation, St. Mary's University, San Antonio.

Fesko, S.L. (2001) Disclosure of HIV status in the workplace: Considerations and strategies. *Health and Social Work*, 26 (4), 235–44.

Friedman, E.G. (2004) The process of self-disclosure of HIV seropositivity to women sexual partners: a qualitative study. Unpublished doctoral disseration, New York University, New York.

Gielen, A.C., O'Campo, P., Faden, R.R. & Eke, A. (1997) Women's disclosure of HIV status: experiences of mistreatment and violence in an urban setting. presented at the American Public Health Association Meeting, San Diego, CA and the HIV and Women Conference, Washington, DC. *Women and Health*, 25 (3), 19–31.

Gielen, A.C., McDonnell, K.A., Burke, J.G. & O'Campo, P. (2000) Women's lives after an HIV-positive diagnosis: disclosure and violence. *Maternal and Child Health Journal*, 4 (2), 111–20.

Goffman, E. (1963) *Stigma: Notes on the Management of a Spoiled Identity*. Aldine, Chicago.

Holt, R., Court, P., Vedhara, K., Nott, K.H., Holmes, J. & Snow, M.H. (1998) The role of disclosure in coping with HIV infection. *AIDS Care*, 10 (1), 49–60.

Jensen, L.A. & Allen, M.N. (1996) Meta-synthesis of qualitative findings. *Qualitative Health Research*, 6, 553–60.

Kimberly, J.A., Serovich, J.M. & Greene, K. (1995) Disclosure of HIV-positive status: five women's stories. *Family Relations*, 44, 316–22.

Klitzman, R.L. (1999) Self-disclosure of HIV status to sexual partners: a qualitative study of issues faced by gay men. *Journal of the Gay and Lesbian Medical Association*, 3 (2), 39–49.

Klitzman, R.L., Kirshenbaum, S.B., Dodge, B. et al. (2004) Intricacies and inter-relationships between HIV disclosure and HAART: a qualitative study. *AIDS Care*, 16 (5), 628–40.

Larkins, S., Reback, C.J., Shoptaw, S. & Veniegas, R. (2005) Methamphetamine-dependent gay men's disclosure of their HIV status to sexual partners. *AIDS Care*, 17 (4), 521–32.

Lincoln, Y.S. & Guba, E.G. (1985) *Naturalistic Inquiry*. Sage, Beverly Hills, California.

MacLeod, J.S. & Austin, J.K. (2003) Stigma in the lives of adolescents with epilepsy: a review of the literature. *Epilepsy & Behavior*, 4, 112–17.

Maman, S., Mbwambo, J., Hogan, N.M., Kilonzo, G.P. & Sweat, M. (2001) Women's barriers to HIV-1 testing and disclosure: challenges for HIV-1 counselling and testing. *AIDS Care*, 13 (5), 595–603.

Murphy, D.A., Roberts, K.J. & Hoffman, D. (2003) Regrets and advice from mothers who have disclosed their HIV+ serostatus to their young children. *Journal of Child & Family Studies*, 12 (3), 307–19.

Myers, K.R. (2004) Coming out: considering the closet of illness. *Journal of Medical Humanities*, 25 (4), 255–70.

Nelson, D. & Harvey, C.B. (1998) The lived experience of HIV and AIDS and first-time disclosure in therapy: implications for counsellors. *Guidance & Counseling*, 13 (3), 34–9.

Noblit, G.W. & Hare, R.D. (1988) *Meta-ethnography: Synthesizing Qualitative Studies*. Sage, Newbury Park, California.

Noone, S.B. (2000) Treading on thin ice: A qualitative study of women with HIV and disclosure. Unpublished doctoral dissertation, The Union Institute.

Ortiz, C.E. (2005) Disclosing concerns of Latinas living with HIV/AIDS. *Journal of Transcultural Nursing*, 16 (3), 210–17.

Parsons, J.T., VanOra, J., Missildine, W., Purcell, D.W. & Gómez, C.W. (2004) Positive and negative consequences of HIV disclosure among seropositive injection drug users. *AIDS Education and Prevention*, 16 (5), 459–75.

Paterson, B. (2001) The shifting perspectives model of chronic illness. *Journal of Nursing Scholarship*, 33 (1), 21–6.

Paterson, B.L. (2003a) Meta-Synthesis: A research method for the study of nursing effectiveness. *Canadian Journal of Nursing Research*, 35 (3), 39–43.

Paterson, B.L. (2003b) The koala has claws: applications of the Shifting Perspectives Model of chronic illness. *Qualitative Health Research*, 13 (7), 987–94.

Paterson, B.L., Thorne, S.E., Canam, C. & Jillings, C. (2001) *Meta-study of qualitative health research: a practical guide to meta-analysis and meta-synthesis*. Sage Publications Ltd., Thousand Oaks, California.

Paterson, B.L., Canam, C., Joachim, G. & Thorne, S. (2003) Embedded assumptions in qualitative studies of fatigue. *Western Journal of Nursing Research*, 25 (2), 1–15.

Paxton, S. (2004) The paradox of public HIV disclosure. *AIDS Care*, 14 (4), 559–67.

Sandelowski, M., Lambe, C. & Barroso, J. (2004) Stigma in HIV-positive women. *Journal of Nursing Scholarship*, 36 (2), 122–8.

Sauka, M.T. & Lie, G.T. (2000) Confidentiality and disclosure of HIV infection: HIV-positive persons' experiences with HIV testing and coping with HIV infection in Latvia. *AIDS Care*, 12 (6), 737–43.

Schrimshaw, E.W. & Siegel, K. (2002) HIV-infected mothers' disclosure to their uninfected children: Rates, reasons and reactions. *Journal of Social and Personal Relationships*, 19 (1), 19–43.

Serovich, J.M., Oliver, D.G., Smith, S.A. & Mason, T.L. (2005) Methods of HIV disclosure by men who have sex with men to casual sex partners. *AIDS Patient Care and STDs*, 19 (2), 823–32.

Sheon, N. & Crosby, M. (2004) Ambivalent tales of HIV disclosure in San Francisco. *Social Science and Medicine*, 58 (11), 2105–19.

Siegel, K., Lekas, H.-M. & Schrimshaw, E.W. (2005) Serostatus disclosure to sexual partners by HIV-infected women before and after the advent of HAART. *Women and Health*, 41 (4), 63–85.

Sowell, R.L., Seals, B.F., Phillips, K.D. & Julios, C.H. (2003) Disclosure of HIV infection: how do women decide who to tell? *Health Education Research*, 18 (1), 32–44.

Stirratt, M.J. (2004) Understanding HIV serostatus disclosure practices with sexual partners among seropositive gay and bisexual men. Unpublished doctoral dissertation, City University of New York, New York.

Strawn, J.M. (1997) Choosing not to tell about human immunodeficiency virus: How and why it happens. Unpublished doctoral dissertation, Teachers College, Columbia University, New York.

Thorne, S. & Paterson, B. (1998) Shifting images of chronic illness. *Image: Journal of Nursing Scholarship*, 30 (2), 173–8.

Thorne, S., Paterson, B., Acorn, S., Canam, C., Joachim, G. & Jillings, C. (2002a) Chronic illness: insights from a qualitative meta-study. *Qualitative Health Research*, 12 (4), 437–52.

Thorne, S.E., Joachim, G., Paterson, B. & Canam, C. (2002b) Influence of the research frame on qualitatively derived health science knowledge. *International Journal of Qualitative Methods* http://www.ualberta.ca/~ijqm/english/engframeset.html (retrieved 28 March 2006).

Vallerhard, A.H., Hough, E., Pittiglio, L. & Marviscin, D. (2005) The process of disclosing HIV serostatus between HIV-positive mothers and their HIV-negative children. *AIDS Patient Care and STDs*, 19 (2), 100–9.

Walsh, D. & Downe, S. (2005) Meta-synthesis method for qualitative research. *Journal of Advanced Nursing*, 50 (2), 204–11.

Walsh, E.R. (2000) Women's decision making experiences regarding disclosure of HIV seropositivity: A qualitative study. Unpublished doctoral dissertation, University of Michigan, Ann Arbor.

Yoshioka, M.R. & Schustack, A. (2001) Disclosure of HIV status: cultural issues of Asian patients. *AIDS Patient Care and STDs*, 15 (2), 77–82.

Zimmer, L. (2006) Qualitative meta-synthesis: a question of dialoguing with texts. *Journal of Advanced Nursing*, 53 (3), 311–18.

Appendix 7.1   Details of primary research reports included in the meta-synthesis.

Research	Discipline of researcher(s)	Focus of study	Research method
Barnes, 1992	Sociology	HIV – disclosure in healthcare settings among asymptomatic people	Qualitative descriptive
Black & Miles, 2002	Nursing	HIV – African American women's experience of disclosure	Qualitative descriptive
Bor et al., 2004	Psychology	HIV – impact of disclosure on family	Qualitative descriptive
Chandra et al., 2003	Psychiatry	HIV – aspects of self-disclosure, including related concerns	Qualitative descriptive
Dane, 2002	Social work	HIV – disclosure by Thai women who had contracted the disease from their spouses	Qualitative descriptive
de Ritter, 2001	Social work	HIV – disclosures in the workplace	Qualitative descriptive
Farmer, 2004	Marriage and family therapy	HIV – Mexican American men's disclosure experiences	Phenomenology
Fesko, 2001	Social work	HIV – disclosure experiences and permanency planning	Qualitative descriptive
Friedman, 2004	Social work	HIV – disclosure to sexual partners by heterosexual men who use illicit drugs	Qualitative descriptive
Gielen et al., 1997	Public health	HIV – women's fears and experiences regarding disclosure	Qualitative descriptive
Gielen et al., 2000	Public health	HIV – role of health care providers in women's disclosure, their experience with disclosure, violence as a consequence of disclosure, and the role of violence in disclosure decisions	Qualitative descriptive
Holt et al., 1998	Medicine	HIV – role of disclosure in living with disease	Qualitative descriptive
Kimberly et al., 1995	Marriage and family therapy	HIV – factors that influence women's intention to disclose	Qualitative descriptive
Klitzman, 1999	Sociology	HIV – self-disclosure to sexual partners by gay men	Grounded theory
Klitzman et al., 2004	Sociology	HIV – how disclosure affects and is affected by antiretroviral treatment	Qualitative descriptive
Larkins et al., 2005	Addictions	HIV – disclosure of gay men who are methamphetamine dependent to their sexual partners	Qualitative descriptive
Maman et al., 2001	Public health	HIV – disclosure of HIV test results with partner	Qualitative descriptive
Murphy et al., 2003	Psychology	HIV – disclosure of mothers to children	Qualitative descriptive
Nelson & Harvey, 1998	Psychology	HIV – first time disclosure to a therapist or counsellor	Phenomenology
Noone, 2000	Sociology	HIV – women's disclosure experiences	Case study

Appendix continues

Appendix 7.1 continued

Research	Discipline of researcher(s)	Focus of study	Research method
Ortiz, 2005	Nursing	HIV – disclosure experiences of Latinas in San Francisco	Qualitative descriptive
Parsons et al., 2004	Unclear	HIV – disclosure behaviour	Qualitative descriptive
Paxton, 2004	Sociology	HIV – personal effects of public disclosure	Qualitative descriptive
Sauka & Lie, 2000	Medicine	HIV – meaning of trust and relationship in disclosure to caregiver	Grounded theory
Schrimshaw & Siegel, 2002	Psychology	HIV – reasons HIV+ mothers give for disclosing or not disclosing	Qualitative descriptive
Serovich et al., 2005	Psychology	HIV – methods of disclosure to casual sex partners for men who have sex with men	Qualitative descriptive
Sheon & Crosby, 2004	Public health	HIV – disclosure practices of men who have anal sex with men	Narrative analysis
Siegel et al., 2005	Social psychology	HIV – reasons for disclosure and non-disclosure among women	Qualitative descriptive
Strawn, 1997	Nursing	HIV – non-disclosure	Grounded theory
Stirratt, 2004	Psychology	HIV – gay and bisexual men's disclosure to sexual partners and its effects on their sexual practices	Grounded theory
Vallerhard et al., 2005	Nursing	HIV – mothers' disclosure to children	Qualitative descriptive
Walsh, 2000	Nursing	HIV – women's decisions regarding disclosure	Grounded theory
Yoshioka & Schustack, 2002	Social work	HIV – how Asian cultural values affect disclosure experiences of Asian American immigrants	Qualitative descriptive

Appendix 7.2   Primary research appraisal tool: a completed example.

Schrimshaw, E.W. & Siegel, K. (2002) HIV-infected mothers' disclosure to their uninfected children: Rates, reasons and reactions. *Journal of Social and Personal Relationships*, 19 (1), 19–43.

Major construct/theory investigated (if applicable):   None.

Purpose/focus of study: To identify the reasons women offer for disclosing or not disclosing their HIV-positive serostatus to their uninfected children.

Genre of Study: (e.g. grounded theory, ethnography) (*Note: if stated genre does not appear to fit with research design, elaborate on lack of fit): Qualitative descriptive (did not explain research approach beyond interviewing).

Nature of sample: 45 HIV-infected mothers selected from larger sample (*N* = 146) of Puerto Rican, African American and non-Hispanic White women's adaptation to living with HIV as a chronic illness.

Appendix continues

Appendix 7.2 continued

- 15 African American
- 15 Puerto Rican
- 15 non-Hispanic White
- 1–5 children (M = 2.4)
- 62% had children living with them
- mean age = 35.4 years
- 38% reported household incomes below US$10 000; 84% less than US$25 000/year
- 67% currently unemployed due to illness (50%) or child care responsibilities (37%)
- 38% divorced and 38% never married
- 31% reported past IV drug use; 78% reported unprotected sex; 18% reported blood transfusion as source of infection
- duration of diagnosis 7 months to 9 years (M = 52.8 months)
- 23% symptomatic; 32% qualified for AIDS diagnosis

Recruitment: Advertisements, flyers and community outreach to health, social and advocacy organisations that serve HIV-infected people in New York. Quota sampling used to obtain equal numbers of each ethnic group.

Inclusion criteria:
- Mothers who tested seropositive for HIV or diagnosed with AIDS; resided in New York metropolitan area; 20–45 years of age; completed 8th grade; had not injected drugs within past 6 months
- If Hispanic, were Puerto Rican and had resided in USA for a least 4 years
- If African American or White, were US-born and non-Hispanic

General description of research approach: Met three times with female research assistant within one-month period. First meeting: demographic information and medical history, and self-administered questionnaire of 'standardised psychosocial measures'. Next two meetings: semi-structured interview about 'various aspects of living with HIV'. Participants given US$25 honorarium. If they indicated they had self-disclosed to children, mothers were asked if they regretted decision.

Ethical considerations: Not discussed.

Major findings:
- Disclosure occurred because wanted to educate children about HIV, wanting children to hear it from them, wanting their children to know before they became very ill, and wanting to be honest with their children
- Reasons for non-disclosure were that child was too young or immature, believing it would be too much of a burden for the child, not wanting children to experience rejection, not wanting children to fear losing their mother, and wanting children to recover from previous losses
- Although some negative responses from children following mothers' disclosure, most participants reported that relationship with children had become closer following disclosure

Research design:
(1) Problem statement
  - Statement of the phenomenon leads directly to the purpose of the study and the research question? *Yes*
(2) Purpose of the research
  - Clearly expressed? *Yes*
  - Significance of research problem clearly indicated? *Yes*
(3) Research questions(s)
  - Explicitly expressed? *Yes*
  - Evidence of flow from the phenomenon? *Yes*
(4) Identification of assumptions
  - Identification of assumptions, preconceptions, and presuppositions of researcher? *No*
(5) Identification of theoretical framework
  - Identification of theoretical framework? *No*
  - If 'yes', name framework (*if not well-known, include brief description).
  - Implied theoretical framework? *No*
  - Clarification of influence of articulated or implied theoretical framework? *No*

Appendix continues

Appendix 7.2 continued

(6)   Researcher credentials
- Documentation of researcher's discipline(s)? *Yes*
- If 'yes', name it. *Public health*
- Any other pertinent information about the researcher (e.g. methodological preference, conceptual preference)? *No*

(7)   Role of researcher
- Non-research relationship of researcher to participants? *Unclear*
- Evidence that researcher has considered the effect of his/her presence as an interviewer on the research findings? *No*
- Evidence that researcher has considered possibility of researcher bias or misinterpretation? *Identified limitations as the reliance on retrospective accounts, the fact that interviews took place before latest antiretroviral drugs. Also said that the finding that mothers differed as to their disclosure preferences according to stage of illness could be explained because end stages of AIDS associated with visible symptoms and visibility of AIDS made disclosure a non-issue*

(8)   Sampling and participants
- Description of type of sampling procedure? *Yes*
- Identification of inclusion criteria? *Yes*
- Discussion of attrition in longitudinal studies? *No*

(9)   Data gathering strategy(ies)
- Clear description of data gathering procedures? *No*
- If 'no', how could the description be improved? *It was unclear what strategies were used to obtain the data for this report and which strategies were for the larger study.*
- Description of gaining access? *Yes*
- Discussion of time frame of data gathering? *Yes*
- If 'yes', what was it? *Three times in one month*

(10) Data analysis strategies
- Description of the method(s) used? *Yes*
- If yes, what was it? *Thematic analysis*
- Identification of categories or common elements found? *Yes*
- Report of the participants' response to the analysis? *No*
- Data analysis presented in clear framework (identification of central themes and categories)? *Yes*
- Analysis well supported by representative quotes/findings? *Yes*
- Provision of evidence as to how representative in the sample the various findings were? *Yes*

(11) Conclusions, discussion, implications, suggestions for further study
- Identification of limitations of the study? *Yes*
- Specific limitations identified? *Retrospective, HAART occurred after data collection; did not include children's accounts; no clear indication of stage of disease*
- Discussion pertains to all significant findings? *Yes*
- Interpretive statements correspond with findings? *Yes*
- Examination of findings with existing body of knowledge? *Yes*
- Clear indication of directions for future research? *Yes*
- If 'yes', indicate directives identified. *Need to obtain children's perspectives; research that determines if mother's reasons for disclosure are actually predictive of disclosure, more in-depth and systematic investigation (qualitative and quantitative)*

Other considerations/thoughts:
- This was the only study to consider how mothers' decisions were affected by the child living with them or away from them
- The mothers are portrayed as essentially protective of their children, even when non-disclosing. This is in contrast to other research involving men that discuss non-disclosers in terms of their cowardice, denial or lack of responsibility

Decision to include in meta-study:
- Meets all inclusion criteria? *Yes*
- If 'no', provide details.
- Recommendation to include in meta-study. *Include*
- If 'undecided', explain why.

8 From Meta-synthesis to Method: Appraising the Qualitative Research Synthesis Report

Margarete Sandelowski

The work featured in this chapter was supported by a grant from the National Institute of Nursing Research, National Institutes of Health (R01 NR04907, 1 June 2000–2 June 2005) awarded to Margarete Sandelowski, Principal Investigator, and Julie Barroso, Co-Principal Investigator.

Portions of this chapter include, in a revised form, material previously published in Sandelowski, M. & Barroso, J. (2005). The travesty of choosing after positive prenatal diagnosis. JOGNN: Journal of Obstetric, Gynecologic, and Neonatal Nursing, 34, 307–18; and in Sandelowski, M. & Barroso, J. (2007). Handbook for Synthesizing Qualitative Research. Springer, New York.

Introduction

The turn to evidence-based practice and the proliferation of qualitative research reports have led to a growing interest in systematic reviews and syntheses of qualitative research. Such projects require a large expenditure of time and resources, and knowledge of an array of qualitative methods and of advanced techniques to integrate findings. Accordingly, most clinicians and researchers are likely to enter the evidence-based practice process at the findings translation stage, where the findings from primary studies that have already been synthesised must be evaluated for their utilisation value (Smaling, 2003) in research or practice. At this point, researchers are generally primarily interested in the theoretical validity of the research synthesis, focusing on the credibility of the synthesis itself (Maxwell, 1992). Clinicians are typically most concerned with its pragmatic and ethical validity (Kvale, 1995), focusing on whether and how to transform research syntheses into such material forms as clinical practice recommendations, guidelines, care standards, appraisal tools, and clinical pathways and protocols.

In this chapter, I offer a template that can be used to read and evaluate qualitative research synthesis reports and, thereby, the studies they represent. To illustrate the components of this template, I draw from a report of a qualitative research synthesis study I conducted with Julie Barroso, 'The travesty of choosing after positive prenatal diagnosis', which was published in *JOGNN: Journal of Obstetric, Gynecologic, and Neonatal Nursing* (Sandelowski & Barroso, 2005), a journal directed toward a largely clinical audience. To make the elements of a qualitative research synthesis report even more transparent, I have revised or added material that does not appear in the *JOGNN* paper. Space restrictions in journals do not allow the publication of all of the information readers may require to appraise such reports.

Components of a qualitative research synthesis report and evaluation criteria

Most journals in the health sciences publishing reports of research syntheses require that they be disseminated in the American Psychological Association (APA)/experimental format (Bazerman, 1988), or a close variation of it. In this style of reporting research, content is typically presented in the third person passive voice and in defined introduction, review of literature, method, results, and discussion sections. In modified experimental/ APA reports of qualitative research, content may be presented in the first person active voice and/or the results may be foreshadowed in the statement of the research purpose or, more typically, are merged with the discussion of these results.

Because of space restrictions in most journals, reviewers will probably not be allowed to include all of the details of their studies. Moreover, journals vary in what components they want included and excluded. For example, some journals do not allow the publication of the list of primary research reports upon which the research synthesis was based, nor much detail on the thinking process behind the method choices made. This can lower readers' evaluations of these reports as, in the research synthesis enterprise, objectivity resides in, and is an achievement of, such reflexive accounting practices. The irony here is that qualitative researchers, especially, are often blamed for not sufficiently articulating their methods, yet continue to be charged with being too wordy or long-winded when they attempt to delineate them. To offset the space problem, many journals now have web sites to house additional information and permit authors to state what additional information is available to readers on request. Accordingly, when appraising a report, readers are well advised to consider the publication practices of the journal in which it appears, so as not to blame authors for 'failing' to include information they were not allowed to include.

Table 8.1 itemises the desired components of experimental/APA style reports of qualitative research syntheses in the order in which they typically appear in such reports, along with criteria that readers may use to evaluate whether:

(1) these elements are sufficiently addressed (i.e. do the authors/researchers provide enough information about them?); and

(2) whether the information offered indicates an accurate understanding of and appropriate use of methods.

Introduction

As indicated in Table 8.1, the experimental/APA style report of a qualitative research synthesis study begins with an introductory section in which the reviewers present the research problem that generated the need for the review and the specific purpose of the review addressing this problem. The most common problem generating qualitative research synthesis projects is the proliferation of studies addressing an experience, but lack of direction for interpreting or using their findings. Accordingly, a common purpose of a research synthesis study is to summarise the knowledge generated in an area in order to draw conclusions directly relevant to practice or to chart directions for future research. Another example of a research problem is the proliferation of primary studies in a common area with apparently discrepant findings. The purpose of a research synthesis study might, therefore, be to account for or to resolve these discrepancies. Other purposes may include clarifying or modelling the relationships among research variables, defining the conditions under which a phenomenon appears, explaining or providing a context for the findings of primary quantitative research or research syntheses, or mapping knowledge fields.

In the prenatal diagnosis study featured here, the original problem that generated the review was a methodological one (Sandelowski & Barroso, 2003e). This is a deviation from the usual category of research problem that addresses a clinical or practice issue or dilemma. In contrast to most research synthesis studies, the 'travesty of choosing' study reported here was not launched to address a clinical problem (e.g. the need to have an evidence base for practice with couples receiving positive prenatal diagnoses), but rather to address a research problem (i.e. the relative lack of techniques for synthesising qualitative research findings). The prenatal diagnosis studies were selected to test the utility of the methods we had developed using studies with HIV-positive women in yet another area in which we had expertise. Reviewers generally

Table 8.1   Components of a report of a qualitative research synthesis project and corresponding evaluation criteria.

Components	Evaluation criteria
I. Introduction	
a. Research problem that generated the study	a1. Is the problem clearly stated? a2. Has the case been made for its existence and significance?
b. Research purpose addressing the research problem	b1. Is the purpose clearly stated? b2. Is it demonstrably linked to the research problem?
II. Methods	
a. Type of review	a1. Is the type of review sufficiently delineated? a2. Is it accurately described?

b.   Search and sampling strategies
    1.   Goals of search strategy
    2.   Parameters for search
        2a.   Topical/thematic boundaries
        2b.   Population boundaries
        2c.   Temporal boundaries
        2d.   Methodological boundaries
    3.   Key definitions and search terms
    4.   Inclusion and exclusion criteria
    5.   Channels of communication and information sources used
    6.   Tools used to conduct searches and track search outcomes
    7.   Profile of reports included (see III a 1–7 below)[a]
	b1. Is it likely that all relevant reports will have been retrieved using these strategies?
	b2. Is it likely that no relevant reports will have been excluded using these strategies?
	b3. Are the search strategies reasonable given the boundaries set for the study and the limitations described?

c.   Appraising reports
    1.   Technique and tools used to extract information from individual reports
    2.   Quality criterion used as covariate or criterion to exclude reports
        2a.   A posteriori analyses of contributions of individual reports to synthesis
    3.   Profile of participants (see III b 1–3 below)[a]
	c1. Are the techniques and tools used sufficiently delineated?
	c2. Are the techniques and tools used accurately described?
	c3. If a quality criterion was used, is the way it was used sufficiently delineated?

d.   Synthesis of findings
    1.   Techniques and tools used to analyse and compare findings
    2.   Techniques and tools used to integrate findings
	d1. Are the techniques and tools used sufficiently delineated?
	d2. Are the techniques and tools used accurately described?
	d3. Are the techniques and tools used appropriate to the study?

e. Techniques and tools used to optimise the validity of study procedures	e1. Are the techniques and tools used sufficiently delineated? e2. Are the techniques and tools used accurately described? e3. Are the techniques and tools used appropriate to the study?
III. Results of review	

a.   Profile of reports
    1.   Number of relevant primary research reports
    2.   Inclusive years of reports
    3.   Primary author disciplinary affiliations
    4.   Geographic location of studies
    5.   Purpose of studies
    6.   Theoretical and methodological orientation of studies
    7.   Identification of related reports (e.g. from same parent study, with identical or overlapping samples)
	a1. Are the relevant characteristics of the included reports sufficiently identified and summarised?

Table continues

Table 8.1 continued

Components	Evaluation criteria

b. Profile of participants represented in reports
   1. Total and mean/median/modal sample size across reports
   2. Age, sex, racial/ethnic, class, national and any other relevant demographic features
   3. Other features of participants relevant to the purpose of the review (e.g. stage of illness or pregnancy, diagnostic tests, treatment modalities)
	b1. Are the relevant characteristics of the participants represented in the included reports sufficiently identified and summarised?

c. Synthesis of findings
   1. Delineation of key findings
   2. Visual displays of findings
	c1. Does the material offered as a synthesis represent an interpretive integration of primary research findings?
	c2. Is the synthesis sufficiently supported by the primary research findings?
	c2. Are the forms (e.g. conceptual model, table, graph) used to present the synthesis appropriate to it?

IV. Discussion of the synthesis produced	
a. Link to existing scholarship	a1. Is relevant scholarship used? a2. Are the links sufficiently delineated?
b. Implications for research	b1. Are the implications drawn from the synthesis? b2. Is the synthesis presented in a form that is translatable for research?
c. Implications for practice	c1. Are the implications drawn from the synthesis? c2. Is the synthesis presented in a form that is translatable for practice?
d. Limitations of the study	d1. Are the limitations identified distinctive to the reported study? d2. Are the limitations sufficiently delineated? d3. Are the distinctive challenges to synthesising the featured body of research sufficiently delineated?
e. Alternative to empirical/analytical reading of primary research findings	e1. Is the alternative reading credible and drawn from the primary research findings? e2. Does the alternative reading conflict with the reading of findings presented as the synthesis?
V. End of text	
a. List of complete citations to primary research reports (may be embedded in one end-of-text reference list with asterisks)	
b. Acknowledgements, including grant support	b1. Do any potential conflicts of interest, or factors shaping the synthesis, exist that are not addressed in the report?

aThis information may appear in either the methods or results sections of a report.

choose topics for research synthesis in areas in which they have expertise and to which they have strong commitments. Moreover, the validity of such studies is optimised when reviewers know the field they are studying. Accordingly, the introduction shown below was modified to communicate a clinical as opposed to methodological research problem. The material contained in it is up-to-date as of 2004, when this paper was originally submitted for review. (The excerpts from the 'travesty of choosing' paper, including modifications made for this chapter, are shown in Boxes 8.1–8.4.)

Methods

As shown in Table 8.1, the methods section that typically follows the introduction in an experimental/APA style report of a qualitative research synthesis should include the type of review conducted, search strategies used, sampling parameters, key definitions and search terms, all the sources of research used, and the tools (e.g. databases created, reference manager program) used to conduct and track search outcomes. In addition, this section should include information on how data were extracted from each report, whether quality judgements were made and how they were used, the analytic and interpretive techniques employed to integrate findings, and the procedures used to optimise the validity of the study.

Qualitative research synthesis is not easy to recognise as a distinctive methodological enterprise because of the highly disparate entities that are presented as reviews of the literature, qualitative research syntheses, qualitative or narrative methods to organise, analyse or interpret bodies of literature, and as qualitative research itself. The distinctions drawn in this section are from Sandelowski & Barroso (2007) and are in the service of clarifying the orientation to qualitative research synthesis featured in this chapter.

Box 8.1   Example of the introduction section in a qualitative research synthesis report – from the prenatal diagnosis review (Sandelowski & Barroso, 2005).

Introduction

Over the past 25 years, prenatal testing has become an increasingly routine event in pregnancy in the United States (Filkins & Russo, 1985; Milunsky, 2004). Pregnancy is no longer divided exclusively in thirds (i.e. in trimesters), but also in halves: before and after obtaining test results. Indeed, women now often experience their pregnancies in the period before receiving test results as 'tentative' (Rothman, 1986), the fate of these pregnancies contingent on whether test results are negative (paradoxically indicating a positive outcome) or positive (paradoxically indicating a negative outcome). When test results are negative, expectant parents feel the usual anxieties associated with childbearing but are generally reassured that their baby will be healthy (Kolker & Burke, 1993). When these results are positive, expectant parents become parents of an impaired child and thereby embark on a journey of adjustment and accommodation once begun only after delivery, before the technology of prenatal diagnosis enabled access to the fetus *in utero* (Rothenberg & Thomson, 1995; Tunis, 1993).

A large body of health and behavioural and social science research now exists exploring expectant parents' experiences with prenatal testing, addressing such areas as how they came to accept or decline testing, their responses to specific tests (e.g. ultrasonography and amniocentesis), and the influence of prenatal testing on parental attachment (e.g. Garcia et al., 2002). Most of these studies were conducted with women receiving negative test results, the most likely outcome of prenatal testing. A significant minority of studies have been conducted with women and couples receiving positive test results, a relatively rare outcome and one assumed to require more specialised professional intervention (e.g. Statham et al., 2000). As more women undergo prenatal testing, and more fetuses are identified as impaired during pregnancy, the need is becoming more urgent to understand their experiences. One means of gaining this understanding is to summarise what is already known about the experience of receiving a positive fetal diagnosis from empirical qualitative research. Accordingly, the purpose of this report is to present a synthesis of findings from this research.

Qualitative research synthesis refers to a process and product of scientific enquiry aimed at systematically reviewing and formally integrating the findings in reports of completed qualitative studies. Qualitative research synthesis projects encompass two large categories of methodological approaches: qualitative meta-summary and qualitative meta-synthesis. *Qualitative meta-summary* is a quantitatively oriented aggregation of qualitative research findings that are themselves in the form of topical or thematic summaries or surveys of data. *Qualitative meta-synthesis* is an interpretive integration of qualitative findings that are themselves in the form of interpretive syntheses of data, including the phenomenologies, ethnographies, grounded theories and other coherent descriptions or explanations of phenomena, events or cases that are the hallmark findings of qualitative research. Qualitative meta-summaries may be an end in themselves, or they may serve as an empirical foundation for, or bridge to, qualitative meta-synthesis, preparing primary survey findings for qualitative meta-synthesis and optimising the validity of the syntheses produced.

Qualitative research synthesis versus other entities

As summarised in Table 8.2, qualitative research synthesis is different from:

- Other reviews of the literature (i.e. the background review, the narrative overview of a research domain)
- Other research syntheses (i.e. quantitative or qualitative syntheses of quantitative research findings)
- Secondary analysis
- Other syntheses found in qualitative inquiry (i.e. constituting the findings within primary studies, constituting an integration or re-interpretation of findings across a programme of research), and from
- Other studies of studies (i.e. meta-study)

Although it has features that overlap with these other forms, qualitative research synthesis is characterised by:

- Systematic and comprehensive retrieval of all of the relevant reports of completed qualitative studies in a target domain of empirical enquiry

- Systematic use of qualitative and quantitative methods to analyse these reports
- Analytic and interpretive emphasis on the findings in these reports
- Systematic use of qualitative methods to integrate the findings in these reports, and the
- Use of reflexive accounting practices to optimise the validity of study procedures and outcomes

In contrast to the background review. In contrast to the background review of literature that is the prelude to a specific study, qualitative research synthesis – by itself – constitutes a form of scientific enquiry. Reviewers conducting qualitative research synthesis studies have the same obligation as researchers conducting studies with human subjects to detail and defend all of the methodological parameters of their studies (e.g. inclusion and exclusion criteria, analytical approaches). The narrative background review of the literature that typically precedes the proposal or report of a primary study is designed to link selected studies in one or more fields in a chain of reasoning (Doyle, 2003). The purpose of this background review is not to synthesise the findings from all of the studies in a domain of inquiry, but rather to make a case for the specific study that it introduces. Writers of such reviews are not obliged to detail the search strategies they used nor the sampling frame for the studies they included. Moreover, what makes this review 'narrative' or 'qualitative' is simply that words are used to conduct the review. This use of the terms 'narrative' and 'qualitative' should not be confused with the actual use of a form of narrative analysis or any one of a host of other specific qualitative methods (e.g. grounded theory) or techniques (e.g. qualitative thematic or content analysis) to study studies (Jones, 2004). Unfortunately, the terms 'narrative' or 'qualitative' are still used to refer to reviews of the literature that are deemed unsystematic or otherwise lacking in the scientific rigour claimed for statistical reviews, or quantitative meta-analysis.

In contrast to the narrative overview. Although they may be systematic and exhaustive in the search, retrieval and analysis procedures used, narrative overviews of research are often wider in scope than background reviews and always less penetrating than qualitative research syntheses, as they merely

Table 8.2   Comparison of research synthesis studies with other reviews of literature.

Type of review or study	Background review	Narrative overview	Qualitative secondary analysis/pooled case comparison	Studies of studies		
				Research synthesis studies		Meta-studies
Purpose	To stage a study To link a study to other research To make a case for the study	To survey topics addressed, and methods used, in a domain of enquiry	To re-analyse data collected in one or more primary studies	To produce a qualitative synthesis of research findings	To produce a quantitative synthesis of research findings	To interpret one or more elements of studies comprising a domain of enquiry
Primary data	Range of literature in relevant domains of enquiry	Reports of empirical qualitative and quantitative research	Original qualitative data	Qualitative and/or quantitative research findings	Qualitative and/or quantitative research findings	e.g. Research traditions, theories, methods
Reading	Empirical/analytical	Empirical/analytical	Empirical/analytical Critical/discursive	Empirical/analytical Critical/discursive	Empirical/analytical	Critical/discursive
Logic	Chain of reasoning	Catalogue	Reframing	Integration	Aggregation Integration	Critique Interpretive comparison
Methods	Selected review of literature	Systematic review	Any qualitative or quantitative methods	Qualitative meta-synthesis (or, meta-data analysis) Modified meta-ethnography Systematic narrative review	Qualitative meta-summary Quantitative meta-analysis	Meta-theory Meta-method Meta-ethnography Meta-narrative

survey the topics and methods used in a field of study. Such 'résumé review(s)' (Kirkevold, 1997:980) offer 'efficient overview(s)' (p. 981) of the research literature for researchers and practitioners.

In contrast to syntheses of quantitative research findings. Both qualitative and quantitative methods can be used to integrate the findings in reports of qualitative or quantitative studies. The differences between qualitative and quantitative synthesis studies lie in the kinds of methods typically used (i.e. meta-analysis in quantitative research synthesis and meta-summary, meta-synthesis, or modified meta-ethnography in qualitative research synthesis) and in the mode of interpretation (i.e. statistical inference versus case-bound and narrative explanation and representation).

In contrast to secondary analysis. In contrast to the emphasis in qualitative research synthesis on qualitative findings is the emphasis in qualitative secondary analysis and pooled case comparisons on qualitative data (Thorne, 1994; West & Oldfather, 1995). In secondary analysis, an original data set is subjected to re-analysis – or two or more such data sets generated in different studies are combined to constitute a new data set – to answer one or more new research questions. The primary data in qualitative secondary analysis studies are the 'raw' interview, observation and other data generated in the field; the primary data in qualitative research synthesis studies are the findings generated from these raw data across a set of primary studies.

In contrast to within-study and within-programme-of-research syntheses. Qualitative research syntheses are also different from the syntheses of data constituting the findings (e.g. the grounded theories, phenomenologies, ethnographies, and the like) in primary qualitative studies. These within-study syntheses (i.e. findings in individual primary qualitative studies) are the primary data in qualitative research synthesis studies. In the borderlands between secondary analyses of qualitative data, within-study syntheses and qualitative research syntheses are projects in which investigators use qualitative research synthesis methods to synthesise or re-interpret findings within and across their own programmes of research (Sandelowski, 1995; McCormick et al., 2003). Both 'raw' data and

findings generated from those data may constitute the primary data in these borderland projects.

In contrast to meta-study. Qualitative research synthesis studies are different from other qualitative studies of studies, such as meta-study, largely by virtue of their focus on actually integrating research findings and of the view of findings as empirically grounded and verifiable interpretations of the lived experiences of research participants. As Noblit & Hare (1988) originally conceived it, meta-ethnography is a form of meta-study that entails the interpretive comparison of study findings, not the integration of them. As Paterson et al. (2001) described it, meta-study is most akin to operations used in intellectual history, history and philosophy of science, information science and other disciplines focused on the evolution and critique of ideas and knowledge development and representation. Meta-studies can be targeted toward the study of findings (meta-data-analysis), methods (meta-method) and theories (meta-theory) in a designated body of research, but they do not necessarily entail any actual combination, assimilation or integration of them in the empirical/analytical sense. Instead, they constitute a critical/discursive engagement with them. Meta-study is arguably better conceived not as a form of research synthesis *per se*, but rather as a method for 'rigorously and systematically deconstructing existing bodies of qualitative research findings' (Thorne et al., 2004:1357). These deconstructions may then be used as a foundation or context for research synthesis, as Greenhalgh et al. (2005) demonstrated in their delineation of the 'meta-narratives', or research traditions characterising diffusion of innovation studies. Meta-studies offer an historical staging and explanatory context for qualitative research synthesis projects that assists reviewers to be more humble in their research integration claims. An example of a qualitative research synthesis study with a discursive disclaimer is our meta-synthesis of motherhood in HIV-positive women in Sandelowski & Barroso (2003c).

Results

This is the heart of a qualitative research synthesis report. This section should include profiles of both the reports themselves and the participants

Box 8.2   Example of the methods section in a qualitative research synthesis report – from the prenatal diagnosis review (Sandelowski & Barroso, 2005).

Methods

The review conducted was a systematic review aimed at integrating the findings from reports of qualitative studies with women and couples receiving positive fetal diagnoses, using both qualitative meta-summary and meta-synthesis techniques (Sandelowski & Barroso, 2003b, d). Any qualitative study involving women and/or their partners living in the United States, of any race, ethnicity, nationality or class, who learned during any time in pregnancy of any fetal impairment by any means of diagnosis were eligible for inclusion. *Qualitative study* was liberally defined as empirical research with human participants conducted in any research paradigm, using what are commonly viewed as qualitative techniques for sampling, data collection, data analysis and interpretation. A *positive prenatal diagnosis study* was defined as including studies conducted with women, men or couples obtaining any diagnosis of fetal impairment, or under suspicion of the existence of a fetal impairment, during pregnancy.

Search and sampling strategies

We used the search strategies described by Bates (1989) and Cooper (1998) to ensure a comprehensive search. The goal of searching was to ensure a high-recall search, in which efforts are directed toward retrieving all of the relevant documents in an area (Marchionini, 1995; Losee, 2000). A relevant report was one in which data were obtained directly *from* women, men or couples obtaining positive fetal diagnoses, not *about* such women, men or couples from any other persons (e.g. nurses, counsellors). Reports of studies in which the research purpose encompassed more than a focus on the personal experience of positive fetal diagnosis (e.g. a study about undergoing prenatal tests including couples receiving positive and negative fetal diagnoses) were considered relevant and included:

(1)   if the findings concerning women, men or couples obtaining positive fetal diagnoses could be distinguished from the findings related to other research participants;

(2)   if they were about any aspect of the experience of obtaining a positive fetal diagnosis; and

(3)   if they were based on data collected directly from women, men or couples obtaining positive fetal diagnoses.

   The search period was December 2002 through March 2003. Table 8.3 shows the search terms we used, truncated where appropriate and including combinations of topic, theme and method terms. Table 8.4 shows the electronic databases searched. We also electronically searched the entire reference collection in our university library for books and anthologies in the areas of prenatal testing, reproductive technology and motherhood. We searched by hand those texts whose tables of contents were not displayed on screen or, if displayed, suggested possible relevant papers, as well as key journals, including *JOGNN: Journal of Obstetric, Gynecologic and Neonatal Nursing, Prenatal Diagnosis* and *Qualitative Health Research.* Our search results were directly downloaded into ProCite® through our university's licence.

Appraisal of reports

Each relevant work was analysed using a 14-item reading guide developed specifically to appraise reports of qualitative studies included in research synthesis studies (Sandelowski & Barroso, 2002). The reading guide directs reviewers to extract information in each of 14 categories, no matter where this information might appear in the report. These categories include research problem, research purpose(s)/question(s), literature review, theoretical orientation to the target phenomenon, methodological orientation, sampling plan, sample, data collection, data management, validity, findings, discussion and ethics. The fourteenth category – form – directs reviewers to consider the general style of the report, as reporting style will influence where information in each of the 13 other categories will likely be found. This initial analysis, in addition to all of the work described below, was completed in Microsoft Word and Microsoft Excel using both hard and scanned copies of the research reports.

No report was excluded for reasons of quality, as the evaluation of a study as good or bad is highly idiosyncratic in qualitative research (Sandelowski & Barroso, 2003a). Leading scholars in the research integration field have warned against the a priori exclusion of studies for reasons of quality as a serious threat to the validity of the results of research integration studies (Cooper, 1998; Conn & Rantz, 2003). Defining a valid finding as one that is supported by the data presented in a report, we found no reason to exclude any report meeting the search criteria or any finding in those reports.

Synthesis of primary research findings

Both qualitative meta-summary and meta-synthesis techniques (Sandelowski & Barroso, 2003b, d) were used to lay the descriptive foundation for the research integration that follows. Qualitative meta-summary is a quantitatively oriented aggregation of qualitative research findings that are themselves in the form of topical or thematic summaries or surveys of data. Meta-summaries address the manifest content in findings, reflect a view of language as a neutral vehicle of communication, and show a quantitative logic: to discern the frequency of each finding and to find in higher frequency findings the evidence of replication foundational to validity in quantitative research and to the claim of having discovered a pattern or theme in qualitative research.

Qualitative meta-synthesis is a form of systematic review or integration of qualitative research findings that are themselves interpretive syntheses of data, including phenomenologies, ethnographies, grounded theories, and other integrated and coherent descriptions or explanations of phenomena, events or cases. Meta-syntheses are integrations that are more than the sum of parts in that they offer novel interpretations of findings. These interpretations will not be found in any one research report *per se*, but rather are inferences derived from taking all of the findings in a set of reports as a whole. The validity of meta-syntheses does not reside in a replication logic, but rather in an inclusive logic whereby all findings are accommodated.

A meta-summary of findings was produced by extracting relevant statements of findings from each report, reducing these statements into parsimonious yet empirically faithful statements of abstracted findings, and then calculating frequency effect sizes for each of these meta-findings. The results of this work are shown in Table 8.5. Data extraction entailed separating researchers' findings pertaining to positive prenatal diagnosis from:

(1) the data they had collected, or the quotations, incidents, stories, and case histories researchers used to provide evidence for their findings;
(2) data and findings not about positive prenatal diagnosis (in those studies not exclusively focused on positive prenatal diagnosis);
(3) imported findings, or findings from other studies to which researchers referred;
(4) analytic procedures, or the coding schemes and data displays researchers used to produce and verify their findings; and from
(5) researchers' discussion of the meaning, implications or significance of their findings to research, education, practice or policy making.

These extracted findings were reduced to 39 meta-findings representing a comprehensive inventory of the findings across all reports. Frequency effect sizes (Onwuegbuzie, 2003) were then calculated by dividing the number of reports containing a finding by the total number of reports. In qualitative research, *effect size* refers to the relative presence or prominence of findings, not to their relative importance or significance. The percentages in Table 8.5 mean nothing by themselves, but acquire meaning only in relation to all of the other percentages shown. The calculation of effect sizes is a quantitative transformation of qualitative data that allows reviewers to extract more meaning from qualitative data, to verify the presence of patterns or themes, and to ensure that findings are neither over- nor underweighted.

The results of the work shown in Table 8.5 laid the empirical foundation for qualitative meta-synthesis. Qualitative content analysis (Morgan, 1993) was used to ascertain the prevailing topical and thematic foci of the findings. Reciprocal translation (Noblit & Hare, 1988) resulted in the linking of findings around the controlling image or metaphor of paradox. Constant comparison analysis (Strauss & Corbin, 1998) was used to clarify the defining and shared features of the experience of positive prenatal diagnosis *vis-à-vis* other ostensibly similar experiences, such as miscarriage, elective abortion and selective fetal reduction.

Procedures for optimising validity

The procedures we used to optimise the validity of this study included: (1) the maintenance of an audit trail (Rodgers & Cowles, 1993); (2) ongoing negotiation of consensual validity in regularly scheduled research team meetings (Eisner, 1991; Belgrave & Smith, 1995); and (3) expert consultation and peer review (Sandelowski, 1998).

Table 8.3   Search terms used in the prenatal diagnosis study.

Topic	Theme	Method
Amniocentesis	Decision making	Case study
Chorionic villus sampling	Parental decisions	Constant comparison analysis
Fetal abnormality	Psychology/psychological	Content analysis
Fetal diagnosis	aspects	Conversation analysis
Fetal malformation	Psychological sequelae	Descriptive study
Fetal screening	Sociocultural aspects	Discourse/discourse analysis
Fetoscopy		Ethnography
Genetic pregnancy		Exploratory study
abortion/termination		Field observation
Genetic testing		Field study
Genetic screening		Focus group
Genetic counselling		Grounded theory
Maternal serum alpha-fetoprotein		Hermeneutic study
screening/MSAFP		Interview/interview study
Positive fetal/prenatal diagnosis		Narrative/narrative analysis
Pre-implantation diagnosis		Naturalistic enquiry
Prenatal diagnosis		Participant observation
Prenatal screening		Phenomenology
Prenatal testing		Purposeful/purposive sample
Selective abortion/termination		Qualitative study/research
Therapeutic abortion		Semiotics/semiotic analysis
Ultrasound/ultrasonography		Thematic analysis

Table 8.4   Electronic databases searched in the prenatal diagnosis study.

Academic Search Elite	MEDLINE
AIDS Information Online (AIDSLINE)	PsycInfo
Anthropological Index Online	Public Affairs Information Service (PAIS)
Anthropological Literature	PubMed
Black Studies	Social Science Abstracts (SocSci Abstracts)
Cumulative Index to Nursing and Allied Health Literature	Social Science Citation Index (SSCI)
(CINAHL)	Social Work Abstracts
Digital Dissertations	Sociological Abstracts (Sociofile)
Dissertation Abstracts Index (DAI)	Women's Resources International
Educational Resource Information Center (ERIC)	Women's Studies

Table 8.5   Frequency effect sizes of synthesised findings.

Findings	Effect sizes (%)
1. A positive or suspicious prenatal diagnosis set into motion a series of nested and time-sensitive decisions, most notably: (1) whether to continue or terminate an affected pregnancy and, if terminating, (2) the mode of termination, (3) whether to view fetal remains, (4) how to handle fetal remains, and (5) whether and what to tell others (Alteneder et al., 1998; Bryar, 1997; Furlong & Black, 1984; Helm et al., 1998; Kolker & Burke, 1993; Matthews, 1990; Menary, 1987; Oustifine, 1990; Rapp, 1988, 2000; Redlinger-Grosse et al., 2002; Rillstone, 1999; Rillstone & Hutchinson, 2001; Rothman, 1986; Sandelowski & Jones, 1996a, b; Vantine, 2000)	100
2. Couples obtaining positive prenatal diagnoses managed information coming in to them pertaining to the diagnosis and the decisions they had to make by: (1) seeking information to make these decisions, affirm a decision already made, come to terms with the diagnosis, and to learn about or verify the diagnosis; and by (2) avoiding information that might undermine or cause them to regret a decision already made or acted on (Alteneder et al., 1998; Bryar, 1997; Furlong & Black, 1984; Helm et al., 1998; Matthews, 1990; Menary, 1987; Oustifine, 1990; Rapp, 1988, 2000; Redlinger-Grosse et al., 2002; Rillstone, 1999; Rillstone & Hutchinson, 2001; Rothman, 1986; Vantine, 2000)	80
3. Although difficult for men, positive prenatal diagnosis was devastating for women as it – and its aftermath – were embodied experiences for women, i.e. prenatal testing, quickening, the continuation or termination of a pregnancy with an impaired fetus, and postpartum leaking of breast milk happen in women's bodies (Bryar, 1997; Furlong & Black, 1984; Kolker & Burke, 1993; Menary, 1987; Oustifine, 1990; Rapp, 1988, 2000; Rillstone, 1999; Rillstone & Hutchinson, 2001; Rothman, 1986; Vantine, 2000)	60
4. Regardless of the specific diagnosis, mode and timing of prenatal testing, or the ultimate outcome of the affected pregnancy, couples experienced positive prenatal diagnosis as a traumatic life event with positive and negative effects often lasting through a subsequent pregnancy and beyond (Bryar, 1997; Furlong & Black, 1984; Kolker & Burke, 1993; Menary, 1987; Oustifine, 1990; Rapp, 1988, 2000; Rillstone, 1999; Rillstone & Hutchinson, 2001; Sandelowski & Jones, 1996a,b; Vantine, 2000)	60
5. Limited by the options available and acceptable to them, couples perceived themselves to be actively or passively choosing for or against a pregnancy, or as having no choice at all, in order to explain or explain away their choices to themselves and others (Menary, 1987; Rapp, 1988, 2000; Redlinger-Grosse et al., 2002; Rillstone 1999; Rillstone & Hutchinson, 2001; Rothman, 1986; Sandelowski & Jones, 1996b; Vantine, 2000)	47
6. Positive prenatal diagnosis engendered an existential crisis in couples because it demanded that they choose the fate of their unborn child and, in the process, confront, reconcile and subsequently act on their beliefs about human imperfection and disability, the obligations of parenthood and the acceptability of abortion (Bryar, 1997; Menary, 1987; Rapp, 1988, 2000; Rothman, 1986; Sandelowski & Jones, 1996b; Vantine, 2000)	40
7. Factors contributing to couples' decision to terminate a pregnancy with an impaired fetus included: (1) the acceptability of abortion; (2) certain prognosis of fetal death; (3) ambivalence about the ability to parent an impaired child; and (4) altruistic concerns for the impaired child and for the effect of the impaired child on other children, marriage and family life (Bryar, 1997; Menary, 1987; Rapp, 1988, 2000; Rillstone, 1999; Rillstone & Hutchinson, 2001; Sandelowski & Jones, 1996a; Vantine, 2000)	40
8. Couples obtaining positive prenatal diagnoses perceived healthcare providers to be both supportive and informative, and judgmental and misinformed, while imparting the diagnosis, during the decision-making process, during the termination event, or during affected and subsequent pregnancies (Helm et al., 1998; Kolker & Burke, 1993; Menary, 1987; Oustifine, 1990; Redlinger-Grosse et al., 2002; Rillstone, 1999; Rillstone & Hutchinson, 2001)	40
9. The role specific diagnoses played in couples' decision making depended on the knowledge they already had or could get about diagnoses and their compatibility with life (Furlong & Black, 1984; Helm et al., 1998; Oustifine, 1990; Rapp, 1988, 2000; Rillstone, 1999; Rillstone & Hutchinson, 2001; Sandelowski & Jones, 1996b)	40

Table continues

Table 8.5 continued

Findings	Effect sizes (%)
10. Positive prenatal diagnosis confronted couples with distinctions normally effaced in everyday practice: i.e. between (1) diagnosis and treatment; (2) diagnosis and prognosis; (3) a wanted pregnancy and a wanted baby; and between (4) a fantasy baby and an actual baby (Menary, 1987; Rapp, 1988, 2000; Rothman, 1986; Sandelowski & Jones, 1996a,b; Vantine, 2000)	33
11. Whether deciding to continue or terminate pregnancies, couples felt pulled to make the opposite decision and obliged to justify their decisions to themselves and others (Helm et al., 1998; Rapp, 1988, 2000; Redlinger-Grosse et al., 2002; Sandelowski & Jones, 1996b; Vantine, 2000)	33
12. Positive prenatal diagnosis entailed a variety of losses for couples, including loss of the joy of pregnancy, possibilities inherent in pregnancy, the dream child, of innocence, and of the world as they knew it (Bryar, 1997; Menary, 1987; Rillstone, 1999; Rillstone & Hutchinson, 2001; Sandelowski & Jones, 1996a; Vantine, 2000)	33
13. Although they may have initially been ambivalent, most couples wanted to (and regretted if they did not) see or hold the fetus, mourn its passing, or preserve or bury material remnants of its existence, including sonogram pictures (Bryar, 1997; Matthews, 1990; Rapp, 1988, 2000; Rillstone, 1999; Rillstone & Hutchinson, 2001; Vantine, 2000)	33
14. Couples experienced the decisions facing them following positive prenatal diagnosis as both already made and yet to be made (Oustifine, 1990; Rapp, 1988, 2000; Rillstone, 1999; Rillstone & Hutchinson, 2001; Vantine, 2000)	27
15. Couples obtaining positive prenatal diagnoses experienced both pressure and relief that the time frame available to make and act on decisions was short, and experienced the waiting period between deciding to terminate and the termination itself as too long (Oustifine, 1990; Rillstone, 1999; Rillstone & Hutchinson, 2001; Rothman, 1986; Vantine, 2000)	27
16. Factors contributing to couples' decision to continue a pregnancy with an impaired fetus included: (1) not having the option to terminate; (2) diagnostic and prognostic uncertainty; (3) religious training against abortion; (4) personal experience with other people with disabilities; (5) viewing the fetus on screen; (6) history of infertility; (7) support from friends and family; (8) anticipating feeling guilty if they aborted; and (9) hope that the child would be normal (Helm et al., 1998; Rapp, 1988, 2000; Redlinger-Grosse et al., 2002; Sandelowski & Jones, 1996a)	27
17. Couples terminating pregnancies following positive prenatal diagnoses managed information going out from them pertaining to the decisions they had made by fully or partially disclosing to, or concealing the diagnosis and its aftermath from, children, other family members, friends and acquaintances, in order to obtain or preserve social support, protect them from the burden of knowledge and avoid social condemnation (Bryar, 1997; Furlong & Black, 1984; Rapp, 1988, 2000; Vantine, 2000)	27
18. Although the foreknowledge enabled by prenatal testing created dilemmas, couples obtaining positive prenatal diagnoses generally viewed prenatal testing as a positive development and anticipated choosing to undergoing testing again in future pregnancies (Matthews, 1990; Rapp, 1988, 2000; Rillstone, 1999; Rillstone & Hutchinson, 2001; Sandelowski & Jones, 1996a)	27
19. **In contrast to #18**, couples obtaining positive MSAFP results and negative amniocentesis results doubted they would choose to have MSAFP testing in future pregnancies (Alteneder et al., 1998)	6
20. Couples experienced selective termination as a technologically induced, historically unique and paradoxical form of suffering entailing the intentional loss of a desired pregnancy and killing to care (Kolker & Burke, 1993; Menary, 1987; Rapp, 1988, 2000; Vantine, 2000)	27
21. Complicating decision making was that all prenatal diagnoses are, in the end, prognostically and socially ambiguous (Rapp, 1988, 2000; Rothman, 1986; Sandelowski & Jones, 1996a)	20

Table continues

Table 8.5 continued

Findings	Effect sizes (%)
22. Because of the uniqueness of their suffering and the potential for social condemnation, couples felt alone and avoided others (Menary, 1987; Rapp, 1988, 2000; Rillstone, 1999; Rillstone & Hutchinson, 2001)	20
23. Couples experienced selective termination as traumatic, regardless of the prenatal test revealing the fetal impairment or stage in pregnancy in which the termination occurred (Furlong & Black, 1984; Kolker & Burke, 1993; Menary, 1987)	20
24. Fetal ultrasonography intensified feelings of attachment to the living fetus and, therefore, feelings of loss following termination or death of the fetus (Helm et al., 1998; Kolker & Burke, 1993; Oustifine, 1990)	20
25. Couples tended to agree on decisions, with men tending to defer to their female partners and to view these decisions as theirs to make (Furlong & Black, 1984; Rillstone, 1999; Rillstone & Hutchinson, 2001; Rothman, 1986)	20
26. Women terminating pregnancies following positive prenatal diagnosis sought to disassociate themselves from women who aborted unwanted pregnancies and to associate themselves with women losing wanted pregnancies (Kolker & Burke, 1993; Sandelowski & Jones, 1996b; Vantine, 2000)	20
27. Religion had a variable influence on decision making, having some or no influence at all (Bryar, 1997; Rapp, 1988, 2000; Rillstone, 1999; Rillstone & Hutchinson, 2001)	20
28. The language of positive prenatal diagnosis intensified the ambiguity of couples' experiences as *cells, karyotypes, embryos, fetuses,* and *specimens* vied with *babies; abortion* vied with *selective termination;* and *positive diagnosis* meant negative news, but the way couples used this language reflected their view of the fetus/baby and their relationship to it, and their efforts to make sense of, come to terms with, and to distance themselves from the pain of termination (Menary, 1987; Oustifine, 1990; Rapp, 1988, 2000)	20
29. Obtaining a positive prenatal diagnosis was initially shocking because couples tended to see prenatal testing as routine (and, in the case of fetal ultrasonography, even as enjoyable) and as confirming their belief that everything was normal (Oustifine, 1990; Sandelowski & Jones, 1996b)	13
30. Couples deciding to continue pregnancies felt pressure from their providers to terminate those pregnancies (Helm et al., 1998; Redlinger-Grosse et al., 2002)	13
31. Factors contributing to women's decision to have an induction of labour included the desires to: (1) have time with the baby; (2) parent the baby, if only briefly; (3) ensure acknowledgement of the existence of the baby; (4) have actual body remains of a baby to preserve, bury and mourn; (5) have time to come to terms with the decision; (6) make amends to the baby; and to (7) atone for the decision to terminate by suffering the pains of labour (Rillstone, 1999; Rillstone & Hutchinson, 2001; Vantine, 2000)	13
32. For couples who had obtained positive prenatal diagnoses, to contemplate conceiving another pregnancy was to contemplate another loss (Bryar, 1997; Rillstone, 1999; Rillstone & Hutchinson, 2001)	13
33. Women who terminated pregnancies following positive prenatal diagnosis, especially by CVS, wanted to mourn but felt they did not deserve to mourn (Kolker & Burke, 1993; Vantine, 2000)	13
34. Women deciding to terminate pregnancies found the embodiment of pregnancy to be unwelcome and sought to minimise its impact by asking the fetus to stop moving and ceasing to observe special dietary and other practices to protect fetal well-being (Oustifine, 1990; Vantine, 2000)	13
35. Contributing to women's decision to have a D & E was the availability of the option (Rillstone, 1999; Rillstone & Hutchinson, 2001)	6

Table continues

Table 8.5 continued

Findings	Effect sizes (%)
36. The strategies women used to reconcile conflicts engendered by selective termination – denying the personhood of the baby, limiting the information they sought about the baby, transferring agency for choice to others, adopting a stance of moral relativity, avoiding disclosing or selectively disclosing the event to others – worked briefly but ultimately felt as if they were betraying themselves and their babies (Menary, 1987)	6
37. Couples, healthcare providers, family and friends underestimated the intensity and duration of feelings of loss following selective termination (Kolker & Burke, 1993)	6
38. Attachment to the fetus intensified grief, but facilitated mourning and recovery (Kolker & Burke, 1993)	6
39. Women sought to relieve themselves of the burden of decision making by ensuring their partners' participation in the process, by looking for divine signs that they had made the right decision, and by hoping for a spontaneous fetal demise that would take the decision to terminate out of their hands (Vantine, 2000)	6

MSAF, maternal serum alpha-fetoprotein; CVS, chorionic villus sampling; D & E, dilatation and evacuation.

Box 8.3   Example of the results section in a qualitative research synthesis report – from the prenatal diagnosis review (Sandelowski & Barroso, 2005).

Results

Profile of reports

Seventeen relevant research reports (marked with an asterisk in the reference list) were retrieved during the search period. (These and other 'travesty of choosing' references are embedded in the reference list for this chapter.) Among these 17 reports were 13 published works (10 journal articles, 2 books and 1 book chapter) and 4 unpublished works (3 doctoral dissertations and 1 Master's thesis), appearing between 1984 and 2001. Table 8.6 contains a profile of these reports. As indicated there, 3 sets of 2 reports each involve the same authors and the same or overlapping samples (Rapp, 1988, 2000; Rillstone, 1999; Rillstone & Hutchinson, 2001; Sandelowski & Jones, 1996a, b). Rapp's (1988) chapter contains early findings from the extensive multi-year ethnographic study she described fully in her book (Rapp, 2000). The Rillstone & Hutchinson (2001) article is an abbreviated version of Rillstone's (1999) dissertation. Each of these sets of works was, therefore, treated analytically as if they were one work. Although the two Sandelowski & Jones (1996a, b) reports (written by the first author of this article) were based on the same sample of women and couples, they were each directed toward different research purposes and thus contain largely different findings. Accordingly, they were treated as two reports except when the same finding appeared in both reports.

As shown in Table 8.6, the primary disciplinary affiliation of these works is nursing, and the most frequently stated methodology is phenomenology. The predominant research purpose was to explore the personal experience of pregnancy termination after positive fetal diagnosis. The primary mode of data collection was the interview; women or couples were interviewed one or more times 11 days to 10 years after the events featured. No explicit theoretical orientation to the experience of positive diagnosis guided any of the studies. The geographic locations of the studies were large urban areas, most notably, Boston and New York.

Profile of research participants

Women obtaining positive prenatal diagnoses comprised the entire sample in 10 of the reports. The remaining reports also included other participants, most notably women's male partners (usually husbands) and, less often, professional providers, such as genetic counsellors. No study was conducted with men alone. Only findings derived from women or couples are included in this review.

The profile of participants presented below is limited by the information reported. Categories in which the information offered precluded meaningful summary include employment, income, education, religion, pregnancy trimester at diagnosis, trimester at termination, mode of pregnancy termination and number of women with healthy children. We inferred from the findings that participants were largely middle class and Christian.

Sample sizes ranged from 3 to 52 women and from 4 to 10 men, with a total of 214 women and 35 of their male partners studied. The majority of women or couples were married and white. Across studies, an array of fatal and non-fatal positive fetal diagnoses were made, largely via amniocentesis. The most common diagnosis was Down syndrome and the most common pregnancy outcome, termination of pregnancy.

Synthesis of primary research findings

As shown in Table 8.5, in which all of the meta-findings are arranged by their frequency, the four most prominent findings across all reports concerned:

(1)   the series of nested and time-sensitive decisions couples were forced to make following positive prenatal diagnosis (point 1. in Table 8.5, hereafter #1);
(2)   their efforts both to obtain and avoid information in the making of these decisions (#2);
(3)   the greater devastation women (as opposed to men) felt following positive diagnosis (#3); and
(4)   the traumatic and reverberating effects of diagnosis, regardless of the specific diagnosis, mode and timing of diagnosis, or whether couples ultimately chose to continue or terminate the affected pregnancy (#4).

These long-term effects were evident not only in findings pertaining to couples' experiences of pregnancies following the affected pregnancy, but also in the fact that women recalled in vivid detail, and even relived and sometimes regretted, events that had occurred up to 10 years prior to being interviewed. These effects encompassed both positive outcomes, such as personal growth and improved marital relationships, and negative outcomes, such as chronic loss and regret.

Also prominent were the findings pertaining to the existential crisis positive prenatal diagnosis engendered in couples by virtue of the life-and-death choices they were compelled to make (#5–6), the divergent views of healthcare providers that couples held as they made and then acted on their decisions (#8), and the variable role diagnosis played in deciding whether to terminate or continue pregnancy (#9). The different and even conflicting views of the role of specific diagnoses, healthcare providers and religion (#27) evident across studies and even in the same study suggest the unique confluence of circumstances shaping individual couples' experiences.

Couples elected to continue their pregnancies for reasons that included the unavailability or unacceptability of the option to terminate and the hope that their babies might yet be normal (#16). In contrast, couples elected to terminate their pregnancies for reasons that included the availability and acceptability of termination and the perceived certainty of fetal death (#7). Factors contributing to the choice to continue pregnancy included past reproductive history, religious training, experience with persons with disabilities, viewing the fetus on ultrasound and social support. Factors contributing to the choice to terminate pregnancy included ambivalence about the ability to parent an impaired child and altruistic concerns for the fetus, other children, and marriage and family life. No matter what they ultimately chose to do, couples felt pulled to make and justify the opposite decision to themselves, close and distant members of their social network, and to healthcare providers (#11). Couples continuing pregnancies felt pressure from providers to terminate their pregnancies (#30), and couples felt the need to explain or explain away their choices (#5). (This finding may also be an artefact of the research interview whereby couples were asked to explain their choices.)

Topical focus on genetic termination

As shown in Table 8.6, the most prevalent topical focus of the findings is the termination of pregnancy following positive prenatal diagnosis, also referred to as selective or genetic termination to differentiate it from elective terminations for reasons other than fetal health. Indeed, in most of the reports reviewed here, the experience of positive prenatal diagnosis is depicted as the experience of genetic termination. The title of Menary's (1987) dissertation report – 'the amniocentesis–abortion experience' – exemplifies the close identification of positive prenatal diagnosis with pregnancy termination evident in the majority of studies.

Moreover, in these studies, it is pregnancy termination, not the positive prenatal diagnosis *per se*, which accounts for the suffering or 'anguish' (Rillstone & Hutchinson, 2001) researchers depicted as unique to the women and couples interviewed. Couples continuing pregnancies following positive prenatal diagnosis suffered the same losses (e.g. the loss of the dream baby) as couples who learn only after birth that their child is impaired. The difference between these couples lay not in their responses to their child, or in the adjustments and accommodations they had to make to that child's care, but rather in the timing of discovery that their child was, or would be, impaired: in *pre*natal as opposed to *post*natal diagnosis (Sandelowski & Jones, 1996a). What made positive prenatal diagnosis experientially distinctive was the availability of the option (to those couples who could readily access termination services and whose fetus was diagnosed early enough in pregnancy to allow it) to terminate a pregnancy with an impaired fetus, and the shifting onto parents of the obligation to accept or refuse that option.

Thematic focus on chosen loss and lost choices

Whereas the most prevalent topic addressed in the findings is genetic termination, the most prevalent theme concerns the dilemmas and consequences of choosing newly engendered by the advent of prenatal testing, i.e. by the knowledge now obtainable during pregnancy that a baby will either die or be impaired and that little or nothing can be done to save or treat the baby. More than half of the findings shown in Table 8.5 are in the area of choice and decision making. A secondary theme concerns the losses couples incurred as a consequence of a positive prenatal diagnosis, no matter what choice they made.

The metaphoric links we discerned between choice and loss are paradox and irony. For couples receiving positive prenatal diagnosis, the experience was one of both chosen losses and lost choices. Vantine's (2000) delineation of 20 paradoxes associated with genetic termination following positive prenatal diagnosis is the most explicit expression of this metaphor, but paradox, contradiction and irony are implicit in the findings of most of the other studies by virtue of the topical emphasis on genetic termination. The key paradox in Vantine's (2000) findings lay in women's experiences of pregnancy termination as an act of both loving – in sparing the impaired fetus/baby further suffering – and killing, in ending the life of the fetus. Rapp (2000:225) referred to the irony of 'chosen loss' that defined genetic termination. Referring to the title of William Styron's 1976 novel, Rothman (1986:179) described women's choices following positive prenatal diagnosis as a 'Sophie's choice' to signify the paradoxical lack of choice that made a 'mockery' or travesty of choosing.

Central to the paradox of positive prenatal diagnosis was that women and their partners were forced to contemplate choosing against a wanted pregnancy. Yet although the pregnancy was wanted, couples had to confront the fact that the impaired baby was not. Wanting to be parents, couples had to acknowledge that they did not necessarily want to be parents of any baby. Positive prenatal diagnosis brought to the surface distinctions normally effaced in everyday practice (#10). A positive prenatal diagnosis emphasised the difference between actual pregnancies and virtual babies. When a diagnosis of an impairment was made, virtual babies (i.e. babies who could be any baby), became actual females with Down syndrome, males with heart defects, live females with spina bifida, or dead, or soon-to-be dead, males with hydrops. Diagnosis, not birth, was the dividing line between *any* baby and a specific impaired but irreplaceable baby: between fantasy and reality, and potentiality and actuality. Regardless of whether couples actually terminated their pregnancies, these pregnancies were figuratively or emotionally terminated as soon as the virtual baby became an actual baby with a specific impairment. The irony of positive prenatal diagnosis is that in forecasting the future, it foreclosed the possibilities inherent in the very word *pregnant*.

Positive prenatal diagnosis also made the embodiment that defines pregnancy as a uniquely female experience a source of anguish for women choosing to terminate their pregnancies. The termination event was profoundly at odds with the fetal life pregnant women felt and the signs of fetal life after termination (i.e. breasts leaking milk; #3). Women sought to minimise or maximise the embodiment of pregnancy to reduce the suffering resulting from this life/death contradiction (#31, 34). Women sought to ignore their pregnancies, or to undergo the pain of labour as a way to acknowledge fetal life and atone for fetal death.

Positive prenatal diagnosis vis-à-vis *other comparable events*

By virtue of the topical and thematic emphasis of the meta-findings, the experience of positive prenatal diagnosis is comparable to other experiences involving choice and loss that nurses encounter every day no matter where and with what populations they practise. Positive prenatal diagnosis is most like other perinatal events perceived as losses, i.e. miscarriage, stillbirth and neonatal death, which expectant and new parents frequently suffer and which have been the focus of a large body of nursing and other research (e.g. Peppers & Knapp, 1980; Savage, 1989; Kavanaugh, 1997; Swanson, 1999; Layne, 2003). Ten of the meta-findings in Table 8.5 (#12, 13, 20, 24, 26, 31–33, 37, 38) address the losses couples suffered largely because of their prior attachment to the pregnancy and fetus. Maintaining this attachment following the pregnancy loss – via seeing or holding the baby after death, and saving material mementos and participating in funeral services to acknowledge its life – was largely instrumental in facilitating the recovery of parents. Reinforcing the irony of perinatal loss is that it is both intensified and mitigated by attachment.

Indeed, women who terminated pregnancies following positive prenatal diagnosis sought to emphasise their kinship with women who had lost babies and to de-emphasise kinship with women choosing to abort babies, on the basis of the attachments and losses they presumably did or did not share (#26). Yet these women had to struggle against the volition that experientially separated them from women having *involuntary* perinatal losses but that united them with women having *voluntary* terminations. Unlike women suffering involuntary losses, these women chose their loss. The choice may have been a Sophie's choice – a paradoxically involuntary choice – but it was nevertheless a choice that women recognised as undermining their claim to kinship with women suffering miscarriages, stillbirths or other catastrophic perinatal events considered to be beyond the control of women and their partners. A positive prenatal diagnosis forced couples to decide whether their babies would die or, at least, in the case of a lethal anomaly, when they would die.

Yet despite this volition, the *wantedness* of pregnancy separated these women from other women having elective terminations whom they perceived as *not wanting* their pregnancies. The volition and wantedness defining the experience of positive prenatal diagnosis are what make it comparable also to the experiences of parents confronted with the choice of selective fetal reduction for multi-fetal pregnancies, and of family members confronted with the choice of removing the life-support of a relative. In all of these cases, an existential crisis is engendered by the ironic combination of volition and desire leading to coercion, i.e. by being forced to choose both for and against something both wanted and not wanted.

The volition inherent in positive prenatal diagnosis is also what makes it comparable to conditions and circumstances considered to be stigmatising. Having an impaired child is by itself a stigmatising event in a culture that values physical perfection, regardless of when an impairment is diagnosed (Rothman, 1986; Rapp, 2000). Yet it is volition, or fear of what others might think of them because they had chosen to terminate their pregnancies, which was the primary motivation for the studied couples' efforts to manage information about those pregnancies (#17, #22). Information management is a key component of stigma management (Goffman, 1963). Acutely aware of the intense feelings in American society concerning abortion, couples choosing to terminate pregnancies struggled with whether, when and how to disclose their choice to others, including their children, other family members, friends and others less close to them. This struggle around disclosure of a potentially stigmatising event makes positive prenatal diagnosis experientially comparable to the struggles of other persons with stigmatising conditions, such as HIV-positive persons (Parker & Aggleton, 2003).

Information management was also a key component of couples' efforts to reduce cognitive dissonance (Festinger, 1957), or the psychological discomfort felt at a discrepancy between what couples knew or believed, and new information. In contrast to stigma management, where the emphasis is on controlling information flowing from couples to others, in dissonance management, the focus is on controlling information flowing to couples from others. Couples either sought or avoided information both to make decisions yet to be made and to uphold decisions they had already made (#2, #14). Their desire to take in information was complicated by the frequent lack of information available about the fetal diagnoses they were given and the ambiguity surrounding all such diagnoses (#21). For example, although expectant parents were most familiar with Down syndrome, no one could predict how impaired their Down syndrome baby would be. Couples recognised the wide gap that existed between prenatal diagnosis and post-natal prognosis (#10).

Table 8.6   Profile of reports and samples.

Report	Discipline	Stated method	Event line and/or topical focus	Sample
Alteneder et al., 1998	Nursing	Phenomenology	From positive MSAFP through negative amniocentesis	16 women: 12W; 3A; 1H
Bryar, 1997	Nursing	Phenomenology	From positive diagnosis to short-term aftermath of termination	3 W women
Furlong & Black, 1984	Social work	None stated	From positive diagnosis to long-term aftermath of termination/Children's responses	4 couples, 9 mothers, and 2 fathers; all W
Helm et al., 1998	Social work	None stated	From positive diagnosis to delivery of baby with Down syndrome	10 W women
Kolker & Burke, 1993	Social science	None stated	From termination to short-term aftermath	24 women, race not stated[a]
Matthews, 1990	Nursing	Phenomenology	From positive diagnosis to short-term aftermath of loss of malformed fetus	20 women: 16W, 4H
Menary, 1987	Education	Grounded theory; phenomenology	From positive diagnosis to long-term aftermath of termination	11 women, race not stated
Oustifine, 1990	Nursing	Exploratory/ descriptive	From positive diagnosis to long-term aftermath of termination	6 W women
Rapp, 1988, 2000[b,c]	Anthropology	None stated	Prenatal testing	52 women obtaining positive diagnoses: mixed race sample, racial distribution not stated[a]
Redlinger-Grosse et al., 2002	Genetics, medicine, public health	Descriptive	Continuation of pregnancy after diagnosis of holoprosencephaly	10 couples and 4 mothers: 21W; 2H; 1A/P
Rillstone, 1999; Rillstone & Hutchinson, 2001[b]	Nursing	Grounded theory	From positive diagnosis to long-term aftermath of termination/Subsequent pregnancy	13 women and 9 partners: 20W; 1H; 1Turkish[a]
Rothman, 1986[c]	Sociology	Exploratory	Prenatal testing	14 women after genetic termination, race not stated[a]
Sandelowski & Jones, 1996a[d]	Nursing	Qualitative description	Evaluation of foreknowledge obtained from positive diagnosis	15 women and 12 partners: all W, except 1AA couple, 1AA woman, and 1 As-A woman
Sandelowski & Jones, 1996b[d]	Nursing	Qualitative	Constructing choices after decision to continue or terminate pregnancy	See Sandelowski et al., 1996a
Vantine, 2000	Psychology	Phenomenology	From positive diagnosis to long-term aftermath of termination	3 W women

W, white; AA, African American; H, Hispanic or Latino; As-A, Asian American; A/P, Asian Pacific Islander.
[a]These studies included participants, e.g. genetic counsellors, women, and couples receiving positive fetal diagnoses, who were not included in this figure nor in the presentation of findings.
[b]The two Rapp works and two Rillstone works were each treated as one work.
[c]These are book-length ethnographies and sociologies, respectively, of prenatal testing and thus contain findings in areas other than positive prenatal diagnosis.
[d]These two works are from identical samples, but involved different analyses. They were treated as two works.

Box 8.4   Example of the discussion section in a qualitative research synthesis report – from the prenatal diagnosis review (Sandelowski & Barroso, 2005).

Discussion

Positive prenatal diagnosis is distinctive among catastrophic perinatal events by virtue of the chosen losses and lost choices it engenders. Because it is both like and unlike other perinatal losses, practice and future research must address the distinctive combination of choice and loss that experientially defines positive prenatal diagnosis.

Clinical implications

Existing guidelines for caring for couples after perinatal losses (e.g. Hutti, 1988; Ryan et al., 1991; Association of Women's Health, Obstetric and Neonatal Nurses, 1998; Workman, 2001) can be adapted to ensure the accommodation of differences among perinatal losses and the experiential variations in individual parents' encounter with any one of these events. Although the integration of findings presented here emphasises shared experiences, it also indicates the variable factors and combinations of factors constituting these experiences. In the end, there is no one experience of positive prenatal diagnosis, but rather as many experiences of it as there are expectant parents.

Specific adaptations to existing guidelines for care should focus on several key areas. Among these are attending to the particular constructions of choice couples receiving positive prenatal diagnoses use both to communicate and to come to terms with the event. This assessment of couples' narrative coping is key to nurses assisting couples to develop narrative strategies conducive to recovery and healing and to nurses adopting a language that does not undermine these coping efforts. In narrative terms, nurses' efforts to understand how couples 'story' their encounter with positive diagnosis is a form of diagnosis. Nursing intervention is then directed toward assisting couples to construct stories of choosing they can comfortably live with (Sandelowski, 1994).

Also of particular importance is the determination of the contents and timing of delivery of information most supportive of couples' desires. Information both consonant and dissonant with prior knowledge or belief can make choosing more painful. Moreover, couples will sometimes want to delay or avoid information that might undermine a decision already made or desired. Accordingly, *when* information is offered is as important as *what* information is offered. For example, couples may be initially reluctant to see the remains or read reports of autopsies of their babies, but later decide they want this information. The timing of information is necessarily influenced by the small window of time parents have to avail themselves of all of their options. Expert practice with couples receiving positive prenatal diagnoses is attentive to these subtle differences in information and timing. Other subtleties include discerning the motivation behind and direction for couples' information management efforts. Couples sought to control information going *out* largely to minimise stigmatisation, but they sought to control information coming in largely to reduce cognitive dissonance.

Research implications

These adaptations to existing clinical guidelines should be the focus of research to evaluate their impact on couples' well-being. Future research should also be directed toward examining more closely the frequently fine differences among perinatal events (e.g. miscarriage, genetic termination, birth of impaired child, neonatal death) and the couples who experience them. Although such events may all be conceived as losses, other conceptualisations may be warranted that capture their distinctive meaning to socio-economically, culturally and ethnically diverse couples. Relatively few studies have addressed couples continuing pregnancies after they have learned their baby will be impaired, or the ethnic minority couples who are often prominent among expectant parents continuing pregnancy after positive fetal diagnosis.

Limitations of research and alternative explanations

Several caveats exist to the research synthesis presented here. This synthesis is limited to qualitative studies of women's and couples' experiences of positive prenatal diagnosis in which the primary topical and thematic foci were the ethical dilemmas raised by having to choose for or against pregnancy termination, rather than positive diagnosis *per se*. In other words, the experience of positive prenatal diagnosis was defined by this dilemma, which may be viewed as either an accurate definition of the experience or an artefact of who participated in the studies reviewed and when in the history of prenatal diagnosis these studies were conducted. The continuing relevance of this integration will depend on advances in fetal diagnosis and therapies, and the continuing availability of pregnancy termination in the United States. Earlier diagnosis and new fetal therapies may reduce the need for terminations after the first trimester, and continuing legal modifications of women's right to choose abortion and reduction in the number of agencies offering them will affect women's experiences.

In order to produce a comprehensive synthesis of evidence to serve as the foundation for evidence-based practice with women and couples receiving positive prenatal diagnoses, the findings from quantitative studies must also ultimately be integrated and combined with the findings reported here and then placed into the larger context of the 'normalisation of prenatal diagnostic screening' as a critical milestone in contemporary Western pregnancy (Browner & Press, 1995).

(As the prenatal diagnosis study was generated to test methods for synthesising qualitative research, and not to add to the evidence base for practice with childbearing couples per se, quantitative studies were automatically excluded from consideration.)

Finally, any integration of qualitative research is comprised of one or more reviewers' interpretations of a selected group of researchers' interpretations of a selected group of research participants' interpretations of selected events in their lives. Although we worked to remain faithful to the findings in the reports reviewed, the synthesis we present here is inescapably a product of a series of complex and dynamic social interactions and interpretive transformations. As such, it can be read as a reasonably accurate index of events in the lives of the women and couples who participated in the studies reviewed. An alternative reading is that the findings reflect researchers' desire to showcase the negative consequences of advances in reproductive technology, primarily manifested in the ethical dilemmas that women and couples undergoing prenatal diagnosis face. An alternative explanation of the finding that choice and loss define women's and couples' experiences of positive fetal diagnosis may be that choice and loss pervade researchers' depictions of women's and couples' experiences of positive fetal diagnosis. In the end, qualitative research syntheses always have multiple existences: as evidence and as discourse.

represented in the studies featured in those reports (although some journals prefer this information be placed in the methods section instead), in addition to the verbal delineation and visual display of the synthesised findings. Depending on their nature and what reviewers want to emphasise about them, synthesised findings may be presented narratively, thematically, conceptually, graphically or in any other form best suited to them.

Discussion of synthesis produced

In this section, reviewers should link the syntheses they produced with existing scholarship and discuss the implications of them for research and practice. This section should be tailored to the audience likely to be reading it. For example, if published in a clinical journal, this section should emphasise the utility of the findings and how they might be trans-

lated for use in practice. Reviewers should address in this section the distinctive limitations of the study and the distinctive challenges synthesising the results of the primary studies posed for them. They may also choose to offer alternative readings of the findings (which may foreshadow a more detailed treatment of them in a future paper).

Conclusion

Understanding reports of qualitative research synthesis is vital to preserving the utility of qualitative research for knowledge advancement in nursing, to moving qualitative research to the centre of the evidence-based practice process, and to developing the soundest evidence base for nursing practice. The template featured here is in the service of that understanding. But such appraisal templates are most useful in the hands of readers of research willing and able to accommodate them to the research literature under review, knowledgeable about the constraints of publication, and mindful of the complexities of qualitative research and of the qualitative research synthesis enterprise.

References

This list includes all references cited in this chapter. References marked with an asterisk (*) indicate reports included in the prenatal diagnosis study.

*Alteneder, R.R., Kenner, C., Greene, D. & Pohorecki, S. (1998) The lived experience of women who undergo prenatal diagnostic testing due to elevated maternal serum alpha-fetoprotein screening. *MCN: American Journal of Maternal–Child Nursing*, 23, 180–6.

Association of Women's Health, Obstetric and Neonatal Nurses (1998) Guideline for providing care to the family experiencing perinatal loss and fetal death. In: *Standards and Guidelines for Professional Nursing Practice in the Care of Women and Newborns*, 5th edn, pp. 20–2. Association of Women's Health, Obstetric and Neonatal Nurses, Washington, DC.

Bates, M.J. (1989) The design of browsing and berry-picking techniques for online search interface. *Online Review*, 13, 407–24.

Bazerman, C. (1988) *Shaping Written Knowledge: The Genre and Activity of the Experimental Article in Science*. University of Wisconsin Press, Madison.

Belgrave, L.L. & Smith, K.J. (1995) Negotiated validity in collaborative ethnography. *Qualitative Inquiry*, 1, 69–86.

Browner, C.H. & Press, N. (1995) The normalization of prenatal diagnostic screening. In: *Conceiving the New World Order: The Global Politics of Reproduction* (Ginsburg, F.D. & Rapp, R., eds), pp. 307–22. University of California Press, Berkeley.

*Bryar, S.H. (1997) One day you're pregnant and one day you're not: Pregnancy interruption for fetal anomalies. *JOGNN: Journal of Obstetric, Gynecologic, & Neonatal Nursing*, 26, 559–66.

Conn, V.S. & Rantz, M.J. (2003) Research methods: Managing primary study quality in meta-analyses. *Research in Nursing and Health*, 26, 322–33.

Cooper, H. (1998) *Synthesizing Research*, 3rd edn. Sage, Thousand Oaks, California.

Doyle, L.H. (2003) Synthesis through meta-ethnography: Paradoxes, enhancements, and possibilities. *Qualitative Research*, 3, 321–45.

Eisner, E.W. (1991) *The Enlightened Eye: Qualitative Inquiry and the Enhancement of Educational Practice*. Macmillan, New York.

Festinger, L. (1957) *A Theory of Cognitive Dissonance*. Stanford University Press, Stanford, California.

Filkins, K. & Russo, J.F. (eds) (1985) *Human Prenatal Diagnosis*. Marcel Dekker, New York.

*Furlong, R.M. & Black, R.B. (1984) Pregnancy termination for genetic indications: The impact on families. *Social Work in Health Care*, 10, 17–34.

Garcia, J., Bricker, L., Henderson, J., Martin, M., Mugford, M., Nielson, J. et al. (2002) Women's views of pregnancy ultrasound: A systematic review. *Birth*, 29, 225–50.

Goffman, E. (1963) *Stigma: Notes on the management of spoiled identity*. Prentice-Hall, Englewood Cliffs, New Jersey.

Greenhalgh, T., Robert, G., Macfarlane, F., Bate, P., Kyriakidou, O. & Peacock, R. (2005) Storylines of research in diffusion of innovation: A meta-narrative approach to systematic review. *Social Science and Medicine*, 61, 417–30.

*Helm, D.T., Miranda, S. & Chedd, N.A. (1998) Prenatal diagnosis of Down Syndrome: Mothers' reflections on supports needed from diagnosis to birth. *Mental Retardation*, 36, 55–61.

Hutti, M.H. (1988) A quick reference table of interventions to assist families to cope with pregnancy loss or neonatal death. *Birth*, 15, 33–5.

Jones, K. (2004) Mission drift in qualitative research, or moving toward a systematic review of qualitative studies, moving back to a more systematic narrative review. *The Qualitative Report*, 9 (1), 95–112. Online journal, www.nova.edu/ssss/ QR/QR9-1/jones.pdf (retrieved 29 August 2004).

Kavanaugh, K. (1997) The parental experience surrounding the death of an infant born at the margin of viability. *JOGNN: Journal of Obstetric, Gynecologic, and Neonatal Nursing*, 26, 43–51.

Kirkevold, M. (1997) Integrative nursing research: An important strategy to further the development of nursing science and nursing practice. *Journal of Advanced Nursing*, 25, 977–84.

*Kolker, A. & Burke, B.M. (1993) Grieving the wanted child: Ramifications of abortion after prenatal diagnosis of abnormality. *Health Care for Women International*, 14, 513–26.

Kvale, S. (1995) The social construction of validity. *Qualitative Inquiry*, 1, 19–40.

Layne, L.L. (2003) *Motherhood Lost: A Feminist Account of Pregnancy Loss in America*. Routledge, New York.

Losee, R.M. (2000) When information retrieval measures agree about the relative quality of document rankings. *Journal of the American Society for Information Science*, 51, 834–40.

Marchionini, G. (1995) *Information Seeking in Electronic Environments*. Cambridge University Press, New York.

*Matthews, A.L. (1990) Known fetal malformations during pregnancy: A human experience of loss. *Birth Defects: Original Article Series*, 26 (3), 168–75.

Maxwell, J.A. (1992) Understanding and validity in qualitative research. *Harvard Educational Review*, 62, 279–300.

McCormick, J., Rodney, P. and Varcoe, C. (2003) Reinterpretations across studies: An approach to meta-analysis. *Qualitative Health Research*, 13, 933–44.

*Menary, J.E. (1987) The amniocentesis–abortion experience: a study of psychological effects and healing process. Unpublished doctoral dissertation, Harvard University, Cambridge, Massachusetts.

Milunsky, A. (ed.) (2004) *Genetic Disorders and the Fetus: Diagnosis, Prevention, and Treatment.* Johns Hopkins University Press, Baltimore, Maryland.

Morgan, D.L. (1993) Qualitative content analysis: A guide to paths not taken. *Qualitative Health Research*, 3, 112–21.

Noblit, G.W. & Hare, R.D. (1988) *Meta-ethnography: Synthesizing Qualitative Studies.* Sage, Newbury Park, California.

Onwuegbuzie, A.J. (2003) Effect sizes in qualitative research: A prolegomenon. *Quality and Quantity*, 37, 393–409.

*Oustifine, J.M. (1990) Abortion after amniocentesis: women's lived experiences. Unpublished Master's thesis, MGH Institute of Health Professions, Boston, Massachusetts.

Parker, R. & Aggleton, P. (2003) HIV and AIDS-related stigma and discrimination: A conceptual framework and implications for action. *Social Science and Medicine*, 57, 13–24.

Paterson, B.L., Thorne, S.E., Canam, C. & Jillings, C. (2001) *Meta-study of Qualitative Health Research: A Practical Guide to Meta-analysis and Meta-synthesis.* Sage, Thousand Oaks, California.

Peppers, L.G. & Knapp, R.J. (1980) *Motherhood and Mourning.* Praeger, New York.

*Rapp, R. (1988) The power of 'positive' diagnosis: Medical and maternal discourses on amniocentesis. In: *Childbirth in America: Anthropological Perspectives* (Michaelson, K.L., ed.), pp. 103–16. Bergin & Garvey, South Hadley, Massachusetts.

*Rapp, R. (2000) *Testing Women, Testing the Fetus: The Social Impact of Amniocentesis in America.* Routledge, New York.

*Redlinger-Grosse, K., Bernhardt, B.A., Berg, K., Muenke, M. & Biesecker, B.B. (2002) The decision to continue: The experiences and needs of parents who receive a prenatal diagnosis of holoprosencephaly. *American Journal of Medical Genetics*, 11, 369–78.

*Rillstone, P. (1999) Prenatal diagnosis of fetal abnormalities: managing catastrophic psychic pain in a subsequent pregnancy. Unpublished doctoral dissertation, University of Florida, Gainesville.

*Rillstone, P. & Hutchinson, S.A. (2001) Managing the reemergence of anguish: Pregnancy after a loss due to anomalies. *JOGNN: Journal of Obstetric, Gynecologic, and Neonatal Nursing*, 30, 291–8.

Rodgers, B.L. & Cowles, K.V. (1993) The qualitative research audit trail: A complex collection of documentation. *Research in Nursing and Health*, 16, 219–26.

Rothenberg, K.H. & Thomson, E.J. (1995) *Women and Prenatal Testing: Facing the Challenges of Genetic Technology.* Ohio State University Press, Columbus.

*Rothman, B.K. (1986) *The Tentative Pregnancy: Prenatal Diagnosis and the Future of Motherhood.* Viking, New York.

Ryan, P.F., Coté-Arsenault, D. & Sugarman, L.L. (1991) Facilitating care after perinatal loss: A comprehensive checklist. *JOGNN: Journal of Obstetric, Gynecologic, and Neonatal Nursing*, 20, 386–9.

Sandelowski, M. (1994) We are the stories we tell: narrative knowing in nursing practice. *Journal of Holistic Nursing*, 12, 23–33.

Sandelowski, M. (1995) A theory of the transition to parenthood of infertile couples. *Research in Nursing and Health*, 18, 123–32.

Sandelowski, M. (1998) The call to experts in qualitative research. *Research in Nursing and Health*, 21, 467–71.

Sandelowski, M. & Barroso, J. (2002) Reading qualitative studies. *International Journal of Qualitative Methods*, 1 (1), Article 5. Online journal available at http://www.ualberta.ca/~ijqm/english/engframeset.html

Sandelowski, M. & Barroso, J. (2003a) Classifying the findings in qualitative studies. *Qualitative Health Research*, 13, 905–23.

Sandelowski, M. & Barroso, J. (2003b) Creating meta-summaries of qualitative findings. *Nursing Research*, 52, 226–33.

Sandelowski, M. & Barroso, J. (2003c) Motherhood in the context of maternal HIV infection. *Research in Nursing and Health*, 26, 470–82.

Sandelowski, M. & Barroso, J. (2003d) Toward a metasynthesis of qualitative findings on motherhood in HIV-positive women. *Research in Nursing and Health*, 26, 153–70.

Sandelowski, M. & Barroso, J. (2003e) Writing the proposal for a qualitative research methodology project. *Qualitative Health Research*, 13, 781–820.

Sandelowski, M. & Barroso, J. (2005) The travesty of choosing after positive prenatal diagnosis. *JOGNN: Journal of Obstetric, Gynecologic, and Neonatal Nursing*, 34, 307–18

Sandelowski, M. & Barroso, J. (2007) *Handbook for Synthesizing Qualitative Research.* Springer, New York.

*Sandelowski, M. & Jones, L.C. (1996a) Couples' evaluations of foreknowledge of fetal impairment. *Clinical Nursing Research*, 5, 81–96.

*Sandelowski, M. & Jones, L.C. (1996b) 'Healing fictions': Stories of choosing in the aftermath of the detection of fetal anomalies. *Social Science and Medicine*, 42, 353–61.

Savage, J.A. (1989) *Mourning Unlived Lives: A Psychological Study of Childbearing Loss*. Chiron, Wilmette, Illinois.

Smaling, A. (2003) Inductive, analogical, and communicative generalization. *International Journal of Qualitative Methods*, 2 (1), Article 5. Online journal available at http://www.ualberta.ca/~ijqm/backissues/2_1/html/smaling.html

Statham, H., Solomon, W. & Chitty, L. (2000) Prenatal diagnosis of fetal abnormality: psychological effects on women in low-risk pregnancies. *Balliere's Clinical Obstetrics and Gynecology*, 14, 731–47.

Strauss, A. & Corbin, J. (1998) *Basics of Qualitative Research: Techniques and Procedures for Developing Grounded Theory*, 2nd edn. Sage, Thousand Oaks, California.

Swanson, K.M. (1999) Research-based practice with women who have had miscarriages. *Image: Journal of Nursing Scholarship*, 31, 339–45.

Thorne, S. (1994) Secondary analysis in qualitative research: Issues and implications. In: *Critical Issues in Qualitative Research Methods* (Morse, J.M., ed.), pp. 263–79). Sage, Thousand Oaks, California.

Thorne, S., Jensen, L., Kearney, M.H., Noblit, G. & Sandelowski, M. (2004) Qualitative metasynthesis: Reflections on methodological orientation and ideological agenda. *Qualitative Health Research*, 14, 1342–65.

Tunis, S.L. (1993) Prenatal diagnosis of fetal abnormalities: Psychological impact. In: *Essentials of Prenatal Diagnosis* (Simpson, J.L. & Elias, S., eds), pp. 347–64. Churchill Livingstone, New York.

*Vantine, H.S. (2000) Terminating a wanted pregnancy after the discovery of possible fetal abnormalities: An existential phenomenological study of making and living with the decision. Unpublished doctoral dissertation, Duquesne University, Pittsburgh, Pennsylvania.

West, J. & Oldfather, P. (1995) Pooled case comparison: An innovation for cross-case study. *Qualitative Inquiry*, 1, 452–64.

Workman, E. (2001) Guiding parents through the death of their infant. JOGNN: *Journal of Obstetric, Gynecologic, and Neonatal Nursing*, 30, 569–73.

9 Role Development in Acute Hospital Settings: A Systematic Review and Meta-synthesis

Myfanwy Lloyd Jones

Introduction

In this chapter I discuss the process of undertaking a meta-synthesis to explore factors that act as barriers and facilitators to effective practice in clinical nurse specialist, nurse practitioner, advanced nurse practitioner and nurse consultant roles in acute hospital settings. The impetus to undertake this meta-synthesis arose from my involvement in the ENRiP (Exploring New Roles in Practice) project commissioned by the United Kingdom Department of Health (Read et al., 2001a). As part of that project, I was involved in case studies of nurses working in roles that were considered locally to be innovative. The case studies identified that a range of factors acted as barriers and facilitators to effective practice in those innovative roles. These factors included characteristics of the organisation, characteristics of the postholder (both personal qualities and previous experience), attitudes of key players, teamworking, inadequate resources and increasing clinical workload (McDonnell et al., 2001).

It is clearly important, in order to optimise the use of limited health service resources and to reduce stress for the individuals, that nurses should be able to work effectively in innovative roles. I was therefore interested to know whether the ENRiP findings were paralleled elsewhere. Because I had experience of systematic reviewing, I chose to pursue this question by undertaking a system-

atic review using meta-study techniques. I subsequently discovered that such a course of action is not unusual: Finfgeld (2003) has noted that most researchers who undertake meta-syntheses have done preliminary qualitative research in the same area of interest, and suggests that they see meta-synthesis as an alternative strategy for moving their work forward.

As the results of my systematic review and meta-synthesis have been published elsewhere (Lloyd Jones, 2005), I will concentrate here on the methodological issues I encountered while carrying out the review, in the hope that my experience may be of interest and assistance to other researchers who intend to undertake meta-syntheses of qualitative research.

Overview of the methods used in the meta-synthesis

Aim

The aim of my meta-synthesis was to address the pragmatic health services research question: What factors do nurses in advanced and specialist roles, or other stakeholders in the roles, identify as facilitating or impeding role development and/or effective practice, both in the UK and elsewhere? I wished to draw on the experiences of a wider range of participants than could be included in any single qualitative study, to identify as many relevant barriers and facilitators as possible and then attempt to generate explanatory hypotheses. I was also interested to see whether differences could be identified between the UK and countries such as the USA, which have different systems of nurse education and healthcare delivery.

In the ENRiP project, innovative roles were defined as those in which the postholder was undertaking direct clinical work with patients which was *either* beyond the generally accepted scope of his or her professional group's work *or* completely new to that professional group in the local context (Read et al., 2001b). Clearly, this definition was too flexible to use as an inclusion criterion in a systematic review of published research. However, a substantial majority of the innovative nursing roles identified using that definition were specialist or advanced roles. I therefore limited the meta-synthesis to qualitative studies of roles identified by the study authors as clinical nurse specialist (CNS), nurse practitioner (NP), advanced nurse practitioner (ANP) or nurse consultant (NC) roles. This had the incidental effect of excluding the ENRiP case studies themselves.

I also limited the meta-synthesis to roles based in acute hospitals because of the possibility that the barriers and facilitators encountered by specialist and advanced nurses based in primary care and community services might differ from those encountered in the acute sector. For reasons of comparability, I also excluded midwifery roles, since standard UK midwifery roles would be regarded as advanced roles in the USA. I also excluded roles in mental health and learning disabilities, even if they were based in acute hospitals, because of the possibility that they might differ significantly from other acute specialties.

Methods

I chose to follow the meta-study methodology of Paterson et al. (2001) because this provided the most rigorous means of reviewing research on the topic of interest. As I wanted to minimise the likelihood of weakening my findings by excluding important information or views (Sherwood, 1999), I undertook an exhaustive literature search in which

I attempted to identify all primary qualitative research studies which provided data relevant to the question: 'What factors facilitate or impede role development and/or effective practice as a clinical nurse specialist, nurse practitioner, advanced nurse practitioner or nurse consultant based in acute hospital settings?' (the full inclusion and exclusion criteria are set out in Table 9.1). Because of time constraints, I restricted the searches to published material. However, I did not use language restrictions.

I searched the most relevant electronic databases, and also searched the internet via Copernic. I hand searched key specialist journals (*Clinical Nurse Specialist* and *Journal of Advanced Nursing*), and pursued all relevant references from the reference lists of those studies that met the review inclusion criteria. I then attempted to triangulate these methods by citation searching, using the Web of Science citation search facility. Fuller details of these searches have been published elsewhere (Lloyd Jones, 2004).

I sought to include relevant studies that used any qualitative methodology, including studies that had both qualitative and quantitative components, provided they presented their qualitative findings separately from their quantitative findings. I had to exclude one mixed qualitative/quantitative study (Irvine et al., 2000) because the findings drawn from the qualitative interview data were integrated with those derived from other components of the study.

As noted in Chapter 6 of this book, some researchers recommend excluding studies which otherwise satisfy the meta-synthesis's inclusion and exclusion criteria if their methodological quality is poor. I did not wish to exclude otherwise relevant studies for reasons of quality, unless these were indeed fundamental. I therefore decided that I would only exclude studies in which either the researchers' 'political' agenda was evident throughout, or the depth and breadth of the data supplied were insufficient to suggest that the findings were trustworthy (Paterson et al., 2001). I also bore in mind Paterson et al's concerns about studies with unusual or skewed samples, especially when those samples are very small (Paterson et al., 2001) (see Chapter 7 for further discussion of this point).

My review was neither framed by a theoretical framework nor intended to test or evaluate a pre-existing theory. However, it was shaped by several

Table 9.1   Inclusion and exclusion criteria (adapted and reproduced by permission from Lloyd Jones, 2005).

	Inclusion criteria	Exclusion criteria
Participants	Clinical nurse specialists Nurse practitioners Advanced nurse practitioners Nurse consultants	Studies that included participants working in midwifery, mental health or learning disabilities Studies that included staff groups other than, or additional to, the populations of interest
Setting	Acute hospitals	Studies that included participants working in primary care or other community locations
Outcome measures	Data relating to factors that facilitate or impede role development and/or effective practice in the listed roles	
Methodology	Primary qualitative research studies (any type)	Studies considered methodologically unsound (i.e. studies in which either the researchers' 'political' agenda was evident throughout or the depth and breadth of the data supplied were insufficient to suggest that the findings were trustworthy)
Findings	Barriers and facilitators affecting role development or effective practice in the relevant nursing roles either stated by the authors or appearing from the published data to be an important element of the study findings	

assumptions or 'claims' (Paterson et al., 2001). The most fundamental of these was the assumption, based on the findings of the ENRiP case studies, that factors do exist which may act as barriers and facilitators to specialist and advanced nursing practice (McDonnell et al., 2001). However, I did not search specifically for, or focus exclusively on, the factors identified in the ENRiP case studies, but made every effort to identify all the relevant factors identified in the included studies. The second assumption that defined the review's limits was the assumption, noted above, that the barriers and facilitators affecting specialist and advanced practice nurses working in mental health and learning disabilities, and in primary and community care, may differ from those encountered in hospital-based acute care. I subsequently found support for this assumption in research on advancing nursing practice, which identified that tensions about work content tended to be solved more quickly and easily in 'small enterprises' than in the larger acute/general healthcare providing organisation, where

self-directed role developments were more strongly resisted (Wilson-Barnett et al., 2000).

Results

I identified 14 relevant studies. The populations of interest were not evenly represented: CNSs were the best represented, by nine studies, while only one study focused on NCs. The studies included participants in new and more established posts (Lloyd Jones, 2005). Surprisingly, despite the longer history and larger numbers of specialist and advanced nursing roles in the USA, most of the studies came from the UK.

The study authors claimed to use a range of methods, including case study methodology, phenomenology, grounded theory and naturalistic inquiry (see Table 9.2). Although, as published, the methodological quality of the included studies seemed variable, none were excluded for reasons of quality. The only apparent 'political' agenda was

Table 9.2 Characteristics of included studies, alphabetically by type of study.

Study	Time period of study	Country of study	Research question	Method used – author's description	Number of postholders	Brief summary of major findings
Glen & Waddington, 1998	Not stated	England	What factors facilitate and impede transition from staff nurse to CNS?	Case study	2	Team and organisational factors affected the amount of discretion the CNSs felt able to exercise
Tye & Ross, 2000	March–June 1998	England	What are the perceived benefits and constraints of providing an ENP service?	Case study	2	Different staff groups had different views of the potential consequences of shifting boundaries between professional groups. Uncertainty had negative effects at an individual and organisational level. Individual ENPs varied in their approach to the role. It was difficult to balance quality and quantity in the ENP role. The organisational context could have an adverse effect on the role
Wong, 1997	Jan 1995– Dec 1995	Hong Kong	What are the main features of the work of CNSs?	Case study	4	The five major areas of CNS work were client care, project work, staff development, research, and management and communication. The balance of these varied from post to post; none of the CNSs interviewed was engaged in all five activities. The three distinctive features of CNS work were: • being outside the normal nursing management hierarchy • managing to claim autonomy and ownership of their expertise despite having their work mainly generated from referrals from other professionals • enjoying more freedom and autonomy than other nurses, with work not subject to routinisation
Woods, 1999	Jan 1996– Jan 1998	England	What issues are faced by staff nurses as they make the transition to ANP?	Case study (longitudinal)	5	Practitioners who move from experienced nurse to ANP apparently have to 'reconstruct' their practice and professional frame of reference. This is a contingent process (i.e. it is shaped by the multiple interpretations of the concept of advanced practice which are socially constructed by dominant stakeholders within an organisation). Consequently, the practice and roles of individual ANPs develop in different ways as they respond to the needs and resources of the institution

Table continues

Table 9.2 continued

Study	Time period of study	Country of study	Research question	Method used – author's description	Number of postholders	Brief summary of major findings
Marsden, 1999	Not stated	England	How do NPs make telephone triage decisions?	Unspecified; data analysis method consistent with case study methodology	7	NPs involved in telephone triage make clinical decisions using an identifiable process of hypothesis testing, taking into account contextual factors as well as clinical information. Questioning skills are critical to this decision-making process. 'Intuition' may be explained by the rapid synthesis of (perhaps unrecognised) expert knowledge
Marsden, 2000	Not stated	England	What problems and anomalies surround telephone triage decision making in ophthalmic A&E? (This question was part of a wider evaluation)	Unspecified; (mixed methods consistent with case study methodology)	7	NPs cannot always obtain from healthcare professionals, especially general practitioners, accurate information on which to base a truly informed decision
Bamford & Gibson, 1998a, b, 1999a–e, 2000; Gibson & Bamford 2001	Aug–Dec 1996	England	What are the role and development needs of CNSs in acute care hospitals?	Exploratory descriptive; consistent with basic qualitative description (Sandelowski, 2000)	25	Identifies a wide range of characteristics, resources and support which CNSs need both for their role and for role development
Ball, 1999	Not stated	Multinational (UK, Australia, New Zealand, USA)	What is advanced about advanced nursing practice?	Grounded theory	30	'Advanced' or 'higher' level practice is characterised and differentiated from 'customary' practice by: • the ability to improve and enhance patient care • the ability, knowledge and experience necessary to engender trust • possession of the personal characteristics needed to promote and survive in the role
McCreaddie, 2001	Not stated	Scotland	What is the current work and role of the CNS?	Grounded theory	20	CNS roles are ill-defined and unsupported. The principal CNS role, and main source of job satisfaction, is the communicator–carer role, but growing workloads impinge on this role

Author, year		Country	Research question	Methodology		Findings
Flanagan, 1998	Not stated	England	What is tissue viability CNSs' experience of, and response to, UK healthcare reforms?	Naturalistic/ descriptive, consistent with basic qualitative description (Sandelowski, 2000)	18	In their struggle to survive the system, tissue viability CNSs are developing a facilitative expert practitioner style associated with the development of coping strategies, including forming coalitions with key stakeholders. However, some coping strategies are incongruent with postholders' values, and thus exacerbate role conflict. Lack of organisational support is detrimental both to patient care activities and to the research and education components of the role
Waters, 1998	Not stated	USA	What is the role of the NP in the gastroenterology setting?	Naturalistic enquiry/case study	1	The NP needs advanced skills, higher education, a knowledge base relating to the discipline and the setting, and practice experience, to formulate a successful practice partnership in a specialised area such as gastroenterology
Arslanian-Engoren, 1995	Not stated	USA	What is it like for CNSs enacting their roles as clinical experts to experience nurse/ physician collaboration?	Phenomenology	4	CNSs who experience nurse/physician collaboration: ● experience mutual respect and trust ● define the practice role as a complex process ● establish collegial relationships with the physician ● maintain a nursing perspective ● live a positive experience (i.e. enjoy their role) They regard collaboration as crucial to their clinical role component, but as not always easy to achieve
Bousfield, 1997	Not stated	England	What is the personal meaning of the role of the CNS in the 1990s?	Phenomenology	7	CNSs are experienced practitioners who seek to occupy positions in which they influence patient care and utilise advanced knowledge, expertise and leadership skills. They try to humanise their lived experience by personal enthusiasm for leadership and knowledge, but suffer lack of support, isolation, inter- and intra-role conflict, disempowerment and burn-out
Loftus & McDowell, 2000	Not stated	Scotland	What is important and what is unique in the experience of the oncology CNS?	Phenomenology	8	Relationships and boundaries are important to OCNS, who can find it difficult to manage boundaries and limit their involvement with patients and relatives. It is difficult to capture what is unique in their experience, but prominent elements of expertise in this group include knowing the patient, information giving and reflective practice

CNS, Clinical Nurse Specialist; ENP, Emergency Nurse Practitioner; OCNS, Oncology Clinical Nurse Specialist; NP, Nurse Practitioner; A&E, Accident & Emergency; NP, Clinical Nurse Specialist.

that all the researchers had nursing backgrounds, but this affected all the studies equally. Some studies had apparent shortcomings relating to the depth and breadth of the data, but these might have been due simply to the constraints imposed by journal word limits, and did not seem sufficiently severe to warrant the exclusion of otherwise useful studies. Some studies had small, and possibly unusual, samples, but these did not seem sufficiently perverse to justify exclusion: it seemed more appropriate to bear their nature in mind when analysing and synthesising the study findings.

Barriers and/or facilitators to role development and/or effective practice formed a major theme in 12 studies (Arslanian-Engoren, 1995; Bousfield, 1997; Flanagan, 1998; Glen & Waddington, 1998; Waters, 1998; Ball, 1999; Marsden, 1999; Woods, 1999; Bamford & Gibson, 2000; Loftus & McDowell, 2000; Tye & Ross, 2000; McCreaddie, 2001), although only one (Glen & Waddington, 1998) took such barriers and facilitators, in this case to the transition from staff nurse to CNS, as its only research question. In the remaining two studies, barriers and facilitators formed either a relatively minor theme (Wong, 1997) or a prominent theme in relation only to a very specific element of the specialist role (Marsden, 2000).

Ideally, I would have liked to explore barriers and facilitators to specialist and advanced nursing practice from the viewpoint not only of the postholders themselves but also of other relevant stakeholders, such as doctors, nursing staff and managers. However, only three reports included the views of other relevant staff groups in addition to the postholders (Waters, 1998; Woods, 1999; Tye & Ross, 2000). In most of the remaining studies, it would not have been relevant to the main study question to interview other healthcare professionals. I found no relevant studies that focused solely on the views of other staff groups: studies of physicians' attitudes towards emergency nurse practitioners (ENPs) (Cairo, 1996) and nurses' perceptions of CNSs (Dowling, 2000) did not specify that these attitudes and perceptions formed barriers or facilitators affecting practice.

Findings

Because the findings of this meta-synthesis have already been published (Lloyd Jones, 2005), it is inappropriate to do more than summarise them very briefly here. Essentially, the meta-synthesis identified a range of factors that could hinder or facilitate the implementation and development of specialist and advanced nursing roles. The most important of these related to relationships with others, and to role ambiguity.

Issues that arose while carrying out the meta-synthesis

Identifying potentially relevant studies

The decision to undertake an exhaustive literature search was appropriate to the study question, but was also resource-intensive. Exhaustive searching of electronic databases is a complex and time-consuming iterative process: scoping searches are carried out and relevant studies identified, keywords from those studies are then used to refine the search strategy (Sindhu & Dickson, 1997), and the searches are repeated. It may be necessary to repeat this process more than once to develop a satisfactory search strategy. Searching for qualitative studies is particularly complex both because it can be difficult to identify appropriate keywords (Evans, 2002; Lloyd Jones, 2004), and because the search must permit the identification of negative or disconfirming cases. In this review, I found by trial and error that, to avoid excluding potentially relevant studies, the final search strategy had to incorporate a very broad approach (Lloyd Jones, 2004).

Retrieving relevant studies

The final electronic literature searches identified 3162 potentially relevant unique references. To identify the studies that satisfied my inclusion and exclusion criteria, I sifted this list using Meade & Richardson's three-stage approach: in other words, I reviewed first the titles, then the abstracts, and finally the full articles, excluding at each step those that did not meet one or more of the selection criteria (Meade & Richardson, 1997). This sifting process is more time-consuming and less efficient at identifying qualitative studies on a particular topic than when its objective is to identify clinical trials of a specific intervention. As it is often impossible to determine from its title whether an article reports a qualitative research study (Lloyd Jones, 2004), it may not be possible to exclude many articles at the title stage. Moreover, many articles have no abstracts, or abstracts that are poor or misleading (Hawker et al., 2002); some abstracts fail to indicate the specific qualitative methods, or even the research paradigm, used (Lloyd Jones, 2004). Consequently, I had to retrieve 132 papers for a full reading, of which only 20 then appeared potentially relevant. In several cases, I then had to seek clarification from the authors because it was not clear from the full text whether the study included participants working in midwifery, mental health or learning disabilities, or based in community services or primary care. I subsequently excluded three studies which had been provisionally included: in two of these, the authors clarified that they included participants working in either midwifery (Cox & Ahluwalia, 2000) or primary care (Torn & McNichol, 1998), while in the third (Walters, 1996), in which the participants were said to have worked in a range of services, clarification was impossible because the author had died. Thus, an initial list of over 3000 papers yielded 17 relevant papers relating to 14 studies (see Figure 9.1).

Despite my best efforts, the electronic searches may have missed some studies as they only identified 4 of the 9 articles in which one of the included studies was published (Bamford & Gibson, 1998a, 1999a, 2000; Gibson & Bamford, 2001). I identified the remainder (Bamford & Gibson, 1998b, 1999b, c, d, e) using an author search in the Cumulative Index of Nursing and Allied Health Literature (CINAHL). Hand searching and searching the internet did not identify any relevant studies not already identified by the electronic searches. Although citations indicated five potentially relevant studies that I had not identified by other means (Bradford, 1989; Johnson, 1992; Bass et al., 1993; Bajnok et al., 1994; Giacalone et al., 1995), two of these were actually not research studies (Johnson, 1992; Bass et al., 1993); a third (Bajnok et al., 1994) sought the views of a range of hospital staff prior to the possible introduction of NP posts. I could not retrieve the remaining two citations (Bradford, 1989; Giacalone et al., 1995) in time for possible inclusion in the review.

Ideally, following Finfgeld (1999), I would only have included studies in which the expressed a priori purpose was to study barriers and facilitators to specialist and advanced nursing practice, and in which such data were not collected incidentally. This would have ensured that those barriers and facilitators were deliberately described and labelled by the participants rather than arbitrarily labelled by the researchers. However, I only found three studies in which the questions specifically included the identification of such barriers and/or facilitators (Glen & Waddington, 1998; Woods, 1999; Bamford & Gibson, 2000). The remainder identified such factors while pursuing other remits. I therefore included all studies in which barriers and facilitators were clearly identified as such, and were prominent in the study findings, even if they were not necessarily a primary focus of the research.

Overall, therefore, the sifting of retrieved studies was more time-consuming than in a systematic review of quantitative studies. This was largely because it was often difficult to determine a study's relevance from its title or abstract (Lloyd Jones, 2004), but was also partly due to the need to determine not only whether the studies retrieved for a full reading referred to barriers and facilitators but also whether that reference was sufficiently substantial to warrant inclusion.

Because only 14 relevant studies were identified, I could include them all in the meta-synthesis, and did not need to use sampling.

Data extraction and study appraisal

I subjected each study that fulfilled the inclusion criteria to repeated readings during which I summarised and appraised its findings using a customised appraisal and data extraction form which I developed from the primary research appraisal tool proposed by Paterson et al. (2001) and from Sandelowski & Barroso's guide for reading qualitative studies (2002). My primary aim in appraising the studies was to achieve an understanding of each study on its own terms (Sandelowski et al., 1997) and to consider how the methodologies used shaped understandings about barriers and facilitators to specialist and advanced nursing practice (Paterson et al., 2001).

For some research questions, it may not be appropriate to combine data from studies with different underlying philosophies. However, given

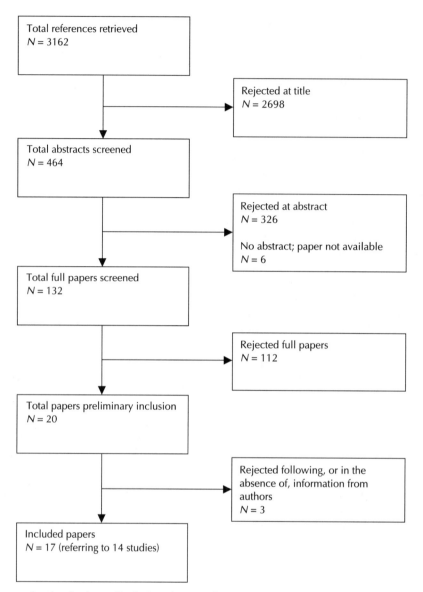

Figure 9.1   Summary of study selection and inclusion: electronic literature searches.

the pragmatic nature of my specific research question, it seemed appropriate to include qualitative studies of any type if they met my inclusion criteria. Unsurprisingly, the phenomenological studies had a narrower focus than those using other methodologies: no phenomenological study identified barriers or facilitators relating to material resources, organisational culture, or the participants' previous experiences. It was thus particularly important to my research question to include studies that pro-

vided political and contextual explanations, as well as those concentrating on specialist and advanced nurses' personal experiences (Porter & Ryan, 1996).

Meta-data-analysis and meta-synthesis

It has been variously claimed that the ideas and themes included in a meta-synthesis should be only the findings presented by the primary researchers

(Noblit & Hare, 1988; Estabrooks et al., 1994) or the themes *and textual quotations* from the included studies (Sherwood, 1999). In this meta-synthesis, I only analysed those ideas and themes presented as findings by the primary researchers. I adopted this approach because it was impossible to determine whether concepts that appeared to be encompassed in the supporting quotations, but that the primary researchers did not identify as findings, would actually have been borne out given full knowledge of the relevant data (e.g. access to the full transcript of the relevant interview). Thus, although illustrative material such as quotations from study participants had an important function in demonstrating that the authors' interpretations and explanations were grounded in the raw data, it seemed risky to use such material as a source of themes and concepts not otherwise identified or substantiated by the authors' interpretations. However, it seemed legitimate to view the quotations as findings when the primary researchers referred specifically to them as providing details of the broader points they wished to make.

As noted in Chapter 6, in the meta-study approach of Paterson et al. (2001), data analysis and synthesis can be undertaken using any systematic interpretive approach used in primary qualitative research. Because of the pragmatic nature of my research question, I used Ritchie & Spencer's 'Framework' approach. This systematic approach to the analysis of qualitative data was developed specifically for applied qualitative research (Ritchie & Spencer, 1994), but is also well suited to the meta-synthesis of qualitative studies which address a pragmatic question.

'Framework' involves five stages (Ritchie & Spencer, 1994):

- Familiarisation with the range and diversity of the material (in meta-synthesis, this overlaps with the process of data extraction and quality appraisal)
- Identification of a thematic framework
- Indexing – the systematic application of that thematic framework to all the data
- Charting, in which the data are lifted from their original context and rearranged according to the appropriate thematic reference
- Mapping and interpretation, in which a structure is identified which illuminates the dynamics of the phenomena under investigation.

When 'Framework' is used in primary research, the preliminary thematic framework is likely to be based largely on a priori issues derived from the original research aims; emergent issues raised by the research participants and analytical themes arising from the recurrence or patterning of particular views or experiences will become more prominent in later versions (Ritchie & Spencer, 1994). However, the preliminary framework does not have to be based on a priori issues. As my meta-synthesis was not designed to test or evaluate a pre-existing theory, I derived my preliminary thematic framework, Framework 1 (see Box 9.1), from the themes and subthemes I identified during familiarisation with selected studies. I then modified this framework following familiarisation with the remaining studies. To consider different possible ways of grouping and categorising themes and subthemes, I then undertook a literature review of studies that identified barriers and facilitators affecting specialist and advanced nursing practice in the acute sector but that did not meet my inclusion criteria; this included surveys (Hupcey, 1993; McFadden & Miller, 1994; Boyle, 1997; van Soeren & Micevski, 2001) and qualitative or mixed-method studies (Walters, 1996; Woods, 1998; Cox & Ahluwalia, 2000; Irvine et al., 2000; McDonnell et al., 2001; McMillan, 2001). This review did not result in any changes to the framework.

I then indexed all the included studies by recording indexing references in their margins using the numerical system used in the thematic framework. During this process, I also undertook the activity described by Noblit & Hare (1988) as translation, standardising and comparing each study's findings using common codes (Sherwood, 1999). I also further modified the framework at this stage.

Once I had indexed all the studies using the modified thematic framework, I developed charts using headings and subheadings drawn from the thematic framework. For this purpose, I collapsed some of the subthemes and sub-subthemes which had emerged during the process of familiarisation and indexing, although I retained them within the thematic framework. I abstracted data from their original contexts, entering each item in the relevant chart with a reference to the original text so that its source could be traced and the process of abstraction examined (for a sample chart, see Table 9.3). Although Ritchie & Spencer (1994) recommend

Box 9.1   Framework 1.

1   Factors that facilitate effectiveness

    1.1   Characteristics of postholder
        1.1.1   assertiveness
        1.1.2   confidence
        1.1.3   enthusiastic leader
        1.1.4   able to deal with conflict and resistance
        1.1.5   politically astute
        1.1.6   flexible
        1.1.7   clear vision
        1.1.8   negotiation skills
        1.1.9   change management skills
        1.1.10   consistency (especially in values and behaviour)
        1.1.11   good communicator (especially in terms of keeping doctors informed)
        1.1.12   good at selling the role
        1.1.13   good interpersonal skills, especially with doctors
        1.1.14   time management/prioritising skills

    1.2   Previous experience
        1.2.1   substantial experience in the specialty
        1.2.2   induction into role

    1.3   Educational/professional issues
        1.3.1   educational preparation for role
        1.3.2   maintaining clinical competence
        1.3.3   use of a log/journal
        1.3.4   constructive criticism from other professionals
        1.3.5   continuous self-evaluation
        1.3.6   appraisal and supervision
        1.3.7   clearly articulated career pathways and professional development

    1.4   Managerial/organisational issues
        1.4.1   clear role boundaries
        1.4.2   professional autonomy (including the freedom to choose colleagues to work with to get the job done)

    1.5   Support:
        1.5.1   from other CNSs
        1.5.2   from 'colleagues'
        1.5.3   unspecified support

2   Factors that act as barriers to effectiveness

    2.1   Characteristics of postholder
        2.1.1   poor time management
        2.1.2   failure to share information
        2.1.3   lack of confidence

    2.2   Lack of previous experience
        2.2.1   lack of experience in the specialty
        2.2.2   lack of clinical expertise
        2.2.3   lack of induction into role
        2.2.4   lack of understanding of organisation culture
        2.2.5   lack of networks within the organisation

2.3   Educational/professional issues
    2.3.1   lack of training in the specialty
    2.3.2   lack of knowledge and skills
    2.3.3   lack of preparation for role
    2.3.4   lack of appraisal and supervision
    2.3.5   lack of clearly articulated career pathway and professional development
    2.3.6   perceived ambivalence of professional regulatory bodies
    2.3.7   absence of educational standardisation
    2.3.8   fear of litigation
    2.3.9   lack of clarity around/limitations of nurse prescribing under local protocol

2.4   Managerial/organisational issues
    2.4.1   organisational culture
        2.4.1.1   differing cultures within the organisation
        2.4.1.2   organisational politics
        2.4.1.3   lack of true teamworking
    2.4.2   lack of role clarity
        2.4.2.1   varying role expectations (of organisation, medical staff, selves)
        2.4.2.2   conflict between PH's goals, targets and priorities and those of the MDT
        2.4.2.3   inter/intra-role conflict (? = lack of clear role definition)
        2.4.2.4   lack of clarity in terms of managerial structures
        2.2.2.5   lack of clarity re. why have employed the PH
    2.4.3   lack of authority
        2.4.3.1   not always able to exercise autonomy

2.5   Lack of support
    2.5.1   lack of support from managers
    2.5.2   lack of support from medical staff
    2.5.3   lack of peer support
    2.5.4   isolation

2.6   Opposition from key players
    2.6.1   hospital staff
        2.6.1.1   doctors
            2.6.1.1.1   fear of deskilling junior doctors
        2.6.1.2   nursing staff
            2.6.1.2.1   resistance to link nurse scheme

2.7   Reluctance to relinquish non-specialist aspects of role
    2.7.1   postholder's fear of losing generalist skills

2.8   Inadequate resources
    2.8.1   accommodation
    2.8.2   nursing staff

2.9   Volume of work

2.10   Burn out

2.11   Conflict between personal and professional needs and expectations and the demands of the job and organisational culture

2.12   Lack of role model

Table 9.3　Sample chart.

Study	Framework Code: Facilitators: managerial/organisational issues				
	1.4.1 clear role definitions/boundaries	1.4.2 autonomy	1.4.3 only CNS in specialty	1.4.4 institution values clinical expertise	1.4.5 able to focus on current role components
Glen & Waddington, 1998	'clear role definitions and boundaries' cited as factors facilitating transition (p. 12)	'the CNSs felt that the ability to practise autonomously was an important aspect of their role' (p. 5) 'the opportunity and ability to choose colleagues with whom to carry out the job is an aspect of autonomous practice . . . can be a factor in establishing and maintaining supportive interpersonal relationships' (p. 6)			
Tye & Ross, 2000					
Wong, 1997					
Woods, 1999					
Ball, 1999		Seen as a most important characteristic of advanced nursing roles, and fundamental to enhancing patient stay (p. 69)		'it also appears to be important that clinical expertise is valued by the employing institution, for without this advanced nursing practice is unlikely to flourish' (p. 72). This may be demonstrated 'through a demonstrable willingness to allow advanced practice nurses to practise, and to update knowledge and skills' (p. 72)	

McCreaddie, 2001

Bamford & Gibson, 2000

'being an independent practitioner facilitated role development, in that the CNS had an ability to be creative and to take responsibility for the progression of the post' (Bamford & Gibson, 2000:8) 'independence and responsibility for the development of their role were also highlighted as being important' (Gibson & Bamford, 2001:8)

'being the only CNS within a specialty was recognised as both an advantage and a disadvantage, in that the role could be very isolating, whilst also allowing for individual role development' (Bamford & Gibson, 1999d:46)

'having the opportunity to focus on the present components of their role was important to their future development' – in particular, the research component (Bamford & Gibson 2000:11)

Marsden, 2000

Flanagan, 1998

Waters, 1998

Arslanian-Engoren, 1995

Bousfield, 1997

CNSs considered it 'important for the future development of the role that clinical nurse specialists argue for the right to exercise professional autonomy and are able to function as independent practitioners' (p. 249)

Loftus & McDowell, 2000

Sense of the boundaries of one's role (p. 517)

Marsden, 1999

entering summaries of the data within the charts, I retained verbatim quotations when they encapsulated the point being made. During the charting process, I undertook a final check to ensure that all themes entered in the charts were adequately substantiated by the data.

Finally, when I had summarised and charted all the relevant data, I began the process of mapping and interpretation. This involved comparing the different accounts, searching for patterns and connections and for explanations for these patterns that were derived directly from the data (Ritchie & Spencer 1994). During the processes of charting, mapping and interpretation, I further modified the framework until it reached its final form (see Box 9.2). The whole process met Paterson et al's description of meta-synthesis as 'a dynamic and iterative process of thinking, interpreting, creating, theorising and reflecting' (Paterson et al., 2001:112).

I found the 'Framework' approach particularly useful because of its explicit and visible methodology, and because it facilitates the maintenance of records of all coding structures (including initial codes, and decisions to collapse codes and categories) and of the locations of relevant data in the primary research. It thus addresses the major problem identified by Sandelowski et al. (1997), of developing usable and communicable systematic approaches that synthesise composite findings and yet maintain the integrity of individual studies. In addition, it is not dependent on achieving data saturation. This was crucial to me: I could not achieve data saturation because so few studies took barriers and facilitators as their primary focus.

Box 9.2   Final framework.

Factors whose presence or absence affected effective working or role development in specialist and advanced nursing practice

1   Characteristics of postholder
    1.1   self-confident, optimistic
    1.2   able to make decisions and accept responsibility
    1.3   able to deal with conflict and resistance
            1.3.1   able to identify issues of real importance
            1.3.2   flexible
            1.3.3   assertive
            1.3.4   negotiation skills
            1.3.5   change management skills
            1.3.6   stamina
    1.4   flexible, adaptable (as in able to learn from others)
    1.5   politically astute, knowing whom to influence
    1.6   motivated, self-directed
    1.7   creative, forward-looking
    1.8   consistent (especially in values and behaviour)
    1.9   good interpersonal skills, good communicator, good at selling the role
    1.10   facilitative expert practitioner style
    1.11   emotional over-involvement with patient
    1.12   individual characteristics match job

2   Previous experience
    2.1   substantial experience in the specialty
    2.2   clinical expertise
    2.3   worked in the same hospital prior to taking up advanced nursing role
    2.4   familiar with the specific service (enough to identify gaps and what needed to improve the service)

3   Educational/professional issues
   3.1   national professional and educational issues
       3.1.1   perceived ambivalence of professional regulatory bodies towards advanced nursing roles
       3.1.2   absence of educational standardisation for advanced nursing roles
       3.1.3   clearly articulated career pathways and professional development
       3.1.4   adequate pay/grading
       3.1.5   lack of medico-legal clarity/fear of litigation
   3.2   formal higher education
   3.3   knowledge base in the specialty
   3.4   specific preparation for role
       3.4.1   specialty-specific skills
       3.4.2   generic skills (e.g. research skills, questioning skills, time management skills, stress management, etc.)
   3.5   availability of suitable courses
   3.6   flexible educational pathway relating to the specialty or role
   3.7   reading about the role
   3.8   induction into role, tailored to the needs of the post and the individual
   3.9   training post
   3.10 mentor/role model
   3.11 keeping up-to-date and maintaining clinical competence
       3.11.1 specialist knowledge
       3.11.2 professional development
       3.11.3 reluctance to relinquish non-specialist aspects of role for fear of losing generalist skills
   3.12 adequate appraisal and supervision
   3.13 feedback, including constructive criticism, from other professionals
   3.14 reflective practice
   3.15 performance measurement to facilitate personal and professional development

4   Managerial/organisational issues
   4.1   culture of employing institution
       4.1.1   general
       4.1.2   values clinical expertise
       4.1.3   slow to change
       4.1.4   organisational politics
       4.1.5   use of short-term contracts, lack of forward planning
   4.2   role definitions and boundaries
       4.2.1   need for clear role definitions and boundaries
           4.2.1.1   unclear expectations of role
           4.2.1.2   differing expectations of role
           4.2.1.3   unrealistic expectations of role
       4.2.2   role incompatibility
           4.2.2.1   other people's clear expectations of the role conflict with the postholder's expectations
           4.2.2.2   other people's clear expectations of the role conflict with the postholder's values
           4.2.2.3   postholder under pressure to expand role into areas in which he/she is not yet confident
       4.2.3   work overload
           4.2.3.1   clinical component takes priority over other areas
           4.2.3.2   role too diverse
       4.2.4   growth of job – increase in clinical workload
       4.2.5   growth of job – increase in administrative tasks

4.3　　professional autonomy
    4.3.1　　protocols
4.4　　characteristics of the institution
    4.4.1　　being the only CNS in a specialty/being one of a team
    4.4.2　　larger units reduce the PH's ability to establish a sense of closeness with patients

5　Relationships with others
  5.1　　effective interprofessional relationships
  5.2　　collaborative relationships with key stakeholders (generally senior managers and other specialist nurses)
  5.3　　support – general
  5.4　　attitudes of other healthcare professionals
    5.4.1　　support of other advanced practice nurses inside and outside hospital
      5.4.1.1　　team/group
    5.4.2　　doctors
      5.4.2.1　　doctors in own specialty
        5.4.2.1.1　　support
        5.4.2.1.2　　lack of support
        5.4.2.1.3　　resistance to change
          5.4.2.1.3.1　　lack of understanding of specialist/advanced nursing roles
          5.4.2.1.3.2　　concerns re. deskilling junior doctors
          5.4.2.1.3.3　　fear of encroachment into medical territory
      5.4.2.2　　doctors in other specialties
      5.4.2.3　　GPs
        5.4.2.3.1　　opposition
    5.4.3　　nursing staff
      5.4.3.1　　support
      5.4.3.2　　resistance to change
      5.4.3.3　　opposition
    5.4.4　　managers
      5.4.4.1　　general
        5.4.4.1.1　　support
        5.4.4.1.2　　unsupportive
        5.4.4.1.3　　opposition
      5.4.4.2　　nurse managers
    5.4.5　　formal counsellor
    5.4.6　　other
      5.4.6.1　　workplace (e.g. lab staff, finance staff)
      5.4.6.2　　professional organisations
      5.4.6.3　　family members and church
      5.4.6.4　　unspecified
  5.5　　isolation

6　Inadequate resources
  6.1　　general
    6.1.1　　inadequate preparation to balance high-quality care against dwindling resources
  6.2　　accommodation
  6.3　　nursing staff
  6.4　　administrative support (secretarial support, computers, etc.)
  6.5　　insufficient funding/staffing to work full-time in role/provide role on all relevant shifts
  6.6　　for research (including academic preparation, time, computers, statistical support and library services)
  6.7　　to access educational opportunities (financial support and time)

Paterson et al. (2001) identified four factors that determine the rigour of a meta-synthesis:

- Truth (the extent to which the data presented are contained in the primary research reports rather than in the researcher's prior conceptions)
- Consistency (the extent to which the conclusions follow logically from the research processes and analytic steps – typically determined by the auditability of a study)
- Neutrality (freedom from bias in the process and outcome of the meta-synthesis), and
- Applicability (consistency between the conclusions of the meta-synthesis and the domains within which the interpretations may have impact)

Because it is explicit and auditable, the 'Framework' approach facilitates the achievement of the first three of these factors. It ensures that the data presented are grounded in the primary research reports; it demonstrates the extent of support in the data for the codes and categories which have been developed, thus helping to determine the adequacy of those codes and categories, and whether the emphasis placed upon them is consistent with their representation in the primary data; and it facilitates the clear documentation of all procedures used and decisions made throughout the review, thus helping to ensure auditability. As Paterson et al. (2001) note, the remaining factor, applicability, can best be judged by those working in the relevant field.

Interpretation of results

The meta-synthesis identified a range of barriers and facilitators which affect role development and/or effective practice in specialist and advanced nursing (Lloyd Jones, 2005). Although some of these factors were not mentioned in those studies in which barriers and facilitators were not the primary focus of the research, this cannot be taken as evidence that they were not relevant to the participants in those studies, but only that they were not seen by the researchers as relevant to their study questions.

Research indicates that specialist and advanced practice nurses' activities are influenced by their length of experience in the role (Burge et al., 1989; Bass et al., 1993). It is thus plausible that they may experience different barriers and facilitators,

depending upon their length of time in the role. Unfortunately, there were relatively few studies in which all participants had clearly been in post for either more (Arslanian-Engoren, 1995; Ball, 1999) or less (Glen & Waddington, 1998; Waters, 1998; Woods, 1999; Tye & Ross, 2000) than 3 years. It was therefore impossible to claim with confidence that factors cited only in studies whose participants were relatively new to the role were irrelevant to established practitioners, or vice versa. However, some factors were mentioned by both groups and therefore cannot be dismissed as inevitable stages of role transition.

Sandelowski (2004) has noted that a meta-synthesis should be more than the sum of its parts, and should offer a novel interpretation which is not contained in any one of the constituent studies but which is derived from all of those studies together. In this meta-synthesis I not only identified a range of barriers and facilitators affecting specialist and advanced nursing practice, but also established that the factors most widely identified as important related to relationships with other key personnel, and to role definitions and expectations. Moreover, these key factors appeared to apply both to relatively new and to well-established roles, and to CNS and NP roles, and appeared to be interlinked. Consequently, it was possible to suggest that the likelihood of negative responses to specialist and advanced nursing roles may be reduced if role ambiguity is reduced by developing clear role definitions and objectives, and communicating them to relevant groups (Lloyd Jones, 2005). Thus, through the meta-synthesis I achieved insights that were not to be found in any one of its constituent studies, and fulfilled Sandelowski's criterion that a meta-synthesis should have immediate utility for clinical practice (Sandelowski, 2004).

Limitations

Some of the limitations of the study derive from its origins as an unfunded MSc dissertation. Ideally, meta-synthesis should be a team effort, because of the different areas of expertise required, and because of the desirability of providing multiple perspectives and countering bias (Paterson et al., 2001) (see also Chapter 7). The independent appraisal of each study by two or more reviewers, and the application of multiple perspectives to the processes of coding, charting, mapping and interpretation, may result in additional insights, more refined interpretations and explanations, and a more comprehensive and conceptually productive review (Cutcliffe & McKenna, 1999; Barbour & Barbour, 2003). However, I was working alone. I would have particularly valued the contribution of an expert in qualitative research in appraising the impact of the various qualitative methodologies on the findings of the primary studies.

I was also working to a strict timetable. Because of the time constraints, I had to limit the literature searches to published material, and rely on published versions of the included studies rather than more detailed project reports which presumably underlay most, if not all, of the published papers. I did not think that I had time to seek additional information from the primary researchers other than that needed to clarify whether a study met my inclusion criteria. However, further contact with the primary researchers might have been useful. Although it does not seem appropriate to request missing data, since the 'data' synthesised in meta-studies are the findings (themes, interpretations and explanations) of the primary studies rather than the raw data collected by the primary researchers (Noblit & Hare, 1988), it does not seem theoretically inappropriate to seek clarification of aspects of study findings (Lloyd Jones, 2004). Thus, some reports mentioned issues that had been identified elsewhere as barriers or facilitators, but did not specify that they were regarded as such by the study participants. Because I could not seek clarification within the limits of this review, I did not include those issues in the meta-synthesis.

In principle, both of the above limitations may be overcome if funding is available to support enough researchers for an adequate period of time. In practice, however, primary researchers cannot always be contacted to obtain additional information. For example, in this meta-synthesis, the single author of one potentially relevant study (Walters, 1996) had died. Wider experience of systematic reviewing indicates that requests for additional data do not meet with universal success.

The third limitation, failure to achieve data saturation, is outside the researcher's control as it depends on the volume of research already undertaken in the area of interest. As in primary qualitative research, failure to achieve data saturation may result in a limited emerging theory (Paterson et al., 2001). None the less, a meta-synthesis that does not achieve data saturation is still valuable as an intellectually rigorous means of identifying and combining existing research on a topic, and as a pointer to areas to be explored in future research.

Conclusion

The most important implication of this meta-synthesis for nursing practice is that it suggests that the likelihood of negative responses to specialist and advanced nursing roles may be reduced by developing clear role definitions and objectives and communicating these to relevant groups.

The meta-synthesis identified factors relating to relationships with others and to role ambiguity as the most important barriers affecting specialist and advanced practice. Because these barriers were reported in studies in which the postholders were established in their roles, they cannot be attributed entirely to unfamiliarity with the roles. However, since few studies included only relatively new *or* more established postholders, it would be interesting to carry out a relatively large qualitative study comparing the barriers and facilitators associated with a specific specialist or advanced nursing role in a number of settings, in some of which the role is new and in others well established.

The meta-synthesis was limited to specialist and advanced practice nursing roles based in acute settings. A similar meta-synthesis of research relating to the barriers and facilitators affecting specialist and advanced practice nurses based in community services or primary care would allow interesting comparisons to be made.

As the discussion of limitations indicates, the process of undertaking the meta-synthesis suggested several major lessons for future similar reviews. These are simple in principle, although they may be more difficult to achieve in practice. Ideally, researchers wishing to undertake a meta-synthesis should work in a team, allow plenty of time for the process, and use full reports, if these are available, rather than published papers.

Acknowledgements

This chapter is based on work undertaken as part of the requirements for the MSc in Health Services Research and Technology Appraisal in the University of Sheffield School of Health and Related Research (ScHARR). I am grateful to ScHARR for funding my participation on that course, and to my supervisor for the dissertation, Mr Andrew Booth, Director of Information Resources and Senior Lecturer – Evidence Based Healthcare Information. Any shortcomings remain my own.

References

Arslanian-Engoren, C.M. (1995) Lived experiences of CNSs who collaborate with physicians: a phenomenological study. *Clinical Nurse Specialist*, 9 (2), 68–74.

Bajnok, I., Grinspun, D., Hubley, P. & Shamian, J. (1994) *Articulating the Nurse-practitioner Role of the 1990s in the Hospital Setting.* Mount Sinai Hospital Department of Nursing, Toronto.

Ball, C. (1999) Revealing higher levels of nursing practice. *Intensive and Critical Care Nursing*, 15 (2), 65–76.

Bamford, O. & Gibson, F. (1998a) The clinical nurse specialist role: key role components identified. *Managing Clinical Nursing*, 2 (4), 105–9.

Bamford, O. & Gibson, F. (1998b) The clinical nurse specialist: staking their claim on a place within the advancing clinical practice arena. *Managing Clinical Nursing*, 2, 99.

Bamford, O. & Gibson, F. (1999a) The clinical nurse specialist role: development strategies that facilitate role evolution. *Advancing Clinical Nursing*, 3 (4), 143–51.

Bamford, O. & Gibson, F. (1999b) The clinical nurse specialist role: criteria for the post, valuing clinical experience and educational preparation. *Advancing Clinical Nursing*, 3, 21–6.

Bamford, O. & Gibson, F. (1999c) The clinical nurse specialist role: personal qualities identified. *Advancing Clinical Nursing*, 3, 109–11.

Bamford, O. & Gibson, F. (1999d) The clinical nurse specialist role: supportive strategies that facilitate role development. *Advancing Clinical Nursing*, 3, 45–8.

Bamford, O. & Gibson, F. (1999e) The clinical nurse specialist: future role development. *Advancing Clinical Nursing*, 3, 152–5.

Bamford, O. & Gibson, F. (2000) The clinical nurse specialist: perceptions of practising CNSs of their role and development needs. *Journal of Clinical Nursing*, 9 (2), 282–92.

Barbour, R.S. & Barbour, M. (2003) Evaluating and synthesizing qualitative research: the need to develop a distinctive approach. *Journal of Evaluation in Clinical Practice*, 9 (2), 179–86.

Bass, M., Rabbett, P.M. & Siskind, M.M. (1993) Novice CNS and role acquisition. *Clinical Nurse Specialist*, 7 (3), 148–52.

Bousfield, C. (1997) A phenomenological investigation into the role of the clinical nurse specialist. *Journal of Advanced Nursing*, 25 (2), 245–56.

Boyle, D.M. (1997) Lessons learned from clinical nurse specialist longevity. *Journal of Advanced Nursing*, 26 (6), 1168–74.

Bradford, R. (1989) Obstacles to collaborative practice. *Nursing Management*, 20 (4), 72I–72P.

Burge, S., Crigler, L., Hurt, L., Kelly, G. & Sanborn, C. (1989) Clinical nurse specialist role development: quantifying actual practice over three years. *Clinical Nurse Specialist*, 3 (1), 33–6.

Cairo, M.J. (1996) Emergency physicians' attitudes toward the emergency nurse practitioner role: validation versus rejection. *Journal of the American Academy of Nurse Practitioners*, 8 (9), 411–17.

Cox, C.L. & Ahluwalia, S. (2000) Specialist nursing. Enhancing clinical effectiveness among clinical nurse specialists. *British Journal of Nursing*, 9 (16), 1064–73.

Cutcliffe, J. & McKenna, H. (1999) Establishing the credibility of qualitative research findings: the plot thickens. *Journal of Advanced Nursing*, 30 (2), 374–80.

Dowling, M. (2000) Nurses' perceptions of the clinical nurse specialist (CNS) role. *Nursing Review (Ireland)*, 17 (4), 96–9.

Estabrooks, C.A., Field, P.A. & Morse, J.M. (1994) Aggregating qualitative findings: an approach to theory development. *Qualitative Health Research*, 4 (4), 503–11.

Evans, D. (2002) Database searches for qualitative research. *Journal of the Medical Library Association*, 90 (3), 290–3.

Finfgeld, D.L. (1999) Courage as a process of pushing beyond the struggle. *Qualitative Health Research*, 9 (6), 803–14.

Finfgeld, D.L. (2003) Metasynthesis: the state of the art – so far. *Qualitative Health Research*, 13 (7), 893–904.

Flanagan, M. (1998) Factors influencing tissue viability nurse specialists in the UK: 2. *British Journal of Nursing*, 7 (12), 690–2.

Giacalone, M.B., Mullaney, D., DeJoseph, D.A. & Cosma, M. (1995) Practice model: development of a nurse-managed unit and the advanced practitioner role. *Critical Care Nursing Clinics of North America*, 7 (1), 35–42.

Gibson, F. & Bamford, O. (2001) Focus group interviews to examine the role and development of the clinical nurse specialist. *Journal of Nursing Management*, 9 (6), 331–42.

Glen, S. & Waddington, K. (1998) Role transition from staff nurse to clinical nurse specialist: a case study. *Journal of Clinical Nursing*, 7 (3), 283–90.

Hawker, S., Payne, S., Kerr, C., Hardey, M. & Powell, J. (2002) Appraising the evidence: reviewing disparate data systematically. *Qualitative Health Research*, 12 (9), 1284–99.

Hupcey, J.E. (1993) Factors and work settings that may influence nurse practitioner practice. *Nursing Outlook*, 41 (4), 181–5.

Irvine, D., Sidani, S., Porter, H. et al. (2000) Organizational factors influencing nurse practitioners' role implementation in acute care settings. *Canadian Journal of Nursing Leadership*, 13 (3), 28–35.

Johnson, N.D. (1992) Collaboration – an environment for optimal outcome. *Critical Care Nursing Quarterly*, 15 (3), 37–43.

Lloyd Jones, M. (2004) Application of systematic review methods to qualitative research: practical issues. *Journal of Advanced Nursing*, 48 (3), 271–8.

Lloyd Jones, M. (2005) Role development and effective practice in specialist and advanced practice roles in acute hospital settings: systematic review and meta-synthesis. *Journal of Advanced Nursing*, 49 (2), 191–209.

Loftus, L.A. & McDowell, J. (2000) The lived experience of the oncology clinical nurse specialist. *International Journal of Nursing Studies*, 37 (6), 513–21.

Marsden, J. (1999) Expert nurse decision-making: telephone triage in an ophthalmic accident and emergency department. *NT Research*, 4 (1), 44–54.

Marsden, J. (2000) An evaluation of the safety and effectiveness of telephone triage as a method of patient prioritization in an ophthalmic accident and emergency service. *Journal of Advanced Nursing*, 31 (2), 401–9.

McCreaddie, M. (2001) The role of the clinical nurse specialist. *Nursing Standard*, 16 (10), 33–8.

McDonnell, A., Lloyd Jones, M. & Read, S. (2001) Innovative nursing roles: effectiveness, economic issues and educational implications – the Sheffield team's case studies. In: *Exploring New Roles in Practice (ENRiP). Final Report* (Read S. et al., eds), pp. 120–60. University of Sheffield School of Nursing and Midwifery, Sheffield. Available at website www.snm.shef.ac.uk/research/enrip/enrip.pdf

McFadden, E.A. & Miller, M.A. (1994) Clinical nurse specialist practice: facilitators and barriers. *Clinical Nurse Specialist*, 8 (1), 27–33.

McMillan, I. (2001) Consultant nurses lack support and resources. *Nursing Standard*, 16 (8), 4.

Meade, M.O. & Richardson, W.S. (1997) Selecting and appraising studies for a systematic review. *Annals of Internal Medicine*, 127 (7), 531–7.

Noblit, G.W. & Hare, R.D. (1988) *Meta-ethnography: Synthesizing Qualitative Studies*. Sage, Newbury Park.

Paterson, B.L., Thorne, S.E., Canam, C. & Jillings, C. (2001) *Meta-study of Qualitative Health Research*, 1st edn. Sage Publications, Thousand Oaks.

Porter, S. & Ryan, S. (1996) Breaking the boundaries between nursing and sociology: a critical realist ethnography of the theory-practice gap. *Journal of Advanced Nursing*, 24 (2), 413–20.

Read, S., Lloyd Jones, M., Collins, K. et al. (2001a) *Exploring New Roles in Practice (ENRiP). Final Report*. University of Sheffield School of Nursing and Midwifery, Sheffield. Available at website www.snm. shef.ac.uk/research/enrip/enrip.pdf

Read, S., Lloyd Jones, M., Collins, K. et al. (2001b) The methodology for stage one of ENRiP. In: *Exploring New Roles in Practice (ENRiP). Final report* (Read S. et al., eds), pp. 22–35. University of Sheffield School of Nursing and Midwifery, Sheffield. Available at website www.snm.shef.ac.uk/research/enrip/enrip.pdf

Ritchie, J. & Spencer, L. (1994) Qualitative data analysis for applied policy research. In: *Analysing Qualitative Data* (Bryman, A. & Burgess, R.G., eds), pp. 173–94. Routledge, London.

Sandelowski, M. (2000) Whatever happened to qualitative description? *Research in Nursing and Health*, 23 (4), 334–40.

Sandelowski, M. (2004) Metasynthesis, metastudy, and metamadness. *Qualitative Health Research*, 14 (10), 1357–60.

Sandelowski, M. & Barroso, J. (2002) Reading qualitative studies. *International Journal of Qualitative Methods*, 1 (1), article 5.

Sandelowski, M., Docherty, S. & Emden, C. (1997) Qualitative metasynthesis: issues and techniques. *Research in Nursing and Health*, 20 (4), 365–71.

Sherwood, G. (1999) Meta-synthesis: merging qualitative studies to develop nursing knowledge. *International Journal for Human Caring*, 3 (1), 37–42.

Sindhu, F. & Dickson, R. (1997) The complexity of searching the literature. *International Journal of Nursing Practice*, 3 (4), 211–17.

Torn, A. & McNichol, E. (1998) A qualitative study utilizing a focus group to explore the role and concept of the nurse practitioner. *Journal of Advanced Nursing*, 27 (6), 1202–11.

Tye, C.C. & Ross, F.M. (2000) Blurring boundaries: professional perspectives of the emergency nurse Practitioner role in a major accident and emergency department. *Journal of Advanced Nursing*, 31 (5), 1089–96.

van Soeren, M.H. & Micevski, V. (2001) Success indicators and barriers to acute nurse practitioner role implementation in four Ontario hospitals. *AACN Clinical Issues: Advanced Practice in Acute & Critical Care*, 12 (3), 424–37.

Walters, A.J. (1996) Being a clinical nurse consultant: a hermeneutic phenomenological reflection. *International Journal of Nursing Practice*, 2 (1), 2–10.

Waters, T. (1998) The role of the nurse practitioner in the gastroenterology setting. *Gastroenterology Nursing*, 21 (5), 198–206.

Wilson-Barnett, J., Barriball, K.L., Reynolds, H., Jowett, S. & Ryrie, I. (2000) Recognising advancing nursing practice: evidence from two observational studies. *International Journal of Nursing Studies*, 37 (5), 389–400.

Wong, F.K.Y. (1997) Work features of clinical nurse specialists. *Hong Kong Nursing Journal*, 33 (4), 7–16.

Woods, L.P. (1998) Implementing advanced practice: identifying the factors that facilitate and inhibit the process. *Journal of Clinical Nursing*, 7 (3), 265–73.

Woods, L.P. (1999) The contingent nature of advanced nursing practice. *Journal of Advanced Nursing*, 30 (1), 121–8.

Part 3

Integrative Reviews of Quantitative and Qualitative Research

10 Overview of Methods

David Evans

Introduction

There is a growing interest in evidence-based practice, which has resulted in a significant increase in the volume of healthcare literature. As a consequence, it is becoming more difficult to ensure that clinical practice is based on the best available research evidence. Part of this difficulty relates to the volume of research that must be identified, appraised and summarised before the best evidence can be identified and implemented. In addition, there has also been a growing awareness that a large proportion of published research is invalid (Rosenberg & Donald, 1995). Evaluations of the standard of statistical analysis of published research have shown that errors are common (Mills, 1993) and findings are often false (Ioannidis, 2005). This problem has been described as 'drowning in information, thirsting for evidence' (Booth, 1996:25). As a result, literature reviews have emerged as a vital component of evidence-based practice.

Much of the interest in reviews of the research literature has focused on systematic reviews of randomised controlled trials (RCTs) to determine the effectiveness of interventions. More recently, there has been a growing interest in methods to identify, appraise and integrate the findings of a range of different types of research. While these integrative reviews are still at an early stage of development, they provide a framework to generate the evidence

to answer many different types of clinical questions. This chapter introduces integrative reviews and some of the methods that are employed during their conduct.

What is an integrative review?

While the term 'systematic review' is widely used to describe reviews of effectiveness, there is little consistency in the names used to describe other types of literature reviews. Some of the names that are encountered include 'structured reviews', 'qualitative reviews', 'critical reviews' and 'integrative reviews'. In addition to the confusion in terminology, these reviews have employed a range of different methods, and vary in their scope and in the type of questions addressed. The proliferation of these reviews has served to contribute to this inconsistency in terminology and methods (Whittemore, 2005). These issues have also made it difficult to evaluate the quality of reviews. Despite these problems, all these types of review share the common goal of attempting to produce a reliable summary of the research.

Integrative reviews provide a much broader summary of the literature than is produced by systematic reviews, and have been described as the broadest category of research reviews, encompassing both empirical and theoretical literature

(Whittemore, 2005). They commonly incorporate the findings from a range of different research designs. However, because their focus encompasses multiple methodological perspectives, the complexity of the review process is increased. This complexity also relates to the difficulty in determining the optimal review method, and this is evident in the many different approaches that have been used in published reviews.

Despite a growing methodological discussion in the healthcare literature, there is currently no widely accepted standard for conducting an integrative review. This lack of a gold standard makes it difficult to distinguish an integrative review from other types of less rigorous reviews. However, the many developments in systematic review methods are also starting to influence how integrative reviews are conducted and reported.

Integrating qualitative and quantitative research in a review

The rise in prominence of systematic reviews has put the RCT at the forefront of healthcare decisions, at the expense of other types of research designs. Qualitative research has tended to be excluded or marginalised in systematic reviews (Evans & Pearson, 2001a). In recent years, however, qualitative research has established an important foothold in health research exploring topics related to decision-making, experience and practitioner–patient interactions (Eakin & Mykhalovsky, 2003).

Qualitative research offers a number of important benefits when included in a research review. It has been suggested that the traditional role of qualitative research has been as a precursor for quantitative work and this has included:

- Identifying and refining the question
- Identifying relevant interventions and outcomes
- Providing data for non-numerical synthesis
- Explaining the findings of quantitative synthesis
- Assisting in the interpretation of the significance and applicability of the review, and
- Assisting in making recommendations (Dixon-Woods et al., 2001:126)

From this perspective, the inclusion of qualitative evidence with that produced by quantitative research provides a more comprehensive investiga-

tion of the topic of interest. The qualitative data provide an added dimension to the review, increasing understanding of the factors that influence the outcomes and helping to shape recommendations for practice.

However, qualitative research extends beyond the role of a precursor for quantitative work, as it has been used to increase our understanding of a range of different phenomena. It also provides a way to identify the priorities and experiences of consumers of healthcare services. Qualitative research addresses issues that are different from those addressed by quantitative research, offering descriptions of experiences, interactions and relationships. The inclusion of both quantitative and qualitative research in a review leads to a more robust and valid evaluation of healthcare issues. In addition, combining the findings from multiple small qualitative studies may broaden their generalisability and clinical application and yield more powerful results than a single study on the topic (Sherwood, 1999; Whittemore, 2005). With research reviews providing the evidence for an increasing number of health decisions, failure to include qualitative research in these reviews means that it is also excluded from the decision-making process.

How best to incorporate both qualitative and quantitative evidence into reviews has proved challenging, and the optimal methods for achieving this synthesis are still at an early stage of development. In recent times, systematic review methods have had an important influence on integrative reviews, providing a framework for their conduct. As a consequence, there has been an improvement in the quality of published integrative reviews, with better reporting of search strategies and the methods used for data synthesis.

Purpose

The purpose of systematic reviews is most commonly that of determining effectiveness, and therefore involves comparison of two or more interventions. The integrative review provides a broader investigation of a topic, and so its focus, purpose and scope are likely to differ from those of the systematic review. During the early development of review methodologies, Cooper (1984) described three different types of reviews:

(1) Integrative reviews, which summarise past research, draw overall conclusions, highlight unresolved issues and provide direction for future research. This type of review focuses on the results of research to integrate the findings from individual studies. The integration of results from a number of different studies enables overall conclusions to be made, and the findings to be generalised to other populations with greater confidence.

(2) Theoretical reviews, which present theories to explain phenomena, compare them in terms of breadth, internal consistency and the nature of their predictions. This type of review provides an opportunity to explore the 'taken-for-granted' issues, and to compare and contrast these beliefs, concepts and boundaries. Theoretical reviews are important in areas of developing knowledge because they allow accepted beliefs to be scrutinised and challenged.

(3) Methodological reviews, which examine and critique the research methods and operational definitions that have been applied to a problem. While part of the systematic review process is the critical appraisal of research, this is usually limited to decisions about the inclusion or exclusion of studies. Many systematic reviews are completed and published with little information given on the results of the critical appraisal, other than how many were excluded. However, for areas of developing research, methodological quality may at times be poor and the definitions used during the study maybe inappropriate, incomplete or inconsistent. Methodological reviews can therefore provide important information to better inform future research endeavours.

While systematic reviews have methodological and integrative components, integrative reviews may address all three. These three differing components of a review help determine its purpose and assist in refining the focus of the review.

A final purpose of all reviews, and one that is often not acknowledged, is that they generate a record of existing research. In effect, the review process provides a stocktake of past research endeavour. While this stocktake most commonly takes the form of a bibliographic record of all research, it may also include a summary of key study characteristics

such as study populations, settings, methods and definitions. Given the growing volume of healthcare literature, this information helps prevent individual studies being lost from sight by the many new publications.

Protocol

The process for undertaking a rigorous and comprehensive review is not very different from that for undertaking primary research. As with all scientific endeavours, the methods for the review of the literature should be established prior to commencement. Without this predetermined plan there is a risk that the review could be driven by anticipated findings and subjective decisions. The protocol is a plan for conducting the review, defining its focus and boundaries, describing each phase of the review process:

● Problem identification
● Location of studies
● Evaluation of studies
● Collection of data from individual studies
● Data analysis

While there are many articles, text and guides giving information on the structure of the protocol for systematic reviews, there is little information on integrative review protocols. Because of their broader focus, these protocols may differ in some aspects from those used during systematic reviews. However, the principles underpinning protocols are the same for both research and reviews, in that they should provide a detailed description of the proposed activity.

Problem identification

One of the most important components of the review process is the identification of the problem and formulation of the review purpose or question. This is important because it defines the focus of the review. Key concepts and variables, such as population, intervention and health problem, must then be determined (Whittemore & Knafl, 2005). A well-formulated question assists all the subsequent review activities because it helps minimise any ambiguity regarding the purpose and expected outcomes of the review. The question must be broad enough to be of interest but small enough to be manageable (Sherwood, 1999). This question forms the basis for the development of selection criteria that are used to select studies for inclusion in the review. Given the enormous volume of healthcare literature, the clear focus provided by the question also helps minimise the number of irrelevant papers that must be screened.

Review question and purpose

For systematic reviews, the suggested format for the review question involves defining the population, intervention and outcomes of interest (Higgins & Green, 2005). In addition, the types of studies that are able to answer the question are also stated. The key components of the question form the basis of the criteria that are used to select studies and inform the development of the strategy that is used to locate relevant research. The question will also influence the analysis of data, in that a narrowly focused question may permit statistical analysis, while a broad question will require the use of tabular and narrative summaries. These activities, starting with the formulation of the problem, help ensure the findings of the review are both rigorous and valid.

Integrative reviews commonly address broader topics than those of systematic reviews and incorporate a broader range of research designs. The risk of the reviewer being overwhelmed by the volume of literature is therefore greater during the integrative review. This is because a large number of irrelevant studies will have to be screened to identify the few that are relevant to the review. Therefore developing a clear focus for the integrative review is just as critical as with the systematic review. Regardless of whether the focus for the integrative review is in the form of a question or purpose, it must describe all the key variables of interest. These key variables will relate to the population of interest, and to the intervention, issue, problem or phenomenon that is to be the focus of the review. Many topics also have multiple possible outcomes, and therefore key outcome variables must be defined if the review is to achieve a clear focus.

Selection criteria

From the many published studies identified during the search, those relevant to the integrative review must be selected, and this process should be based on clear scientific reasoning (Petitti, 1994). While the process of selection will entail a degree of judgement, it should be guided by clearly stated criteria that delineate the area of interest. While the question and purpose define the focus of the review, it is the selection criteria that define its scope and boundaries. The criteria are derived from the review question and, like the question, should provide a clear description of the key variables. These variables form the sampling frame for the review, in that they describe the characteristics of the sample of studies from which the data for the review will be drawn. For studies to be included in the review, they must meet all the criteria. Key variables that may be addressed include:

- Population
- Intervention, condition or phenomenon
- Outcomes or data that are of interest
- Research designs that will produce relevant data, or type of literature of interest
- Other criteria, such as language, geographical location or time frame

The selection criteria are used when making decisions about the inclusion of publications in the review. The characteristics of identified studies are evaluated against the criteria, ensuring a clear rationale for each study included in the review. The use of selection criteria helps to ensure that the process is rigorous, and also helps avoid the inclusion of irrelevant information. It is common practice in systematic reviews for the selection of studies to be undertaken independently by two reviewers.

Selection criteria for qualitative research will differ from those for quantitative research; however, the same principles guide the development process. Important issues related to the selection of qualitative studies suggested by Estabrooks et al. (1994) include:

- Focus on similar populations or themes
- Have a similar research approach
- Reporting of themes and labels must be clear and must be grounded in the data to be able to demonstrate comparability of themes and labels across studies

Integrative reviews commonly include research using a range of different methods, and so selection criteria must allow for this. Ideally, the selection criteria should accommodate those research designs that are considered to provide data of relevance to the integrative review.

The use of selection criteria during integrative reviews appears to be inconsistent, and they are not described in many published reviews. However, the development and use of selection criteria have a number of benefits during the integrative review process. They give an opportunity for the reviewer to identify and document the key variables of interest to the review. Given the broad nature of integrative reviews, the use of selection criteria provides an effective process for screening the literature to identify papers relevant to the review. Criteria also help main rigour and minimise the risk of bias. Finally, the criteria can be listed in the review report, allowing others to evaluate the process and the decisions made during the review.

Locating studies

A systematic and exhaustive search of the literature is the hallmark of the systematic review. The aim of this search is to uncover all studies on the review topic. However, this task is made difficult because the full complement of studies is not known. To improve the likelihood of identifying all relevant studies there has been considerable development of optimal search strategies by organisations such as the Cochrane Collaboration. Electronic databases offer the easiest and least time-consuming way to identify studies (Higgins & Green, 2005). The systematic review search may also cover bibliographies, conference proceedings, government reports, hand searching key journals and contacting experts on the review topic (Jones & Evans, 2000). However, while these activities appear simple, the apparent ease of the search belies the complexities that take place during the search process (Booth, 1996). The risk is that reviewers will find enough citations to be satisfied but be unaware of the many studies they may have missed. To minimise this risk, a search strategy is developed which outlines the intended approach and documents all sources to be searched.

Much of the development of systematic review searches has focused on identifying experimental research, but how useful these strategies are during an integrative review is not really known. Evaluations have demonstrated that database searches for RCTs may only find 30–80% of published studies (Dickersin et al., 1994). However, there is little information on the effectiveness of searches for identifying other research designs, and current methods used to identify quantitative research do not translate easily to qualitative research (Evans, 2002; Jones, 2004). These difficulties relate to the lack of key search terms in the titles of some qualitative studies, the variable information given in abstracts, and inconsistencies in the indexing of these studies across the different databases (Evans, 2002). This means that it is often necessary to screen large numbers of citations to identify a small number of relevant studies. It is therefore important for the reviewer to recognise that the identification of qualitative research in electronic databases is both complex and difficult, and that the development of a search strategy is just as important for the integrative review as it is for other types of reviews.

Strategies that may improve the search process include careful selection of databases and search terms, searching bibliography lists, hand searching relevant journals and searching conference abstracts. Seeking advice from a librarian during the development of the search strategy is likely to improve the final search strategy. A two-stage search strategy has been recommended (Dickersin et al., 1994; Counsell, 1997). The first stage entails a preliminary limited search of databases to identify optimal search terms, which is then followed by a search incorporating all identified search terms. When selecting optimal search terms, it may be helpful to combine methodological terms, such as ethnography, phenomenology, grounded theory, qualitative, focus groups or thematic analysis, with the subject terms to increase the likelihood of finding the studies using the research design of interest (Evans, 2002). Searching the reference lists of identified studies is also a key component of many literature searches. However, this search is complicated by the number of errors found in reference lists (Taylor, 1998) and the fact that the title of some papers listed in reference lists gives little indication of the nature of the paper. Contacting experts may also be helpful because one survey of nurses who had conducted research found that, while 58% had written up their research, only 10% had actually submitted it for publication (Hicks, 1995). Including conference abstracts in the search strategy may be an important search activity because these studies represent the most current research and many would not have reached publication (Kelly, 1998).

Evaluating studies

It has long been recognised that the quality of some published research is poor (Mills, 1993; Anthony, 1996; Ioannidis, 2005). If poor-quality studies are included in a review, they may distort the synthesis and cause difficulties in interpretation (Dixon-Woods et al., 2004). As a result, it is common practice during systematic reviews to critically appraise all studies before inclusion in the review. The aim of this appraisal is to ensure that only rigorous research is included in the review.

In experimental studies, bias or errors occur most often as a result of the methods used during four critical stages of the study (Higgins & Green, 2005). These four types of bias are:

Selection bias   Problems in the allocation of participants to study groups resulting in differences between the groups. Selection bias is minimised by participants being randomised to study groups.

Performance bias   Differences in care provided to participants in the study groups, other than the intervention being evaluated. Performance bias is minimised by blinding study participants and care providers to the treatment group allocation.

Attrition bias   Differences between groups in the number of participants who do not complete the study. Attrition bias is minimised by ensuring all participants who are entered into the study are accounted for in the results. Additionally 'intention to treat' analysis, whereby participants who are lost to follow-up are included in the analysis, is also used to determine if inclusion of these participants could have changed the findings of the study.

Detection bias   Differences in the assessment of outcomes of participants in the different study groups. Detection bias is minimised by blinding the assessors to study group allocation.

Much methodological development in the critical appraisal of research has focused primarily on the RCT. Critical appraisal of qualitative research, in the context of reviews, has received less attention and remains an area of controversy. One barrier to this process has been that the terms 'interpretive' and 'qualitative' are used to refer to a range of different methods such as phenomenology, grounded theory and ethnography. These differing methods are often not differentiated when issues related to quality in qualitative research are addressed (Evans & Pearson, 2001b). Sandelowski (1993:1) has suggested that 'The problem of rigour in qualitative research continues to arouse, beguile and misdirect'. Schwandt (1996) has suggested that if we are to judge the goodness of the undertaking and product of social inquiry, then an alternative to the traditional criteriology must be sought. Lincoln (1995) referred to this debate as a dialogue about emerging criteria, because the entire field of interpretive inquiry is itself still evolving and being defined.

However, despite this controversy, development of methods by which to appraise the rigour of qualitative research has continued and guidelines, criteria and checklists for qualitative research have been developed (Popay et al., 1998; Malterud, 2001; Rychetnik et al., 2002). However, the difficulty in the use of criteria and checklists is that they attempt to evaluate the quality of a study based on the information included in the published paper. Issues such as journal word limits and style may influence the description that is reported. It has even been suggested that, had such checklists been a feature of qualitative research to date, then many of the most influential research papers might not have been selected for publication on the grounds of failing to fulfil all the stated criteria (Barbour & Barbour, 2003).

Many appraisal criteria have been proposed or used to evaluate qualitative research (Malterud, 2001; Rychetnik et al., 2002; Dixon-Woods et al., 2004) and these criteria include:

- Clarity of objectives and research question
- Explicit researcher position and role
- Qualitative methods were suitable for exploration of research question
- Best method was chosen with respect to research question
- Theoretical framework adequate with respect to aim of study

- Clear rationale for sample rationale
- Strategy for data collection clearly stated
- Principles and procedures for data organisation and analysis fully described
- Audit trail in collection and analysis of data
- Clear basis for findings
- Findings relevant with respect to aims of study
- Quotes used adequately to support and enrich the researcher's synopsis
- Data, interpretations and conclusions clearly integrated
- Transferability of findings
- Relevance, importance and usefulness of findings

In published integrative reviews, as with the other phases of the review process, there has been great variability in the approach to critical appraisal and many reviewers have not undertaken any appraisal of research. This may be due in part to the broader range of research included in integrative reviews. The inclusion of multiple research designs means that criteria are needed for each type of research, which serves to increase the complexity of the appraisal process. The lack of agreement on how best to evaluate qualitative research adds to the difficulty. Alternatively, it may be more feasible to have the appraisal process undertaken by experts in the research methodology, using consensus to identify those studies that should be excluded from the review.

However, study quality may not be a critical issue for some integrative reviews. If the focus of the review is not primarily on the study findings, then the process of appraising research may not be appropriate. For example, critical appraisal would not be necessary if the purpose of the review is to investigate theoretical aspects of the topic, determine the nature and scope of existing research or explore the definitions that have been used in past investigations.

Data collection

The data used during the analysis phase of the integrative review are the results from individual studies. These data must first be collected from the study reports. While there are clear guides for this process during systematic reviews (Khan et al., 2001; Higgins & Green, 2005), data collection for integrative reviews has received little attention. In systematic reviews it is common practice to use a data collection form during this process. This form serves as a direct link to the review question, it serves as a record of this phase of the review and is the data from which the analysis will emerge (Higgins & Green, 2005). The details that should be collected are those relevant to the key components of the review question and will vary depending on the subject and nature of the review.

The aim of this phase is to ensure complete documentation of all relevant data from each included study. To minimise the risk of transcription error, it is common practice to have two reviewers extract the data from studies independently. Whenever possible, the aim is to extract raw data, free from any manipulation or transformation. However, this can be challenging for the integrative reviewer given the broader nature of the review questions. This highlights the importance of careful planning of this phase of the review and the need for consideration of what data will be needed for the analysis.

During reviews of qualitative research the data collection phase is less distinct, and has also been described as part of the data synthesis process (Noblit & Hare, 1988). However, regardless of the approach taken for the data synthesis, some information will be required, such as study details, participant demographics, geographical location, time frame and information on the research design. As the number of studies to be included in the review increases, the collection and management of these data will become increasingly difficult. This suggests that, as with systematic reviews, a data collection form is also needed during the integrative review. The use of a data collection form also allows the reviewer to pilot the form and examine the type of data that will be extracted from the studies included in the review.

Problems can be encountered during this phase of the review when studies fail to report relevant data or adequate description of the study method (Pigott, 1994). Poor reporting of method or results has been identified as a common problem in RCT reports (Hahn et al., 2002; Chan et al., 2004). This incomplete reporting may be a significant problem during integrative reviews, given the greater diversity of study designs that may be included in the review. Contacting the authors of the research paper may be a useful strategy for obtaining missing data.

However, this can be a labour-intensive task if a large number of studies is involved. In addition, locating the authors can be very difficult, and may be impossible for older published studies.

Data analysis

While there is a general agreement that a range of different research designs can and should be included in reviews, there is less agreement on how the synthesis of these differing study designs should be undertaken. For systematic reviews, data synthesis can be achieved using descriptive or statistical methods (Khan, 2001). For qualitative research, data synthesis is achieved by a variety of methods, often broadly classified as meta-synthesis.

Descriptive data synthesis

The objective of a descriptive or non-quantitative review is to present the characteristics and results of studies in a meaningful way (Khan, 2001). This summary is best achieved by narrative and tabulation. This approach to data synthesis has received less attention than meta-analysis, and this may be a result of its similarity to the methods used in traditional reviews of the literature. However, descriptive synthesis can adhere to the principles of rigour expected of systematic and integrative reviews. Descriptive synthesis is a means of summarising the characteristics and findings of a body of research in a succinct and coherent manner. Importantly, when meta-analysis is not appropriate, this descriptive approach is a valid alternative. However, this approach is limited in terms of drawing conclusions about effectiveness. Many good examples of this approach can be found in both systematic and integrative reviews.

Statistical data synthesis

Results may also be synthesised statistically using meta-analysis, which is the statistical combination of the results of two or more studies. Meta-analysis is used to combine the results of studies systematically to produce a conclusion about a body of research (Petitti, 1994). In health care, meta-analysis is most closely associated with the RCT, although it has also been used to synthesise the findings of observational studies (Stroup et al., 2000). The aims of meta-analysis are to give an estimate of the average effectiveness of an intervention, to investigate whether the effect is roughly the same in different studies, settings and participants, and if the effect is not the same, to investigate the differences (Higgins & Green, 2005). Meta-analysis is only undertaken when studies address the same question, use a similar population, administer the intervention in a similar manner, measure the same outcomes for all participants, and use the same research design (Jones & Evans, 2000). When studies differ in one or more of these elements, meta-analysis may not be appropriate.

Qualitative data synthesis

The increase in quantitative research has been matched by a similar increase in qualitative research. However, isolated studies do not contribute significantly to the understanding of phenomena (Jensen & Allen, 1996). As a consequence, there is a growing interest in developing approaches to integrate and synthesise the findings of qualitative studies. The strength of this synthesis process is that it offers an understanding that is based on a range of populations, settings and circumstances (Evans & Pearson, 2001b). This broad base for generation of evidence on a phenomenon allows for greater confidence in the evidence and increases its transferability to other settings.

One important principle underpinning meta-analysis, that the synthesis should not attempt to combine data that are fundamentally different, also applies to the synthesis of qualitative data. To undertake a meta-analysis of RCTs, each study should be the same in all important characteristics. This principle applies to integrative reviews so that, regardless of the approach to data synthesis, each study must have similar characteristics. That is, the data synthesis should be both sensible and appropriate.

There is no general agreement on the optimal approach to data synthesis during integrative reviews. However, the descriptive synthesis that is used in systematic reviews is perhaps one of the most common approaches. As in systematic reviews, this descriptive synthesis is achieved through a narrative and tabular summary of study characteristics, methods and findings. Supplementing this synthesis, a variety of other methods has been used to synthesise qualitative data. These methods have been summarised by Dixon-Woods et al. (2005) and include:

Narrative summary   A narrative summary of the literature is perhaps the simplest approach and allows quantitative and qualitative data to be incorporated into the review. However, as with traditional reviews of the literature, the rigour of the review process is more difficult to demonstrate and evaluate. A narrative approach may be more appropriate when a broad perspective is required, rather than an in-depth look at a particular issue (Cook et al., 1997).

Thematic analysis   Identification of prominent themes in the literature and summary of findings under thematic headings is another approach that has been used (Dixon-Woods et al., 2005).

Meta-ethnography   Meta-ethnography is an approach to the synthesis of qualitative research that was proposed by Noblit & Hare (1988) as an analogy to meta-analysis. It differs from meta-analysis, in that it synthesises rather than aggregates the findings of individual studies.

Grounded theory   The constant comparative method of grounded theory has been used as the framework for data synthesis (Dixon-Woods et al., 2005).

Meta-study   Meta-study has been proposed by Paterson et al. (2001) (see also Chapter 7) and provides a framework that focuses on theory, method and data. Synthesis of data can be achieved using a number of different approaches, including grounded theory, meta-ethnography and thematic analysis (Dixon-Woods et al., 2005).

Content analysis   Content analysis is another method used for the synthesis of research. Content analysis is an established research tool that is used to gain knowledge, new insights and a representation of facts (Nandy & Sarvela, 1997). It is a means to obtain simple descriptions of data (Cavanagh, 1997). Content analysis converts qualitative data

into quantitative form, and while this makes it easier to manipulate, the process reduces complexity and context (Dixon-Woods et al., 2005).

Bayesian meta-analysis   Bayesian form of meta-analysis has also been used for data synthesis, as it is able to handle data from different types of studies. Bayesian meta-analysis incorporates prior probability distribution based on subjective opinion or subjective evidence, which is updated in the light of the results of the studies producing an assessment of current evidence (Higgins & Green, 2005; Dixon-Woods et al., 2005). However, this approach is controversial and, like all other approaches to data synthesis in reviews, is still under development.

The data synthesis phase of the review is at an early stage of development and this is reflected in the variability of methods encountered in published integrative reviews. While methods such as the meta-ethnography are able to deal with qualitative studies, they are not able to manage data from quantitative research. Others methods such as Bayesian meta-analysis and content analysis would have a significant impact on the interpretive nature of the qualitative research being analysed, reducing the complexity of the data during the data transformation process. However, even the simplest approach to data synthesis, the narrative summary, has been subject to criticism because of its subjective nature and lack of rigorous processes for data management.

This would suggest that, regardless of the approach taken during the integrative review, it will be important that the principles underpinning systematic reviews guide the process. First, the proposed method of data analysis and synthesis should be documented in a review protocol before commencing the review. As with qualitative and quantitative research, there should be a clear data trail to allow appraisal of the data and comparison between studies. Finally, the method used should be clearly reported to allow others to evaluate the review process adequately.

Integrative review report

Integrative reviews are conducted for the purpose of generating a rigorous summary of research and so should adhere to the principles that guide the primary research they seek to summarise. As with primary research, the report should give an accurate and comprehensive summary of the review method and its findings. There have been concerns raised about the quality of reporting of systematic reviews, resulting in the development of standards for systematic review reports (Moher et al., 1999). However, there has been no formal attempt to standardise the reporting of integrative reviews. As a result, there is great variability in published integrative reviews. This variability is most evident in the completeness of published review reports, with descriptions of the review method often being very limited. Yet, if integrative reviews are to be viewed as a scholarly endeavour, then they must meet the standards expected of primary research and systematic reviews.

The integrative review report should provide sufficient information to allow the quality and relevance to be evaluated, and the findings acted upon. The framework used for reporting systematic reviews also acts as a useful guide for the integrative review (Table 10.1).

Table 10.1   Integrative review report requirement.

Review activity	Information required in published report
Review focus	Purpose and aim of review Rationale for conducting the integrative review Review question

Search strategy	Electronic databases searched
	Key search terms
	Other search activities, such as:
	    bibliography and reference lists searched
	    internet search strategy
	    journals hand-searched
	Results of the search process

Selection criteria	Criteria for selecting studies and articles, including:
	    population or setting
	    intervention, condition, concept or phenomenon
	    outcome or data of interest
	    research designs or type of articles
	    other criteria such as sampling time frame
	Any exclusion criteria such as language or date of publication
	How the criteria were used to select studies and articles
	Results of the selection process

Critical appraisal	Approach to appraisal of study or article quality Criteria used to determine quality How the criteria were used Results of the critical appraisal process
Data collection	Approach to collection of data from articles and study reports Strategies used to minimise transcription error
Data synthesis	Approach to data synthesis Specific methods used for the synthesis of data How the process was managed
Results	Details of studies and articles included in review Findings or key issues from individual papers Results of the synthesis process
Discussion	Major findings Any limitations of review Implications for research and practice

Conclusion

Systematic reviews provide rigorous evidence of effectiveness that help shape and guide health care. However, many issues that are important to consumers, clinicians and healthcare organisations are beyond their scope because they concern issues other than effectiveness. Integrative reviews are starting to emerge as important activities that have the potential to fill the gap that exists between the traditional literature review and the systematic review. However, integrative reviews are still evolving and optimal methods have yet to be determined. Yet, if these reviews are to provide this evidence for practice, then the standard of their conduct and reporting must be as rigorous as those expected of all other research activities.

References

Anthony, D. (1996) A review of statistical methods in the Journal of Advanced Nursing. *Journal of Advanced Nursing*, 24, 1089–94.

Barbour, R.S. & Barbour, M. (2003) Evaluating and synthesizing qualitative research: the need to develop a distinct approach. *Journal of Evaluation in Clinical Practice*, 9 (2), 179–86.

Booth, A. (1996) In search of the evidence: informing effective practice. *Journal of Clinical Effectiveness*, 1 (1), 25–9.

Cavanagh, S. (1997) Content analysis: concepts, methods and applications. *Nurse Researcher*, 4 (3), 5–16.

Chan, A.W., Hrobjartsson, A., Haahr, M.T., Gotzsche, P.C. & Altman, D.G. (2004) Empirical evidence for selective reporting of outcomes in randomised trials. *Journal of the American Medical Association*, 291 (20), 2457–65.

Cook, D.J., Mulrow, C.D. & Haynes, R.B. (1997) Systematic reviews: synthesis of best evidence for clinical decisions. *Annals of Internal Medicine*, 126, 376–80.

Cooper, H. (1984) *The Integrative Research Review: A Systematic Approach.* Sage Publications, Beverly Hills.

Counsell, C. (1997) Formulating questions and locating primary studies for inclusion in systematic reviews. *Annals of Internal Medicine*, 127, 380–7.

Dickersin, K., Scherer, R. & Lefebvre, C. (1994) Identifying relevant studies for systematic reviews. *British Medical Journal*, 309, 1286–91.

Dixon-Woods, M., Fitzpatrick, R. & Roberts, K. (2001) Including qualitative research in systematic reviews: opportunities and problems. *Journal of Evaluation in Clinical Practice*, 7 (2), 125–33.

Dixon-Woods, M., Shaw, R.L., Agarwal, S. & Smith, J.A. (2004) The problem of appraising qualitative research. *Quality and Safety in Health Care*, 13, 223–5.

Dixon-Woods, M., Agarwal, S., Jones, D., Young, B. & Sutton, A. (2005) Synthesising qualitative and quantitative evidence: a review of possible methods. *Journal of Health Service Research and Policy*, 10 (1), 45–53.

Eakin, J.M. & Mykhalovsky, E. (2003) Reframing the evaluation of qualitative health research: reflections on a review of appraisal guidelines in health sciences. *Journal of Evaluation in Clinical Practice*, 9 (2), 187–94.

Estabrooks, C.A., Field, P.A. & Morse, J.M. (1994) Aggregating qualitative findings: an approach to theory development. *Qualitative Health Research*, 4, 503–11.

Evans, D. (2002) Database searches for qualitative research. *Journal of the Medical Library Association*, 90 (3), 290–3.

Evans, D. & Pearson, A. (2001a) Systematic reviews: gatekeepers of nursing knowledge. *Journal of Clinical Nursing*, 10, 593–9.

Evans, D. & Pearson, A. (2001b) Systematic reviews of qualitative research. *Clinical Effectiveness in Nursing*, 5 (3), 111–17.

Hahn, S., Williamson, P.R. & Hutton, J.L. (2002) Investigation of within study selective reporting in clinical research: follow-up of applications submitted to a local research ethics committee. *Journal of Evaluation in Clinical Practice*, 8 (3), 353–9.

Hicks, C. (1995) The shortfall in published research: a study of nurses' research and publication activities. *Journal of Advanced Nursing*, 21, 594–604.

Higgins, J.P.T. & Green, S. (eds) (2005) *Cochrane Handbook for Systematic Reviews of Interventions 4.2.5* (updated May). In: The Cochrane Library, Issue 3. John Wiley & Sons, Chichester.

Ioannidis, J.P.A. (2005) Why most published research findings are false. *PloS Medicine*, 2 (8), e124.

Jensen, L.A. & Allen, M.A. (1996) Meta-synthesis of qualitative findings. *Qualitative Health Research*, 6 (4), 553–60.

Jones, M.J. (2004) Application of systematic review methods to qualitative research: practical issues. *Journal of Advanced Nursing*, 48 (3), 271–8.

Jones, T. & Evans, D. (2000) Conducting a systematic review. *Australian Critical Care Nursing Journal*, 13 (2), 66–71.

Kelly, J.A. (1998) Scientific meeting abstracts: significance access and trends. *Bulletin of the Medical Library Association*, 86 (1), 68–76.

Khan, K.S., Riet, G., Glanville, J., Sowden, A.J. & Kleijnen, J. (eds) (2001) *Undertaking Systematic Reviews of Research on Effectiveness: CRDs Guidance for those Carrying Out or Commissioning Reviews.* CRD Report Number 4, 2nd edn. NHS Centre for Reviews and Dissemination, University of York, York.

Lincoln, Y.S. (1995) Emerging criteria for quality in qualitative and interpretive research. *Qualitative Inquiry*, 1 (3), 275–89.

Malterud, K. (2001) Qualitative research: standards, challenges and guidelines. *Lancet*, 358, 483–8.

Mills, J.L. (1993) Data torturing. *New England Journal of Medicine*, 329 (16), 1196–9.

Moher, D., Cook, D.J., Eastwood, S., Olkin, I., Rennie, D. & Stroup, D.F. (1999) Improving the quality of reports of meta-analyses of randomised controlled trials: the QUOROM statement (statistical data included). *Lancet*, 354, 1896–900.

Nandy, B.R. & Sarvela, P.D. (1997) Content analysis re-examined: a relevant research method for health education. *American Journal of Health Behaviour*, 21 (3), 222–34.

Noblit, G.W. & Hare, R.D. (1988) *Meta-ethnography: Synthesizing Qualitative Studies*, Vol. 11. Sage Publications, Newbury Park.

Paterson, B.L., Thorne, S.E., Canam, C. & Jillings, C. (2001) *Meta-study of Qualitative Health Research*. Sage, Thousand Oaks, California.

Petitti, D.B. (1994) *Meta-analysis, Decision Analysis and Cost-effectiveness Analysis*. Oxford University Press, New York.

Pigott, T.D. (1994) Methods for handling missing data in research synthesis. In: *The Handbook of Research Synthesis* (Cooper, H. & Hedges, L.V., eds). Russell Sage Foundation, New York.

Popay, J., Rogers, A. & Williams, G. (1998) Rationale and standards for the systematic review of qualitative literature in health services research. *Journal of Qualitative Health Research*, 8 (3), 341–51.

Rosenberg, W. & Donald, A. (1995) Evidence based medicine: an approach to clinical problem solving. *British Medical Journal*, 310, 1122–6.

Rychetnik, L., Frommer, M., Hawe, P. & Shiell, A. (2002) Criteria for evaluating evidence on public health interventions. *Journal of Epidemiology and Community Health*, 56, 119–27.

Sandelowski, M. (1993) Rigor or rigor mortis: the problem of rigor in qualitative research revisited. *Advances in Nursing Science*, 16 (2), 1–8.

Schwandt, T.A. (1996) Farewell to criteriology. *Qualitative Inquiry*, 2 (1), 58–72.

Sherwood, G. (1999) Meta-synthesis: merging qualitative studies to develop nursing knowledge. *International Journal of Human Caring*, 3 (1), 37–42.

Stroup, D.F., Berlin, J.A., Morton, S.C. et al. (2000) Meta-analysis of observational studies in epidemiology: a proposal for reporting. *Journal of the American Medical Association*, 283 (15), 2008–12.

Taylor, M.K. (1998) The practical effects of errors in reference lists in nursing research journals. *Nursing Research*, 47 (5), 300–3.

Whittemore, R. (2005) Combining evidence in nursing research: methods and implications. *Nursing Research*, 54 (1), 56–62.

Whittemore, R. & Knafl, K. (2005) The integrative review: updated methodology. *Journal of Advanced Nursing*, 52 (5), 546–53.

11 Rigour in Integrative Reviews

Robin Whittemore

Introduction

Systematic and rigorous methods for synthesising the literature on a specific clinical problem or phenomenon of concern are essential for knowledge development in nursing. Reviews that are of high quality present the state of the science, rate the strength of evidence, resolve conflicting reports of evidence, propose clinical guidelines and/or contribute to theory development. Yet, conducting a review of high quality is complex and challenging. The quantity and variety of literature on any potential topic complicate the ability to synthesise the results objectively and without bias. Significant methodological advancement to improve the rigour of the review process has occurred over the past decade. This methodological development has contributed to a proliferation of reviews of high quality and greater specification of review methods and procedures.

Methods for synthesising the literature in nursing include: systematic, meta-analytic, integrative and qualitative reviews. While there are common elements to these reviews, each has a specific purpose, scope, sample and type of analysis (Table 11.1) (Whittemore, 2005). As a result, each poses unique methodological challenges.

The integrative review is a method that summarises the literature on a clinical problem or phenomenon of concern that incorporates multiple perspectives and types of literature. The diversity of the sampling frame is the hallmark of this type of review. Integrative reviews are the broadest type of review, and include experimental and non-experimental research as well as the theoretical literature if appropriate. Thus, integrative reviews have the potential to contribute to a comprehensive portrayal of the phenomenon of concern. Process, context and a varied perspective can be elucidated (Whittemore & Knafl, 2005).

Because the integrative review has the potential to capture the complexity of varied perspectives and includes diverse approaches to knowledge development, it has been advocated as important for evidence-based practice initiatives in nursing (Kirkevold, 1997; Estabrooks, 1998; Evans & Pearson, 2001; Whittemore & Knafl, 2005). However, the complexity of using a diverse literature base has the potential to contribute to subjectivity, bias and a lack of rigour (Cooper, 1998; Beck, 1999). The purpose of this chapter, therefore, is to highlight the methodological challenges of the integrative review method and to propose guidelines to enhance the rigour of the process and the quality of the results.

Rigour in integrative reviews

In general, reviews of the literature are considered research (of research) and rigour has been defined

Table 11.1 Methods of nursing research reviews.

Type of review and exemplar	Definition	Purpose	Scope	Sampling frame	Analysis
Integrative review (Redeker, 2000)	A summary of the literature on a specific concept or content area whereby the research is summarised, analysed and overall conclusions are drawn	To review methods, theories and/or empirical studies around a particular topic	Narrow or broad	Quantitative or qualitative research; theoretical literature; methodological literature	Narrative
Meta-analysis (Clemmens, 2001)	A summary of past research using statistical techniques to transform findings of studies with related or identical hypotheses into a common metric and calculating the overall effect, the magnitude of effect and subsample effects	To estimate the effect of interventions or relationships	Narrow	Quantitative research of similar methodology	Statistical
Systematic review (Forbes, 1998)	A summary of past research using an objective and rigorous approach of studies with related or identical hypotheses	To summarise evidence regarding a specific clinical problem	Narrow	Quantitative research of similar methodology	Narrative or statistical
Meta-summary, meta-synthesis, formal grounded theory, meta-study (Beck, 2002)	A summary of past research combining the findings from multiple qualitative studies	To inform research or practice by summarising processes or experiences	Narrow or broad	Qualitative research	Narrative

Reprinted with permission from Whittemore, R. (2005) Combining evidence in nursing research. *Nursing Research, 54,* 56–62.

as the extent to which the review meets the standards appropriate for primary research (Ganong, 1987; Cooper, 1998). Methods for formulating the problem, searching the literature, evaluating the data, analysing the data and presenting the results have been proposed (Cooper, 1998; Centre for Reviews and Dissemination, 2005; Cochrane Collaboration, n.d.). Systematic methods aimed at obtaining valid conclusions have become the standards of rigour for all types of research reviews, similar to the standards for quantitative research. However, the integrative review method involves narrative analysis in order to combine diverse data sources, an analysis approach more aligned with qualitative research methods. Therefore, standards of rigour in integrative reviews must also incorporate qualitative standards for rigour, which include evidence of critical appraisal and transparency of the methodological process, particularly the data analysis stage. Thus, it is proposed that criteria for enhancing rigour in integrative reviews include a systematic method, evidence of critical appraisal, and transparency. These criteria will be discussed in more detail.

Systematic methods

To enhance rigour in undertaking an integrative review, a systematic method is necessary. Methodological guidelines for conducting literature reviews have been developed (Cooper, 1998; Centre for Reviews and Dissemination, 2005; Cochrane Collaboration, 2005). While these guidelines are primarily aligned with the systematic review or meta-analysis, anyone conducting an integrative review would benefit from reviewing these resources as there are methodological similarities between the systematic review and the integrative review. Guidelines specific to the integrative review have also been proposed and will be summarised briefly (Ganong, 1987; Kirkevold, 1997; Whittemore & Knafl, 2005).

Problem and purpose

The initial stage of any review method is a clear identification of the clinical or conceptual problem the review is addressing and the purpose of the review. A well-defined problem and purpose delimit the content and the variables of interest, and this

subsequently facilitates the ability to conduct a comprehensive search and accurate data collection process (Cooper, 1998).

Literature search

A comprehensive search of the literature is essential to enhancing the rigour of any review since a representative sample is a critical component for accurate unbiased conclusions (Ganong, 1987; Cooper, 1998; Conn et al., 2003a). Ideally, all of the literature directly relevant to the review purpose is retrieved and included in the review. However, locating all of the existing literature on a particular topic is surprisingly challenging (Oxman & Guyatt, 1988; Conn et al., 2003b). Often multiple strategies such as computerised database searching, ancestry searching, journal hand searching, networking and/or searching research registries are required to obtain a representative sample (Conn et al., 2003a). A well-defined sampling plan inclusive of search terms, selection criteria and search strategies is necessary. Consultation with a reference librarian has the potential to improve the specificity and the comprehensiveness of the search.

The appropriate sample size for an integrative review will vary depending on the purpose, sampling frame and amount of data available to be extracted from primary sources. A small sample size in an integrative review lends itself to less robust and generalisable conclusions, while a large sample size may contribute to considerable variation in findings and difficulty in analysis and synthesis. Large sample sizes can be reduced by further delimiting the inclusion and exclusion criteria; however, any sampling decision must be methodologically justified and made explicit.

Data collection

Once a comprehensive literature search has been completed, a systematic approach to organising and collecting common data from primary sources needs to be undertaken. Data collection in integrative reviews requires a standard and thorough examination of each primary source (Cooper, 1998). Pre-determined relevant data from each primary source need to be extracted, preferably using tables, charts or matrices (Miles & Huberman, 1994; Garrand, 1999). Data extraction forms are ideally piloted with several primary sources and revised to ensure an accurate portrayal of all primary sources. To further ensure accuracy, two independent reviewers may code individual primary sources. Multiple coders allow for errors to be identified, discrepancies to be addressed and inter-rater agreement to be calculated (Brown et al., 2003). A data collection approach that uses tables or matrices provides a succinct organisation of the literature and facilitates visualisation and comparison of primary sources on variables of interest, relationships, or issues. It is important to recognise that data from primary sources can be incorrectly or inadequately extracted. For example, a critique of the literature about therapeutic touch indicated that research with favourable findings were more often cited (O'Mathuna, 2000). Thus, accurate data collection and coding procedures are essential to ensure methodological rigour (Broome, 1993; Brown et al., 2003).

Evaluation of quality of primary sources

When undertaking a systematic or meta-analytic review, evaluation of the quality or internal validity of primary sources is also recommended (Cooper, 1998; Conn & Rantz, 2003). Quality scores are often calculated for each primary source and subsequently incorporated into the data analysis stage. However, the evaluation of quality is complex and there is no gold standard to guide the process (Jadad et al., 1998; Conn & Rantz, 2003). Evaluating the quality of primary sources in the integrative review method where diverse sources, inclusive of empirical and theoretical literature, are included increases the complexity further. Ideally, consideration of the quality of primary sources in an integrative review is addressed in a meaningful way as this greatly influences the credibility of conclusions and the ultimate quality of an integrative review. Suggestions for the evaluation of quality in integrative reviews have been proposed by Whittemore & Knafl (2005). Further practical application and discussion of strategies to evaluate quality in integrative reviews is indicated.

Data analysis

A systematic method for data analysis should be identified explicitly before undertaking an integrative review. Integrative reviews require a narrative analysis of a large repertoire of data, often grouped by themes or variables of interest. Data analysis for integrative reviews, like that for qualitative research, is a complex endeavour and credible methods have the potential to reduce bias and increase the accuracy of conclusions. A major concern with any narrative analysis is that the values or biases of the analyst may influence the interpretive effort (Miles & Huberman, 1994). A common problem is an often unrecognised commitment to an a priori view of the phenomenon of concern, or an inadequate consideration of all of the evidence (Sandelowski, 1995). Whittemore & Knafl (2005) have specifically addressed the complexity of data analysis in integrative reviews and have proposed that the qualitative method developed by Miles & Huberman (1994) assists in obtaining thorough, integrated and accurate conclusions. The method consists of data reduction, data display, data comparison, conclusion drawing and verification (Table 11.2) (Miles & Huberman, 1994).

Counting may be an additional aspect to the data analysis process of integrative reviews that enhances rigour, as counting highlights the recognition of patterns in the data. Findings that are more common are often more important than those that are unusual (Sandelowski, 2001). Brown (1999) suggests that findings should be classified as consistent, moderately consistent or inconsistent across primary sources. Data analysis procedures also need to include the opportunity for the analyst to identify conflicting evidence and tenuous results, as well as to consider several different explanations for interpreting the data. In addition, all conclusions should be verified by re-examining primary sources for accuracy and the reasons for variability (Miles & Huberman, 1994). Eliciting feedback from others also assists in maintaining analytical honesty and decreasing subjectivity during the data analysis phase. More frequently, integrative reviews are undertaken by a team of researchers, and this also has the potential to protect against subjectivity and bias.

Evidence of critical appraisal

Employing systematic methods in undertaking an integrative review is a necessary but insufficient

Table 11.2   Data analysis of integrative reviews.

Data analysis procedure	Explanation
Data reduction	Extracting and coding data from primary sources to simplify, abstract, focus, and organise data in a concise framework
Data display	Developing data display matrices or conceptual maps of data extracted from primary sources creatively around particular variables and subgroups
Data comparison	Examining data displays iteratively to identify patterns, themes or relationships
Conclusion drawing	Isolating patterns, processes, commonalities and differences
Verification	Verifying all conclusions with primary sources for accuracy. Addressing conflicting evidence and alternate hypotheses

Source: adapted from Miles & Huberman (1994).

component for obtaining valid conclusions and implications. Investigators must also demonstrate evidence of critical appraisal – both of the methodical processes and their own potential biases through a self-critical attitude. This implies the necessity for an honest and forthright investigation (Morse et al., 2002) and an ethical component to rigour that involves truthfulness, conscientiousness and attentiveness to all aspects of the investigation (Davies & Dodd, 2002). Evidence of critical appraisal is particularly important during data analysis. Ideally, investigators are critical in searching for alternative hypotheses, exploring variation and identifying negative instances (Marshall, 1990). Recursive and repetitive verification of emerging patterns and themes with primary sources assists in confirming that the interpretation is grounded in the data and that all data sources have been considered (Ambert et al., 1995; Morse et al., 2002). Failure to find supporting evidence for alternative or contrary interpretations of the data provides greater confidence in the original interpretation and explanation (Patton, 1990).

Transparency

As with all qualitative research, transparency or auditability of the research process may enhance rigour as it provides insight into research judgements (Lincoln & Guba, 1985). Methodological decisions and interpretations are explicitly presented, allowing the reader to follow the logic of the decision trail from review aim to data collection, data analysis and conclusions. An audit trail or record should be kept by the investigator during the entire review process, and this should document all decisions, analytical ideas, thoughts, issues or alternative hypotheses that come up (Rodgers & Cowles, 1993; Miles & Huberman, 1994).

Transparency of the research process becomes evident in presenting the results of the integrative review. In presenting the results, the goal is to make clear how the data were collected, how the analysis was carried out, and how the conclusions were derived from the data analysis. Integrative review results should be written using a format similar to primary research, including sections on background, method, results, discussion and conclusions. Methodological procedures, evidence from primary sources and the data analysis process should be reported in detail so that the basis for conclusions can be determined (Oxman & Guyatt, 1988; Slavin, 1995). The literature search process should be clearly documented in the method section, including the search terms, databases used, additional search strategies, and inclusion and exclusion criteria for the determination of relevant primary sources. Any sampling decision should be made explicit and justified (Whittemore & Knafl, 2005). The procedures for data analysis should also be reported in the method section of an integrative review report.

Transparency of the data analysis process is also very important to include in the results of an integrative review report. In general, tables document the evidence of primary sources, allowing the reader to ascertain that conclusions of the review relied on all the relevant evidence (Miles & Huberman, 1994; Oxman, 1994). Multiple tables are often used to show the logical sequence of analysis, explicitly linking conclusions to data displays. Ideally, congruence between the aims, method and findings, as well as logical congruence between the conclusions and previous knowledge, are made transparent.

Lastly, limitations of the integrative review and threats to validity that may undermine results should also be made transparent. Explicitly identifying review limitations and demonstrating that the interpretive effort took into consideration limitations of the review has the potential to assure more accurate and clinically applicable conclusions.

Quality in integrative reviews

The process of combining diverse primary sources in an integrative review is complex and challenging. Bias and error can occur at any stage of the process, since numerous methodological decisions and analytical judgements are required. Specific types of errors and methodological procedures that may protect against these errors are presented in Table 11.3. Systematic methods, evidence of critical appraisal and transparency of the methodological process have the potential to decrease error and improve the quality of integrative reviews. Quality criteria for research reviews in general have been proposed previously and are summarised in Box 11.1 (Whittemore, 2005).

Table 11.3   Sources of error and methodological procedures to decrease error in integrative reviews.

Sources of error	Definition	Methodological procedures
Literature search and sample selection		
Unexplained selectivity	Exclusion of literature within scope of review	Use multiple search strategies
Lack of discrimination	Inattention to quality of primary sources	Evaluate quality of primary sources and include in analytic effort
Data analysis		
Erroneous detailing	Incorrect extraction of data from primary sources	Define coding procedures Use piloted data extraction form Have two independent reviewers extract data from primary sources
Double counting	Multiple reports from one study sample or same authors on same topic	Develop inclusion and exclusion criteria to address this
Non-recognition of faulty author conclusions; unwarranted attribution or overstated author conclusions	Uncritical acceptance of all conclusions of primary sources	Critique primary sources; include quality assessment in analytic effort
Suppression of contrary findings	Lack of acknowledgement of contrary findings	Include all evidence from primary sources in data analysis Explore variability of findings, conflicting findings, and rival hypotheses
Conclusion drawing		
Consequential errors	Inability to accurately draw conclusions due to aforementioned errors	Use systematic and objective methods
Failure to consider all evidence relevant to generalisation		Use well-specified data extraction and analysis procedures

Source: adapted from Dunkin (1996).

Box 11.1   Quality criteria in research reviews (reprinted with permission from Whittemore, R. (2005) Combining evidence in nursing research: Methods and implications. *Nursing Research*, 54, 56–62).

Quality criteria

(1)   Well-defined problem and review purpose
(2)   Explicit identification of review method
(3)   Investigators with expertise in content and methodology
(4)   Clear specification of review process and protocol
(5)   Comprehensive and explicit literature search
(6)   Explicit, unbiased and reproducible data extraction for content and quality
(7)   Primary study quality considered in analysis
(8)   Data analysis is systematic and variability of findings addressed
(9)   Evidence included from primary studies
(10) Conclusions based on evidence and capture complexity of clinical problem
(11) Methodological limitations identified

Conclusions

Systematic and rigorous integrative reviews have the potential to present a comprehensive portrayal of a healthcare problem or topic of concern. Greater attention to methodological rigour in integrative reviews will contribute to more accurate conclusions and a greater applicability of results to research, practice and policy.

References

Ambert, A.M., Adler, P.A., Adler, P. & Detzner, D.F. (1995) Understanding and evaluating qualitative research. *Journal of Marriage and the Family*, 57, 879–93.

Beck, C.T. (1999) Facilitating the work of a meta-analyst. *Research in Nursing and Health*, 22, 523–30.

Beck, C.T. (2002) Mothering multiples: A meta-synthesis of qualitative research. *American Journal of Maternal Child Nursing*, 27, 214–21.

Broome, M.E. (1993) Integrative literature reviews for the development of concepts. In: *Concept development in nursing*. 2nd edn (Rodgers, B.L. & Knafl, K.A., eds), pp. 231–50. W.B. Saunders, Philadelphia.

Brown, S.A., Upchurch, S.L. & Acton, G.J. (2003) A framework for developing a coding scheme for meta-analysis. *Western Journal of Nursing Research*, 25, 205–22.

Brown, S.J. (1999) *Knowledge for Health Care Practice: A Guide to Using Research Evidence.* WB Saunders, Philadelphia.

Centre for Reviews and Dissemination. (2005) *Review methods and resources.* Available at website http://www.york.ac.uk/inst/crd/crdreview.htm (retrieved 12 February 2006).

Clemmens, D. (2001) The relationship between social support and adolescent mothers' interactions with their infants: A meta-analysis. *Journal of Obstetric, Gynecologic, and Neonatal Nursing*, 30, 410–20.

Cochrane Collaboration (n.d.) Available at website http://www.cochrane.org (retrieved 15 August 2004).

Conn, V.S. & Rantz, M.J. (2003) Managing primary study quality in meta-analyses. *Research in Nursing and Health*, 26, 322–33.

Conn, V.S., Isaramalai, S., Rath, S., Jantarakupt, P., Wadhawan, R. & Dash, Y. (2003a) Beyond MEDLINE for literature searches. *Journal of Nursing Scholarship*, 35, 177–82.

Conn, V.S., Valentine, J.C., Cooper, H.M. & Rantz, M.J. (2003b) Grey literature in meta-analyses. *Nursing Research*, 52, 256–61.

Cooper, H. (1998) *Synthesizing Research: A Guide for Literature Reviews*, 3rd edn. Sage Publications, Thousand Oaks.

Davies, D. & Dodd, J. (2002) Qualitative research and the question of rigor. *Qualitative Health Research*, 12, 279–89.

Dunkin, M.J. (1996) Types of errors in synthesizing research in education. *Review of Educational Research*, 66, 87–97.

Estabrooks, C.A. (1998) Will evidence-based nursing practice make practice perfect? *Canadian Journal of Nursing Research*, 30, 15–36.

Evans, D. & Pearson, A. (2001) Systematic reviews: Gatekeepers of nursing knowledge. *Journal of Clinical Nursing*, 10, 593–9.

Forbes, D.A. (1998) Strategies of managing the behavioural symptomatology associated with dementia of the Alzheimer type: A systematic overview. *Canadian Journal of Nursing Research*, 30, 67–86.

Ganong, L.H. (1987) Integrative reviews of nursing research. *Research in Nursing and Health*, 10, 1–11.

Garrard, J. (1999) *Health Sciences Literature Review Made Easy: The Matrix Method*. Aspen Publication, Gaithersburg, MD.

Jadad, A., Moher, D. & Klassen, T. (1998) Guides for reading and interpreting systematic reviews: II. How did the authors find the studies and assess their quality? *Archives of Pediatric and Adolescent Medicine*, 152, 812–17.

Kirkevold, M. (1997) Integrative nursing research – an important strategy to further the development of nursing science and nursing practice. *Journal of Advanced Nursing*, 25, 977–84.

Lincoln, Y.S. & Guba, E.A. (1985) *Naturalistic Inquiry*. Sage, Beverly Hills, CA. Marshall, C. (1990) Goodness criteria: Are they objective or judgment calls? In: *The Paradigm Dialog* (Guba, E.G., ed.). Sage, Newbury Park, CA.

Miles, M.B. & Huberman, A.M. (1994) *Qualitative Data Analysis*. Sage, Thousand Oaks, CA. Morse, J.M., Barrett, M., Mayan, M., Olson, K. & Spiers, J. (2002) Verification strategies for establishing reliability and validity in qualitative research. *International Journal of Qualitative Methods*, 1, article 2. Retrieved February 15,

2006 Available at website http://www.ualberta.ca/~ijqm/english/engframeset.html (retrieved 15 February 2006).

O'Mathuna, D.P. (2000) Evidence-based practice and reviews of therapeutic touch. *Journal of Nursing Scholarship*, 32, 279–85.

Oxman, A.D. (1994) Systematic reviews: Checklists for review articles. *British Medical Journal*, 309, 648–51.

Oxman, A.D. & Guyatt, G.H. (1988) Guidelines for reading literature reviews. *Canadian Medical Association Journal*, 138, 697–703.

Patton, M.Q. (1990) *Qualitative Evaluation and Research Methods*, 2nd edn. Sage Publications, Newbury Park.

Redeker, N.S. (2000) Sleep in acute care settings: An integrative review. *Journal of Nursing Scholarship*, 32, 31–8.

Rodgers, B.L. & Cowles, K.V. (1993) The qualitative research audit trail: a complex collection of documentation. *Research in Nursing and Health*, 16, 219–26.

Sandelowski, M. (1995) Qualitative analysis: What it is and how to begin. *Research in Nursing and Health*, 18, 371–5.

Sandelowski, M. (2001) Real qualitative researchers do not count: The use of numbers in qualitative research. *Research in Nursing and Health*, 24, 230–40.

Slavin, R.E. (1995) Best evidence synthesis: An intelligent alternative to meta-analysis. *Journal of Clinical Epidemiology*, 48, 9–18.

Whittemore, R. (2005) Combining evidence in nursing research: Methods and implications. *Nursing Research*, 54, 56–62.

Whittemore, R. & Knafl, K. (2005) The integrative review: Updated methodology. *Journal of Advanced Nursing*, 52, 546–53.

12 Habit Retraining for Urinary Incontinence in Adults

Joan Ostaszkiewicz and Beverly O'Connell

Introduction

This chapter describes a process used to integrate evidence from different types of research designs to address the research question of the effectiveness of using habit retraining for the management of urinary incontinence (UI) in adults and to identify the contextual factors that need to be considered when designing evaluation studies on habit retraining (HRT). The first section of this chapter describes the background, methods and results of a Cochrane systematic review on the effectiveness of habit retraining. In addition, it describes some of the issues and challenges encountered when undertaking this type of review. Following this, we describe the methods used to integrate information from both randomised controlled trials (RCTs) and other types of study design, extracting information on the contextual factors that need to be considered when designing evaluation studies on HRT. This latter method took a more inclusive approach to evidence by incorporating studies with mixed designs. This resulted in a more comprehensive understanding of the evidence on HRT.

Background

A number of behavioural interventions have been recommended for the management of UI in adults

(Abrams et al., 2005). One such intervention is habit retraining. This is a caregiver-dependent intervention (Fantl et al., 1996), which has been promoted for use among nursing home residents with incontinence, particularly where cognitive and/or motor deficits limit the application of more active behavioural approaches. It is also a useful strategy in community settings to assist caregivers to manage incontinence in care-dependent individuals (Fantl et al., 1996). First described by Clay (1978), HRT involves identifying an incontinent person's toileting pattern and then developing an individualised toileting schedule that pre-empts involuntary bladder emptying, either by decreasing or increasing voiding intervals, while aiming to keep these intervals as long as possible without incontinence.

In 2004, a systematic review was undertaken (Ostaszkiewicz et al., 2004) to examine the evidence base for this intervention. It adhered to the Cochrane Collaboration guidelines (Higgins & Green, 2005) in that it used evidence from randomised controlled trials or quasi-randomised controlled trials. The objective was to assess the effectiveness of HRT for the management of UI in adults.

Systematic review method

The first stage in conducting the systematic review involved developing a research protocol. This defined the methods used to conduct the systematic review and detailed the inclusion and exclusion criteria. Specifically, it addressed the types of studies that were to be considered, as well as the types of participant, intervention and outcome measures. Similarly, the data sources used to identify studies were identified in advance, as were the criteria used to evaluate the quality of these studies. Approaches to data analysis were also determined a priori.

Inclusion/exclusion criteria

Types of studies

Consistent with policy guidelines from the Cochrane Incontinence Review Group, the inclusion criteria were limited to evidence from RCTs and quasi-randomised controlled trials. This is because RCTs are more likely to provide reliable information than other sources of evidence on the differential effects of alternative forms of health care (Kunz et al., 2006).

Types of participant

The review was limited to considering the effectiveness of the intervention amongst adults, and was not confined to particular subgroups or settings.

Types of intervention

The intervention was limited to HRT, delivered either alone or combined with other interventions such as medication, pelvic floor muscle exercises (PFME) and biofeedback. We developed a clear definition of this intervention so that it could be distinguished from other similar interventions.

Types of outcome

We chose a set of outcomes that were based on the International Continence Society Outcomes Standards Reports (Mattiasson et al., 1998) and recommendations of a report on outcome measures for research into lower urinary tract dysfunction in frail older adults (Fonda et al., 1998). These included patient symptoms, perception of improvement or cure (as reported by patient or caregiver), clinical outcomes, number of incontinent episodes in 24 hours, pad changes due to incontinence over 24 hours, pad weight, voided volume, maintenance of skin integrity, health status measures, health economic measures and adherence to the research protocol.

Search strategy

A strategy for conducting the search was developed. This was based on the guidelines of the Cochrane Collaboration in that it was designed to identify all randomised or quasi-randomised controlled trials. However, we also searched for other forms of evidence by hand searching selective journals, checking relevant websites and conference proceedings and checking the reference lists of all topic-relevant publications. Citation chasing was enhanced with the use of a science citation index.

The search was extensive and elicited data from both English and non-English language journals and from published and unpublished data. No arbitrary limitation was placed on the age of the data. To select publications that yielded topic-relevant studies, the keywords used in the search of electronic databases were: urinary incontinence, timed, regular and scheduled voiding/toileting, habit training/retraining, bladder training/retraining, prompted voiding/toileting, behaviour/cognitive/conservative therapy/treatment/modification, toilet training, nursing homes/care and dementia. To search for publications that met the design criteria, the keywords used were: randomised controlled trial/s, controlled trial/s, random allocation, double blind method, single blind method, clinical trials, placebo, random, research design. The electronic databases included in the search were the Cochrane Database of Systematic Reviews, the Cochrane Clinical Controlled Trials Register, Database of Abstracts of Reviews of Effectiveness, MEDLINE, CINAHL, EMBASE, Current Content, Biosis and Psyclit. The date of the most recent search of the trials register for this review was May 2002.

Systematic review results

Search results

The total yield of publications was 1851. Fifty-eight of these were found to be topic-relevant and met

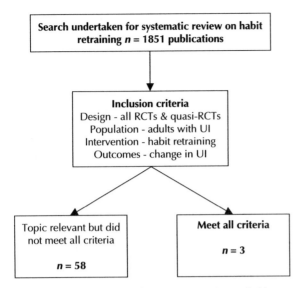

Figure 12.1 Search results for systematic review on habit retraining. UI, urinary incontinence; RCT, randomised controlled trial.

some, but not all, of the inclusion criteria. These studies were briefly reviewed in terms of the population of interest, research methods/design, intervention and rationale for their exclusion and they were then placed in a Table of Excluded Studies. The most common reasons for excluding studies were that (1) they failed to meet the study design criteria or (2) the intervention was more consistent with other forms of toileting assistance than with the review definition of HRT. Four were found to be duplicate publications. Only three studies met all of the criteria that had been predefined for the Cochrane systematic review, and these became the subject matter of the review. For an overview of the results of the search strategy, see Figure 12.1.

Description of studies

The three studies that were eligible for inclusion in the review had a combined sample size of 337 participants. These participants were primarily care-dependent older women with concurrent cognitive and/or physical impairment, and were residing either in residential aged-care facilities or their own homes. These studies evaluated HRT, combined with other approaches, compared with usual care. Outcomes evaluated in these studies were:

- Frequency and/or severity of UI
- Incidence of urinary tract infection
- Skin rash and skin breakdown
- Cost, and
- Caregiver preparedness, role strain and burden

Results of assessment of quality and data analysis

The three studies were appraised for methodological quality using criteria recommended by the Cochrane Collaboration. These criteria are based on the assumption that avoidance of bias is best achieved by secure concealment of random allocation prior to formal entry, few and identifiable withdrawals and dropouts, and analysis based on an intention to treat (Alderson et al., 2003). None of the studies met all of these criteria.

Between-group data that were available for pooling showed no statistically significant differences in the incidence or volume of incontinence between groups. Within-group analyses did, however, show improvements on these measures. Reductions were also reported for the intervention group in one study for skin rash, skin breakdown and in caregivers' perceptions of their level of stress; however, the data could not be analysed further.

The descriptive data suggested that HRT was a labour-intense activity. For example, it was reported that caregivers found it difficult to maintain voiding records and to implement the toileting programme. A 61% compliance rate was reported in one trial where the intervention was tested in a residential care facility and where the implementation was dependent on usual care staff. Electronic loggers, used as an adjunct to caregiver-delivered wet/dry checks, were reported as providing more accurate data than those from caregiver conducted wet/dry checks. To date, no analysis of the time and resources associated with these comparisons is available.

Reviewer conclusion and recommendations

Based on the review methodology, the reviewers concluded that current data on HRT using three studies were limited. Although the systematic review provided information on clinical effectiveness, it yielded limited information on other important contextual and clinical issues (i.e. optimal duration and intensity of voiding records, duration and nature of education, and the most effective method to obtain accurate data).

Dilemmas encountered implementing the Cochrane systematic review criteria

Limiting the review to one form of evidence

Adhering to the Cochrane Incontinence Review Group criteria on types of evidence that should be considered led to a number of studies being excluded. Specifically, those that were not randomised or quasi-randomised controlled trials were excluded. Studies excluded were a mix of reviews of literature, expert opinion papers, case studies, cohort studies and placebo-controlled trials focusing on an intervention requiring an adjustment in a voiding or toileting schedule. The outcome of using this formula resulted in information being limited to fewer studies.

Although Cochrane systematic reviews follow stringent guidelines designed to promote rigour and consistency across reviews, these guidelines restrict the type of evidence that is included and the types of questions that can be answered. In a healthcare discipline that considers both the physical and humanistic aspects of care, and where the context of clinical care does not always lend itself to being controlled or to implementing a randomisation process, reliance on one form of evidence places limits on the development of disciplinary knowledge and may provide only partial information to guide practice. For example, O'Connell & Myers (2001), who conducted a falls prevention study in an acute care setting, highlighted that the complexity and large number of contextual issues within acute care prevented them from designing and conducting a randomised controlled trial. At the same time, the data from the pre-test/post-test design provided useful information to assist clinicians in considering their management and prevention of patient falls. Several authors have recommended that nursing practice should be developed based on different types of research methods, where the empirical data are integrated into other sources of knowledge (i.e. personal and ethical knowledge) (Carper, 1978).

Critical appraisal and establishing levels of quality

Another dilemma that needs to be considered is the usefulness of the Cochrane guidelines for critiquing the quality of studies, which are based on criteria developed within a reductionist paradigm. More specifically, these criteria relate to the potential for selection, performance, attrition and detection bias (Kunz et al., 2006). The application of these guidelines in the present review led to many of the studies being classified as providing low-quality evidence. Nevertheless, the findings of these studies offered valuable information that could be used to guide practice and to assist in the development of future research. In support of using different types of evidence, scholars from social science and health disciplines dispute the hierarchy of evidence model espoused by proponents of evidence-based practice and the assumption that control and the reduction of bias has privilege over other forms of evidence (Upshur et al., 2001). They argue that research findings are seldom presented in research reports as neutral information or facts: they are pre-assigned some degree of truth-value by researchers, who present their work as an argument in favour of their conclusion (Hughes, 1990). According to Hughes, scientific knowledge (positivism) has failed to live up to its aspiration of providing laws of social life equivalent in scope, certainty and predictive capacity to those offered by natural science (Hughes, 1990). Furthermore, he specifies that it is simply 'another belief system with no special claim to absolute superiority over others' (p. 149).

The arguments detailed above provide the basis for considering more inclusive approaches to what constitutes quality evidence. One approach to overcoming these problems is to conduct an integrative review. Integrative reviews are the broadest category of research reviews and can encompass different types of evidence, including theoretical as well as empirical literature, as discussed by Whittemore and Knafl (2005). They argue that, because integrative reviews allow for greater variety in the sampling procedure, they have the potential to answer broad questions that go beyond issues of effectiveness.

In the context of the above-mentioned dilemmas, we decided to revisit the literature identified in the systematic review database and to use content analysis to identify the contextual factors that need to be considered when designing evaluation studies on HRT. The rest of this chapter is concerned with the methods used to undertake this integrative review, its findings and how these both enhanced and challenged the findings from the systematic review on HRT. This is followed by recommendations for the conduct of future similar reviews.

Managing and integrating evidence from mixed design studies

Identifying the source of data and applying the selection criteria

The data source for conducting the integrative review consisted of the three randomised or quasi-randomised controlled trials identified in the original Cochrane systematic review on HRT (Ostaszkiewicz et al., 2004), as well as 58 publications that were excluded as they did not meet all of the inclusion criteria for the above-mentioned review. The total data source, therefore, consisted of 61 publications.

We developed and applied a new set of exclusion/inclusion criteria to these publications. These criteria differed from those used to conduct the Cochrane systematic review on HRT in that they were more inclusive of the findings from different types of study design. We included all publications on HRT except opinion- or discussion-based papers, single-case studies and those not presenting original research (Figure 12.2). Publications that described other behavioural interventions, such as bladder training, prompted voiding, timed voiding, pelvic floor muscle exercises and biofeedback, were excluded unless they also described an HRT component (i.e. a flexible voiding schedule that aims to mimic the person's natural voiding pattern).

Search results

A total of ten publications met these new inclusion criteria and formed the basis of this integrative review. Thus, their application revealed seven more articles than had been identified for the Cochrane systematic review. Four of these were RCTs and the other six used a pre-post test design with a single cohort.

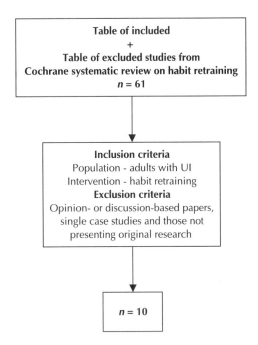

Figure 12.2 Search results for integrative review on habit retraining. UI, urinary incontinence.

Data extraction

Data were extracted from these publications and coded under the same set of headings used to conduct the Cochrane systematic review. These headings were: (1) methods, (2) participants, (3) intervention and (4) outcomes. For the purposes of the integrative review, we collected additional data under the following headings:

- Resources required to implement the intervention (i.e. staffing/caregiver time)
- Assessment and evaluation methods
- Intervention implementation strategies
- Adherence to the study protocol
- Attrition and reasons, and
- Researchers' reflections on barriers and facilitators to the intervention

The data extraction phase was undertaken by two reviewers, who worked independently following a test of inter-rater reliability. Areas of disagreement were resolved by discussion and agreement. The extracted data were converted from their individual sources and displayed in table format (see Appendix 12.1).

Data evaluation

As the purpose of the integrative review was to identify the contextual factors that need to be considered when designing evaluation studies on HRT, our approach to assessing quality was based on guiding principles from The Joanna Briggs Institute (JBI, 2006). These principles include the view that the results of well-designed research studies grounded in any methodological position provide more vigorous evidence than anecdotes or personal opinion. Hence, a quality measure that we adopted was to accept publications that met levels I, II or III of evidence proposed by the Australian National Health and Medical Research Council (NHMRC) Canberra 1999 and adopted by JBI. Specifically, level I evidence is defined as that obtained from a systematic review of all relevant RCTs. Level II evidence is considered to be that obtained from at least one properly designed RCT. Level III-1 is evidence obtained from well-designed pseudo-randomised controlled trials (alternate allocation or some other method). Level III-2 is that obtained from comparative studies with concurrent controls and allocation not randomised (cohort studies), case control studies, or interrupted time series with a control group. Level III-3 is evidence obtained from comparative studies with historical control, two or more single-arm studies, or interrupted time series without a parallel control group (NHMRC, 1999).

Data analysis

To analyse the extracted data, we employed a thematic analysis procedure (Daly et al., 1997). This involved reviewing the data extracted under the six headings above and determining the major findings and themes that related to patient outcomes and other factors that had an impact on the study design.

Results

Population

The total sample size from the combined ten studies was 545 participants, and two major cohorts were represented in these studies. These were the same groups that had emerged from the previously conducted systematic review and included cognitively impaired older people in residential elder care settings and frail, predominantly cognitively impaired older people who lived in the community with a caregiver. There was one exception to this: one study examined the efficacy of HRT with people attending an outpatient clinic. The predominant focus of the intervention was pelvic floor muscle exercise (PFME) with biofeedback, and there was no description of HRT.

Interventions

Descriptive data on HRT from the ten studies indicated that HRT as a toileting assistance approach has been implemented in combination with other strategies. These strategies varied across studies and included: PFME exercises with biofeedback; medical investigation and treatment of underlying disorders; anticholinergic therapy; relaxation techniques; education on dietary modifications; fluid intake and bowel management; changes to the immediate environment to enable people with cognitive impairment to identify the toilet more easily; social or material reinforcement/rewards to patients and/or to those required to implement HRT; education on the protocol and feedback to individuals required to implement HRT; and home visits and telephone support to home based caregivers. These studies are summarised in Table 12.1.

Nine of the ten studies involved usual care staff as well as specifically employed research staff to implement the intervention. The research staff provided the much needed extra human resource time required to coordinate the study, conduct the intervention and collect and analyse the data.

All studies had two parts to their interventions. First, there was an initial assessment period where each participant's usual voiding pattern was monitored and documented. The second part involved implementing the individualised HRT programme. The initial assessment period varied across studies, including checking each person's continence status on an hourly to two hourly basis for a period from 3 days to 1 month. In addition, the type of clinical assessment information collected varied across studies and included physical and mental status testing, specialised investigations (i.e. bladder scan,

Table 12.1   Study interventions and resources required for implementation.

Setting	Study	Intervention/s and resources
Out-patient clinic for people with incontinence	Baigis-Smith 1989	Kegel exercises with biofeedback, relaxation techniques and information on diet modification and bowel regimes provided by research staff in an out-patient clinic
Long-term care setting	Chanfreau-Rona 1984	Changes to the ward environment to enhance residents' ability to access the toilet and social or material reinforcement/rewards. Intervention delivered by usual care staff under the direction of research staff
	Chanfreau-Rona 1986	Changes to the ward environment to enhance residents' ability to access the toilet and verbal and material rewards. Intervention delivered by usual care staff under the direction of research staff
	Colling 1992	Four hours of education on the protocol to residential care staff, reimbursement to wards for staff attendance at education, staff feedback and verbal encouragement. Intervention delivered by usual care staff under the direction of research staff
	Gaitsgori 1998	Anticholinergic therapy to patients with urge incontinence. Intervention delivered by usual care staff under the direction of research staff
	Jirovec 1991	Feedback to staff. Intervention delivered by usual care staff under the direction of research staff
	King 1980	Medical investigation and treatment, changes to the ward environment, social activities delivered by usual care staff under the direction of research staff
	Saltmarche 1991	Social reinforcement, recommendations regarding adequate fluid intake and education to staff. Intervention delivered by usual care staff under the direction of research staff
Home carers	Colling 2003	Home visits, weekly telephone calls, education on the protocol and support to home based caregivers delivered by research staff
	Jirovec 2001	Monthly telephone calls, recommendations regarding adequate fluid intake, changes to the home environment to enhance toilet access, education on the protocol and support to home-based caregivers delivered by research staff

Studies are given by first author and date.

simple cystometry, cystoscopy, etc.). For details see Table 12.2.

Outcomes

Outcome data were extracted and reviewed to determine the extent to which the findings could be aggregated to provide a summary estimate (see Table 12.3). Aggregating the findings proved problematic as statistical outcome data were limited to seven of the ten studies and in these pre- and post-intervention data or between-group data were limited to six studies. In addition, aggregating or summarising the data from these six studies was difficult as they reported different outcome measures (e.g. frequency of urinary incontinence, volume of urinary incontinence, number of individuals improved and urinary incontinence frequency ratio).

A further limitation to summarising the data to determine the clinical effectiveness of HRT was the absence of sensitivity analyses to enable the reader to determine the extent to which the results reflected the unique contribution of HRT. In addition,

Table 12.2 Features of the assessment required for habit retraining.

Setting	Study	Frequency of continence checks	Duration of assessment and monitoring	Human/material resources involved in assessment and monitoring	Details of clinical assessment
Out-patient clinic for people with incontinence	Baigis-Smith 1989	Participants were asked to keep own record every 2 hours	2 weeks	Participant Nurse practitioner/s	Catheterisation for residual urine Bedside cystometrogram Urinalysis Diagnosis of incontinence type History Mini-Mental Status Questionnaire Physical examination – abdominal and rectal examination and, in women, a pelvic exam Perineometer score
Long-term care setting	Chanfreau-Rona 1984	Two hourly checks	2 weeks	Usual care staff Research staff	Clifton Assessment Procedures for the Elderly Perceptions of nursing staff regarding participants' health status Observation of participants' mobility status
	Chanfreau-Rona 1986	Two hourly checks during the daytime	2 weeks	Usual care staff Research staff	Clifton Assessment Procedures for the Elderly
	Colling 1992	One hourly checks	14 × 3 24-hour periods	Usual care staff Specifically employed research assistants Research staff An electronic logger which provided 72 hours of continuous electronic monitoring to establish precise voiding patterns for each subject	A detailed medical record review An assessment of mental, functional, and behavioural status SPMSQ, Katz ADL Index A focused physical examination Urinalysis and culture and sensitivity Simple urodynamics evaluation Post-void residual A stress test Simple cystometry
	Gaitsgori 1998	One hourly checks	3 days	Usual care staff Research staff	Diagnosis of type of UI Exclusion of UTI Exclusion of post-void residual
	Jirovec 1991	Hourly checks from 7 a.m. to 10 p.m.		Usual care staff (nursing aids) Research staff	Mental Status Questionnaire Medical assessment Catheter samples of urine for UTI – MSU

	Study	Checks	Duration	Staff	Assessments
	King 1980	One hourly checks	1 month	Usual care staff (nursing staff) Research nurse	Medical and psychiatric assessments Biochemical and haematological investigations as appropriate Rectal examinations for faecal problems MSU
	Saltmarche 2001		1 week	Usual care staff Research staff	Assessment to exclude obstruction, infection and high post-void residual volume An assessment of functional and behavioural abilities with respect to the toileting ability A detailed urological review An assessment of cognitive and functional levels using standardised indices frequently employed in geriatric assessments Cystoscopy and urodynamics
Home carers	Colling 2002	Two hourly checks	3 consecutive days	Home-based caregivers Research staff An electronic logger which provided 6 × 24 hour periods of continuous electronic monitoring to establish precise voiding patterns for each subject spaced over 3 week intervals	Short Portable Mental Status Questionnaire Katz ADL Index Hadley, Wood McCracken Behavioral Capabilities Scale for Older Adults Bladder scan Voiding diaries Oregon Health Sciences University Skin Rash and Breakdown Tool Urinalysis – MSU Caregiver burden – (Archbold and Steward) Economic Burden Scale Global Role Strain Preparedness for Caregiving scale Physical examination – screening-focused neurological examination, pelvic and rectal examination Assessment of UI type based on UI history and physical examination
	Jirovec 2001		1 week	Home-based caregivers Nurse practitioner Urologist	Physical examinations to establish the functional nature of the incontinence Urinalysis Bladder scan to identify post-void residual Review of medications

Studies are given by first author and date.

MSU, Midstream specimen of urine; ADL, activities of daily living; UI, urinary incontinence; UTI, urinary tract infection; SPMSQ, Short Portable Mental Status Questionnaire.

Table 12.3 Outcome data.

Study	Statistical data	Between group statistical data	Within group statistical data	Descriptive data	Data collection points	Critical appraisal issues
Baigis-Smith 1989	Yes	UI accidents per week t-test for baseline and end of treatment $t(54) = 4.99$ $P < 0.0005$ Peak perineometer readings t-test peak mean $t(54) = -4.8$, $P < 0.0005$ Mean sustained hold $t(54) = -5.6$, $P < 0.0005$			Baseline; baseline to end of treatment; at 1 month; at 3 months; at 6 months; at 1 year	Are these results an outcome of Kegel exercises, biofeedback, adjustment to fluid intake, adjustment to dietary intake, a bowel regime, relaxation techniques or HRT?
Chanfreau-Rona 1984	No	No	No	Improvement for one group and deterioration for other groups	Ward A – Baseline at weeks 1–2, reassessment at weeks 9–10, follow-up at weeks 21–22 Ward B – Baseline at weeks 1–5, reassessment at weeks 12–13 Ward C – Baseline at weeks 1–2, reassessment at weeks 9–10	No statistical data reported Are these results an outcome of environmental changes, removal of pads, social or material reinforcement/rewards or HRT?
Chanfreau-Rona 1986	Yes but limited to a subgroup analysis of high wetters and low wetters	No		No difference between intervention and control groups on frequency of incontinence	Baseline; reassessment – at 7 weeks; follow-up at 3 months	Are these results an outcome of environmental changes, removal of pads, social or material reinforcement / rewards or HRT? No statistical data on between group differences for total sample The data are based on a subgroup analysis of the 30 patients – divided into high wetters and low wetters – i.e. not analysed by groups to which they were assigned

Colling 1992	Yes	Frequency of UI: Gp 1: (51) mean = 4.5 versus Gp 2: (37) mean = 5.5 Volume of UI: Gp 1: (51) mean = 600 cc versus Gp 2: (37) mean = 650 cc No report on statistical significance	UI frequency ratio from 0.7 at baseline to mean 0.57 during treatment ($P > 0.000$) UI volume ratio v. small significant differences in the mean volume over the 14 data collection periods ($t = 2.60$, $P \leq 0.005$)	14 × 24 hour data collection periods over the 32 weeks	Are these results an outcome of education, staff feedback and verbal encouragement or HRT? Is a reduction in 50 cc urine or a reduction in 1.1 p/p episode of UI clinically significant?
Gaitsgori 1998	Yes	No	Initial results 94% of patients improved, 15/35 (43%) totally dry during the day and 6% failed treatment At 10 months: 11/35 (31%) totally dry and 12 (34%) dry during the day	Baseline data collection for 3 days; 10 days intervention; reassessment after 10 days; reassessment at 10 months	With a sample of 35 and a 10 day intervention – then evaluation at 10 months, are the results a true reflection of the intervention?
Jirovec 1991	Yes	No	No significant difference in incontinence when all subjects were compared before and after the toileting programme. $t(13) = .35$, $P > 0.05$ Unit A had significantly less UI post test; $t(5) = 3.46$, $P < 0.02$ (M = 3.66, SD = 2.16 before; M = 1.66, SD = 1.86 after) Unit B – no significant differences post test; $t(7) = -1.69$, $P > 0.05$ (M = 2.75, SD = 1.16 before; M = 2.75, SD = 1.16 after)	Baseline data collection for unstated timeframe; reassessment at the end of 6 week intervention	With a total sample of 14 participants in the study, are the results valid? In Unit A there was a mean reduction in 2 episodes of UI p/p – is this clinically significant?

Table continues

Table 12.3 continued

Study	Statistical data	Between group statistical data	Within group statistical data	Descriptive data	Data collection points	Critical appraisal issues
King 1980	No	No	No	Urinary incontinence: 2 patients were completely cured and 2 were almost cured, 10 patients improved, one patient improved moderately. Faecal incontinence: of 13 incontinent at baseline: 6 were cured, 3 considerable improvement, 2 some improvement, 2 no improvement	1 month of baseline assessment; 4 month intervention	No statistical data and/or definition of improved, moderately improved, considerably improved, some improvement, almost cured
Saltmarche 1991	No	No	No	A significant difference between groups. On further analysis it became evident that while the experimental group did not improve significantly, the control group deteriorated in continence status over the study period	Baseline data based on one week of data collection; 8 week intervention; outcome data – 1 week of data collection	No statistical data reported – study reported as failed by trialist.
Colling 2003	Yes	Frequency of UI: Gp 1: (32) mean = 4.0 episodes/24 hrs [SD 2.63]; Gp 2: (24) mean = 3.43 episodes/ 24 hrs (SD 2.50) $p = 0.23$ Volume of UI: Gp 1: (32) mean = 292 cc 24 hours (SD 202 cc); Gp 2: (24) mean = 193 cc 24 hours (SD 233 cc) $P = 0.02$	UI frequency reduced by an average of 0.9 per 24-hour period from baseline (p = 0.02) UI volume decreased from 480 cc at baseline to 292 cc at the end of treatment ($P = 0.04$)	Skin health: Within group reduction in incidence of skin rash (17.7% at baseline to 9.4% at conclusion of treatment period) Within-group reduction in incidence of skin breakdown (11.6% at baseline to 2.3% at conclusion of treatment period)	Data collection at baseline; following 3 weeks to obtain voiding pattern data. etc.; following a 6-week intervention period; at week 9; at week 12; after a 6-week post-intervention period	Are these results an outcome of the home visits, weekly telephone calls, education on the protocol and support to home based caregivers or HRT? Is 99 ml reduction in volume of UI and/or a reduction of 1.43 episodes of UI per 24 hours clinically significant?

		($P = 0.05$) versus non-significant increase in skin breakdown for control group UTI – *E. coli* at 3 weeks: Gp 1: [5]; Gp 2: [2]; then 1–2 for study duration Caregiver burden – Total reduction from 30% to 18% of caregivers who felt unprepared to care for their care recipient's incontinence Pre intervention – incontinence management third most frequent stressor Post intervention – incontinence management sixth most frequent stressor		
Jirovec 2001	Yes	Baseline UI frequency: Exp gp: M = 0.43, SD 0.23 versus Con gp: M = 0.47, SD = 0.31 6 month UI frequency: Exp gp: M = 0.37, SD 0.28 versus Con gp: M = 0.49, SD 0.36 28/44 in treatment group and 15/30 in control group showed a decrease in incontinence	Baseline – 1 week of voiding diary data; reassessment – at 6 months – 1 week of voiding diary data	Are these results an outcome of the monthly telephone calls, recommendations regarding adequate fluid intake, changes to the home environment to enhance toilet access, education on the protocol and support to home based caregivers or HRT? What is the threshold for a decrease in incontinence and when does a decrease become clinically significant?

Studies are given by first author and date.
UI, urinary incontinence; HRT, habit retraining.

due to the complexity of the intervention and the need for its frequent application (i.e. toileting individuals according to their usual patterns), it was difficult to determine the actual adherence to the study intervention. Therefore it was problematic to draw firm conclusions on the effectiveness of the interventions as the findings may have been directly related to the level of adherence to the intervention rather than to the actual intervention (O'Connell & Warelow, 2001).

Gross analysis of the ten studies revealed that five reported clinical improvements, two had mixed results, one gave results that were difficult to interpret and draw conclusions from, one reported no difference between the intervention and control groups, and one was reported as a failed study and hence did not provide results. Two of the six reports gave outcome data that were comparable. These two trials were the same ones identified in the published Cochrane systematic review. In conclusion, half the studies reported positive findings; however, it was not possible to determine the clinical significance of these results because of variability across studies and the large number of interventions being evaluated at the same time.

Adherence

As implementation of the intervention was dependent on the action of another person/s (i.e. staff working in residential elder care settings, family caregivers and/or research staff), we decided that it was important to acquire information on how easy or difficult it was for them to adhere to the study intervention. Qualitative and quantitative data on adherence were available for six of the ten studies on HRT. Only one study provided statistical data on adherence, reporting that usual care staff adhered to the protocol 61% of the time (Colling et al., 1992) (Table 12.4).

Factors identified as impeding adherence to the study protocol in residential elder care settings included:

- Constant changes in nursing staff
- Daily staff shortages and heavy workloads
- Personality factors and group dynamics among staff
- A preference by usual care staff for their existing routines

- The additional time involved in implementing HRT compared to usual care
- A lack of perceived benefit to the usual care staff
- A belief by usual care staff that the absence of complete cure was not worth the effort or that patients were 'too difficult or demented' to be toileted
- Use of relief staff, bed closures and patient relocations

By contrast, factors that facilitated HRT in residential elder care settings included: staff commitment to maintaining the routines and incorporating individualised toileting procedures into other routine activities.

Factors that impeded adherence to the study protocol amongst community-dwelling care-dependent people included:

- The burden of care for caregivers
- Care-dependent people resistant to being toileted, and
- The requirement to monitor the care-dependent voiding pattern for a consistent period of time

Use of an electronic voiding recorder was suggested as a viable alternative that might mitigate some of the latter barriers.

Discussion

The systematic review on HRT conducted under the guidelines of the Cochrane Collaboration Incontinence Review Group provided sound evaluation data on the clinical efficacy of HRT or lack thereof due to small sample size, insufficient studies, outcomes and follow-up data (see Ostaszkiewicz et al., 2004); however, these guidelines did not offer a model for: (1) synthesising non-clinical outcome data from these studies, and/or for (2) including evidence from mixed design studies. Our integrative review did not alter the findings on the question of clinical effectiveness of HRT reported in the original systematic review on HRT (Ostaszkiewicz et al., 2004). Although a further three studies were identified that reported improved continence results using HRT, the heterogeneity of these studies made it difficult to aggregate the data and draw sound conclusions on clinical effectiveness. The addition of information from non-randomised controlled studies did, however, provide data illustrating the

Table 12.4 Adherence to habit retraining and researchers' reflections on barriers and facilitators to the intervention.

Setting	Study	Adherence	Researchers' reflections
Out-patient clinic for people with incontinence	Baigis-Smith 1989	No data provided.	No comment by researcher on adherence
Long-term care setting	Chanfreau-Rona 1984	'Constant changes in nursing staff, daily staff shortages and heavy workloads resulted in non-completion of follow-up for Groups 2 and 3 and discontinuation of counting wet pants for Gp 1'	'Personality factors and group dynamics among staff in different wards impacts upon the validity of the results. Staff shortages and high workloads impede implementation of the interventions. Final improvement is related to initial level of incontinence, indicating the need to implement interventions as soon as symptoms arise'
	Chanfreau-Rona 1986	No data provided.	No comment by researcher on adherence
	Colling 1992	'Staff adhered to protocol 61% of the time'	'Introducing and maintaining programmes, such as PURT, in nursing homes are complex undertakings. First, there must be careful selection of which residents should receive a particular type of UI management. Second, UI management should be taught to new aides, and the practice of experienced aides teaching new aides should be questioned as it leads to reinforcing the status quo. Many of the nursing staff preferred to maintain their current routines rather than adjust to individual patient needs which may have occurred partly because it took staff an average of 2.5 minutes longer per resident to toilet rather than to change them when they were wet. Thus, nursing aides did not experience a benefit from toileting residents, especially those who were quite immobile. Further, some commented that unless the resident could be trained to be completely continent, it was not worth toileting them. Other reasons given for not following the toileting programme: were too hard to change routines; it is better to change residents than to bother them with toileting; they are too difficult or too demented to be toileted. Finally, a few aides expressed resentment about the project being imposed on them by administration and outsiders. These comments raise the question: who *does* make specific patient care decisions?'

Table continues

Table 12.4 continued

Setting	Study	Adherence	Researchers' reflections
	Gaitsgori 1998	No data provided	'This protocol initially demands instance and persistence and requires more attention and care from the part of the staff. The protocol finally becomes a part of daily routine in the nursing home and is rewarding. Success is due to the tailored individuals scheme and particularly depends on the constant supervision of the nursing staff'
	Jirovec 1991	'In Unit B where no significant change in incontinence occurred, the toileting procedure was poorly implemented'	'Inconsistencies in the staffing environment and the individualised toileting programme in Home B actually resulted in a greater degree of incontinence after the programme.' "The average nursing home with its shortages of professional nursing staff would have difficulty implementing a similar programme unless competent nursing supervision was available to incorporate individualized toileting procedures within other routine activities on the floor'
	King 1980	No data provided.	No comment by researcher on adherence
	Saltmarche 1991	Although the study was well designed using conventional methodology and monitored closely by a full-time research associate utilising manipulation checks for the application of the intervention, the analysis indicated that the Habit Retraining intervention had not been consistently implemented.	'Lack of control of the environment, coupled with nursing shortages, use of relief staff, bed closures and patient relocation are factors negatively impacting upon intervention research.' 'The heterogeneity of the population and the changes in a number of important variables, over this period of time brings into question the use of conventional research design methods, such as randomized controlled studies'
Home carers	Colling 2003	'Comments made to the research nurses when they visited to collect data raised doubts about the consistency of following the PURT prescriptions for some subjects. Data logger information confirmed this concern'	'The use of the electronic voiding recorder uncovered a number of voiding diary recording discrepancies; therefore its use to monitor compliance is superior to relying on voiding diaries alone.' 'Accessing and retaining an adequate sample to conduct this study was challenging.' 'It is possible the prescriptions were only carried out as caregivers had the time and energy to add this new care routine into their already busy lives'
	Jirovec 2001	'Caregivers in both groups found keeping a weeklong record burdensome: thus more frequent measurement of degree of incontinence was not thought to be feasible. Caregivers in the treatment group did not normally keep a record of incontinent episodes'	'Several more severely cognitively impaired elders successfully participated in the programme – most were uncooperative with the toileting protocol and resisted attempts to toilet them.' 'Caregivers are the best judges as to whether the cognitively impaired elder can be toileted on a regular basis'

Studies are given by first author and date.
PURT, patterned urge-response toileting; UI, urinary incontinence.

complexity of conducting this type of trial and the need for further resources to implement and maintain HRT.

Another finding was the variation in timing of measuring patient outcomes. For example, studies varied in:

- Duration of the baseline assessment to establish patients' voiding patterns
- Duration of the intervention, and
- Timing of data collection

While some studies had multiple data collection points, others were limited to pre- and post-intervention data collection. It is likely that this variation in data collection, rather than the intervention itself, could explain the differences in levels of continence (O'Connell & Warelow, 2001). This issue of determining the correct time frames for measurement is another factor that needs to be researched prior to evaluation studies being conducted on HRT.

The findings from this integrative review suggest that there are some key resource issues that need to be considered when implementing and maintaining HRT. Schnelle et al. (1998) noted that clinical intervention protocols are often developed without consideration of future implementation factors and that, even if an intervention is clinically effective, it is not likely to be adopted unless it is also practical to implement and maintain. The practical issues that need to be considered in implementing and maintaining HRT include the ability and preparedness of staff or caregivers to perform the necessary assessment and implementation procedures, receptiveness of patients to receiving the intervention, additional time required for staff or caregivers to conduct the procedures and the frequency and duration of assessment and monitoring. Data from the integrative review revealed different durations and frequencies of collecting assessment and monitoring information on voiding patterns and incontinence. As this process is labour intensive, it is important to establish the optimum time necessary to obtain accurate information on continence status.

In addition, this integrative review identified a number of factors that impede or support adherence to HRT, and this information seems fundamental to the development of future research in this area. A recent review on patient adherence to treatment suggests that poor compliance with therapeutic regimens is a major healthcare problem and, while there is no gold standard for the measurement of adherence to treatment, the absence of this measurement in research can significantly affect the validity and reliability of research findings (Vermeire et al., 2001).

Factors identified from the integrative review that were found to impede adherence to HRT included: the time-consuming nature of the intervention, staff commitment to routinely performing the intervention in the context of a demanding workload and patient resistance to the intervention. These findings are supported by previous research that has consistently reported the difficulties of sustaining rehabilitative or behavioural interventions for continence care in frail older adults in settings that rely on those interventions being implemented by usual care staff or caregivers, even when those interventions have been clinically effective (Schnelle, 1990; Colling et al., 1992). Although the findings from the integrative review reveal the involvement of research staff, this increase in resources did not ensure full adherence. Therefore, it is likely that, when staffing levels return to usual levels and research staff are unavailable, the implementation of HRT may be difficult within the constraints of a usual workload. This is supported by DuBeau (2005:1254), who reported that 'prompted voiding decreases urinary incontinence rates in clinical trials, but its implementation fades once research assistance leave and regular staff take over'. This indicates that current staffing and funding models used in residential elder care settings may be inadequate to support labour-intensive continence management strategies and that funding agencies need to consider this issue in their funding formulas. The recommendation for residential care facilities to be staffed more appropriately to enable residents to receive appropriate continence care is not new. Schnelle et al. (2002), for example, trialled an exercise and incontinence intervention in a nursing home setting and reported improvements in both outcomes. However, this improvement was based on a ratio of five residents to one nursing assistant.

It was also evident that some of the barriers to implementing HRT were similar for both residential care and community settings. These barriers related to the burden of care, care-dependent individuals being resistant to being toileted, and the difficulties associated with the requirement of monitoring voiding patterns for a consistent period of time. These findings are interesting as they indicate that the constant burden experienced by carers in community settings may render the use of HRT difficult as its use may add to this burden. Given that one of the most common reasons for carers to place older dependants in residential care is related to incontinence (Pearson, 2003), it is important that healthcare workers recommend strategies that assist caregivers to provide continence care that is practical to implement and maintain.

Conclusion

The integrative review method outlined in this chapter to examine the evidence from both quantitative and qualitative studies was consistent with the approach used to conduct a systematic review in that it was systematic, explicit and reproducible. It differed, however, from the traditional systematic review as it considered different types and levels of evidence. The key challenge in conducting this integrative review was the task of combining data on clinical effectiveness from different types of studies in which different outcome measures were used. The findings from the original systematic review on HRT (a total of three studies) provided qualified support for the use of HRT. The inclusion of findings from the seven additional studies considered in the integrative review presented conflicting findings on the clinical effectiveness of HRT. Although two of these studies demonstrated positive findings, this outcome was negated by the five studies in which findings were equivocal. Consequently, no firm conclusions could be drawn about the clinical effectiveness of HRT, and further evaluative studies are required.

The integrative review has, nevertheless, offered different and useful insights that extend beyond the clinical effectiveness question. Specifically, it offered a model for systematically analysing descriptive and comparable data on other factors. These data have provided contextual information on a number of important factors that need to be considered in the development of future studies evaluating HRT, including the need for adequate human and material resources to implement and maintain HRT and increase adherence to the protocol. These findings have implications for practice,

demonstrating the labour-intensive nature of conducting HRT and raising questions about the feasibility of implementing HRT against the backdrop of limited human and monetary resources. As this integrative review revealed anomalies in adherence to the research protocol, we question whether the Cochrane review process could be strengthened by considering adherence to the protocol in greater depth.

Another issue highlighted was the different time frames and methods used to conduct baseline assessment and to measure patient outcomes. This lack of standardisation needs to be addressed to minimise the extent to which vulnerable participants are subjected to intense assessment and measurement procedures.

Although conducting this integrative review proved challenging, it offered insights that are not necessarily captured by aggregating statistical data from RCTs. The method used in this integrative review offers one approach to managing data from different types of studies and highlights the benefits of considering different sources of research data. Although we confined the data extracted to a few categories, the potential exists to extract and review an unlimited volume of data from studies that are comparable and to elicit insights that either enhance or challenge the findings from reviews that aim for a single summary estimate.

References

Abrams, P., Cardozo, L., Khoury, S. & Wein, A. (eds) (2005) *Incontinence*, 3rd edn. Health Publication, Plymouth, UK.

Alderson, P., Green, S. & Higgins, J.P.T. (eds) (2004) Assessment of study quality. *Cochrane Reviewers' Handbook 4.2.1*, Section 4. The Cochrane Library, Issue 1. John Wiley & Sons, Chichester.

Baigis-Smith, J., Smith, D.A., Rose, M. & Newman, D.K. (1989) Managing urinary incontinence in community-residing elderly persons. *The Gerontologist*, 29 (2), 229–33.

Carper, B. (1978) Fundamental patterns of knowing in nursing. *Advances in Nursing Science*, 1 (1), 13–23.

Chanfreau-Rona, D., Bellwood, S. & Wylie, B. (1984) Assessment of a behavioural programme to treat incontinent patients in psychogeriatric wards. *British Journal of Clinical Psychology*, 23 (4), 273–9.

Chanfreau-Rona, D., Wylie, B. & Bellwood, S. (1986) Behaviour treatment of daytime incontinence in elderly male and female patients. *Behavioural Psychotherapy*, 14 (1), 13–20.

Clay, E.C. (1978) Habit retraining: a tested method to regain urinary control. *Geriatric Nursing*, 1 (4), 252–4.

Colling, J., Ouslander, J., Hadley, B.J., Eisch, J. & Campbell, E.B. (1992) The effects of patterned urge-response toileting (PURT) on urinary incontinence among nursing home residents. *Journal of the American Geriatric Society*, 40 (2), 135–41.

Colling, J., Owen, T.R., McMcreedy, M. & Newman, D. (2003) The effects of a continence program on frail community dwelling elderly persons. *Urologic Nursing*, 23 (2), 117–31.

Daly, J., Kellehear, A. & Gliksman, M. (1997) *The Public Health Researcher: A Methodological Approach*. Oxford University Press, Melbourne, Australia.

DuBeau, C. (2005) Improving urinary incontinence in nursing home residents: Are we FIT to be tied? *Journal of the American Geriatrics Society*, 53, 1254–6.

Fantl, J.A., Newman, D.K., Colling, J. et al. (1996) *Managing Acute and Chronic Urinary Incontinence*. Clinical Practice Guideline. Quick References Guide for Clinicians, No. 2. U.S. Department of Health and Human Services, Public Health Service, Rockville, MD. Agency for Health Care Policy and Research. Available at website http://www.nlm.nih.gov (retrieved 9 June 2003).

Fonda, D., Resnick, N.M., Colling, J. et al. (1998) Outcome measures for research of lower urinary tract dysfunction in frail older people. *Neurourology and Urodynamics*, 17 (3), 273–81.

Gaitsgori, Y., Gruenwald, I., Zarmi, S. & Michalak, R. (1998) Individual timed voiding as a long term treatment modality for demented patients in nursing homes. Abstracts from the 28th Annual Meeting International Continence Society, Jerusalem, Israel. *Neurourology and Urodynamics*, 17 (4), 323–4.

Higgins, J.P.T. & Green, S. (eds) (2005) *Cochrane Handbook for Systematic Reviews of Interventions 4.3.5*, (updated May 2005). The Cochrane Library, Issue 3. John Wiley & Sons, Chichester, UK.

Hughes, J. (1990) *The Philosophy of Social Research: Aspects of Modern Sociology*, 2nd edn. Longman, London & New York.

JBI (The Joanna Briggs Institute) (2006) Available at website http://www.joannabriggs.edu.au/pubs/approach.php (retrieved 7 November 2006).

Jirovec, M.M. (1991) Effect of individualized prompted toileting on incontinence in nursing home residents. *Applied Nursing Research*, 4 (4), 188–91.

Jirovec, M.M. & Templin, T. (2001) Predicting success using individualised scheduled toileting for memory-impaired elders at home. *Research in Nursing and Health*, 24 (1), 1–8.

King, M.R. (1980) Treatment of incontinence. *Nursing Times*, June, 1006–10.

Kunz, R., Vist, G. & Oxman, A.D. (2006) Randomisation to protect against selection bias in healthcare trials (Cochrane Methodology Review). The Cochrane Library, Issue 4. Update Software, Oxford.

Mattiasson, A., Djurhuus, J.C., Fonda, D., Lose, G., Nordling, J. & Stohrer, M. (1998) Standardization of outcome studies in patients with lower urinary tract dysfunction: a report on general principles from the Standardisation Committee of the International Continence Society. *Neurourology and Urodynamics*, 17 (3), 249–53.

NHMRC (National Health and Medical Research Council) (1999) A guide to the development, implementation and evaluation of clinical practice guidelines. Available at website http://www.nhmrc.gov.au/publications/_files/cp30.pdf (retrieved 4 November 2006).

O'Connell, B. & Warelow (2001) Challenges of measuring and linking patient outcomes to nursing interventions in acute care settings. *Nursing and Health Sciences*, 3, 113–17.

O'Connell, B. & Myers, H. (2001) A failed fall prevention study in an acute care setting: Lessons from the swamp. *International Journal of Nursing Practice*, 7, 126–30.

Ostaszkiewicz, J., Johnston, L. & Roe, B. (2004) Habit retraining for the management of urinary incontinence in adults. *The Cochrane Database of Systematic Reviews*, (2), CD002801.

Pearson, A. (2003) *Incidence of Incontinence as a Factor in Admission to Aged Care Homes*. Publications Production Unit Report No. 42. Australian Government, Canberra, Australia.

Saltmarche, A., Pringle, D.M., Reid, D.W. & Zorzitto, M. (1991) Habit retraining: an incontinence study that leaked. *Neurourology and Urodynamics*, 10 (4), 413–14.

Schnelle, J.F. (1990) Treatment of urinary incontinence in nursing homes by prompted voiding. *Journal of the American Geriatrics Society*, 38, 356–60.

Schnelle, J.F., Cruise, P.A., Rahman, A. & Ouslander, J.G. (1998) Developing rehabilitative behavioral interventions for long-term care: technology, transfer, acceptance and maintenance issues. *Journal of the American Geriatrics Society*, 46 (6), 771–7.

Schnelle, J.F., Alessi, C.A., Simmons, S.F., Al-Samarrai, J.R., Beck, J.C. & Ouslander, J.G. (2002) Translating clinical research into practice: A randomized controlled trial of exercise and incontinence care with nursing home residents. *Journal of the American Geriatrics Society*, 50, 1476–83.

Upshur, R.E.G., Van Den Kerkhof, E.G. & Goel, V. (2001) Meaning and measurement: An inclusive model of evidence in health care. *Journal of Evaluation in Clinical Practice*, 7 (2), 91–6.

Vermeire, E., Hearnshaw, H., Van Royen, P. & Denekens, J. (2001) Patient adherence to treatment: three decades of research. A comprehensive review. *Journal of Clinical Pharmacy and Therapeutics*, 26, 331–42.

Whittemore, R. & Knafl, K. (2005) The integrative review: updated methodology. *Journal of Advanced Nursing*, 52 (5), 546–53.

Appendix 12.1   Table of included studies for integration of evidence from mixed design studies on habit retraining

A. **Baigis-Smith, J., Smith, D.A., Rose, M. & Newman, D.K. (1989) Managing urinary incontinence in community-residing elderly persons. *The Gerontologist*, 29 (2), 229–33.**

Participants	Methods	Intervention	Outcomes	Intervention implementation strategies	Resource requirements	Assessment and evaluation methods	Attrition and reasons	Adherence to protocol
54 volunteers aged 60 or over	Before and after study with a single group	Kegel exercises with biofeedback + intervention called habit retraining combined with relaxation techniques, and information on habit training, diet modification and bowel regimes. 2 weekly visits until improvement seen	Mean number of urinary accidents per week At baseline: 17 (median 8; SD 26; range 0.5–140) (n = 54) At end of treatment: 4 (median 0.8, SD 8; range 0–42) (n = 54) At follow-up 1-month: 3 (median 0.5; SD 7; range 0–36) (n = 46) 3-month: 6 (median 0.5; SD 13; range 0–56) (n = 39) 6-month: 4 (median 1; SD 9; range 0–35) (n = 33) 1-year: 1 (median 0; SD 2; range 0–7) (n = 19) t-test for baseline and end of treatment: t(54) = 4.99, P < 0.0005 Mean peak perineometer readings At baseline: 7 (median 6; SD 4; range 2–19) End of treatment: 10 (median 8; SD 3; range 4–34)	Kegel exercises augmented by biofeedback, habit training and relaxation techniques	Nurse practitioner care, mean number of visits: 3 Perineometer	Mini-Mental State Questionnaire (MMS) to assess cognitive status. Self-reported. Bladder record: 2 hourly record of voiding and fluid intake, including normal urination and episodes of urinary incontinence, amounts of leakage, and cause of accidents, for the duration of the treatment (mean treatment duration 3 × 2 weekly visits) and for 2 weeks prior to each follow-up at 1, 3, 6 and 12 months.	25% Data not collected on reason	No data provided

Perineometer readings of pubococcygeal muscle strength (reliability established by manufacturer) mean of 3 readings each of peak and hold readings at baseline, at each treatment visit, end of treatment and 1, 3, 6 and 12 month follow-up

At follow-up
1-month: 10 (median 8; SD 6; range 4–31)
3-month: 11 (median 8; SD 8; range 2–32)
6-month: 10 (median 8; SD 6; range 4–27)
1-year: 10 (median 7; SD 7; range 4–25)
Mean sustained hold perineometer readings
At baseline: 3 (median 3; SD 2; range 0.3–10)
End of treatment: 6 (median 5; SD 3; range 2–15)

At follow-up
1-month: 6 (median 5; SD 3; range 0.9–5)
3-month: 6 (median 5; SD 3; range 0.4–5)
6-month: 6 (median 5; SD 3; range 2–13)
1-year: 7 (median 5; SD 5; range 2–17)
t-test peak mean: $t(54) = -4.8$, $P < 0.0005$
Mean sustained hold: $t(54) = -5.6$, $P < 0.0005$

Appendix continues

Appendix 12.1 continued

B. Chanfreau-Rona, D., Bellwood, S. & Wylie, B. (1984) Assessment of a behavioural programme to treat incontinent patients in psychogeriatric wards. *British Journal of Clinical Psychology*, 23 (4), 273–9.

Participants	Methods	Intervention	Outcomes	Resource requirements	Intervention implementation strategies	Assessment and evaluation methods	Attrition and reasons	Adherence to protocol
24 females from 3 psychogeriatric wards	Cohort study with purposive selection based on levels of UI and usual care control group	Changes to the ward environment to enhance residents' ability to access the toilet for all groups. Ward A: HRT + social reinforcement for 4 weeks and then partial reinforcement for 2 weeks, reassessment, followed by 9 weeks usual care, reassessment. Ward B: Usual care (4-hourly toileting) for 6 weeks. Ward C: Usual care (4-hourly toileting) + emphasis on environmental changes	Mean frequency of incontinence: Ward A: Baseline, 13; weeks 9 and 10, 11; 9 weeks later, 12. Ward B: Baseline, 17; weeks 12 and 13, 24. Ward C: Baseline, 24: (weeks 9 and 10)	Assessment and implementation procedures implemented by usual care staff with research staff supervision	Weekly meetings with ward staff to discuss problems and provide feedback, including data on numbers of incontinence aids used	Baseline 2 week period of 2 hourly checks by nursing staff. Clifton Assessment Procedures for the Elderly (CAPE) conducted by researchers and nursing staff at baseline and at the end of reassessment. Nurse's subjective assessment of the patient's incontinence. Numbers of incontinence aids used each month – not reported	No data provided	'Constant changes in nursing staff, daily staff shortages and heavy workloads resulted in non completion of follow-up for Groups 2 and 3 and discontinuation of counting wet pants for Gp 1' 21-week follow-up not completed

Researchers' reflections: 'Personality factors and group dynamics among staff in different wards impacts upon the validity of the results. Staff shortages and high workloads impede implementation of the interventions. Final improvement is related to initial level of incontinence, indicating the need to implement interventions as soon as symptoms arise.'

C. Chanfreau-Rona, D., Wylie, B. & Bellwood, S. (1986) Behaviour treatment of daytime incontinence in elderly male and female patients. *Behavioural Psychotherapy*, **14** (1), 13–20.

Participants	Methods	Intervention	Outcomes	Resource requirements	Intervention implementation strategies	Assessment and evaluation methods	Attrition and reasons	Adherence to protocol
30 females and males from 4 psychogeriatric wards	Cohort study with purposive selection based on levels of UI and usual care control group	2 weeks baseline followed by environmental changes to all wards. Gp 1: 2 weeks habit retraining + verbal and material rewards followed by 3 weeks of partial reinforcement followed by 2 weeks of full reinforcement. Gp 2: Usual care	No significant difference between intervention and control groups on frequency of incontinence. Results stratified by baseline level of incontinence (Low Wetters, wet 7 or less times per week and High Wetters, wet 8 or more times per week) showed that for Low Wetters the intervention group were significantly better on level of continence than the control group at follow-up. For Higher Wetters the control group did better than the intervention group. Differential rate of response between patients with different degrees of incontinence was supported	3 × 2 weeks at baseline, end of intervention and follow-up by usual care staff. Painting of toilet doors, placing of signs on doors and plastic footsteps on floors. Rescheduling of usual care to 'peak times' for toileting, with reinforcers (i.e. sweets)		2-hourly checks for 2 weeks at baseline, at end of intervention and at 3-month follow-up. Clifton Assessment Procedures for the Elderly (CAPE). Conducted by researchers and nursing staff at baseline and at the end of intervention and at 3-month follow-up	3 patients died, 1 in intervention group, 2 in control group	No information provided

Appendix continues

Appendix 12.1 continued

D. Colling, J., Ouslander, J., Hadley, B.J., Eisch, J. & Campbell, E.B. (1992) The effects of patterned urge-response toileting (PURT) on urinary incontinence among nursing home residents. *Journal of the American Geriatric Society*, 40 (2), 135–41.

Participants	Methods	Intervention	Outcomes	Resource requirements	Intervention implementation strategies	Assessment and evaluation methods	Attrition and reasons	Adherence to protocol
$n = 113$ elderly nursing home residents. Gp 1: (51) Gp 2: (37)	Cluster RCT	Individualised scheduled toileting versus usual care	Between-group data on frequency of UI: Gp 1: (51) mean = 4.5 versus Gp 2: (37); mean = 5.5. Volume of UI: Gp 1: (51) mean = 600 cc versus Gp 2: (37); mean = 650 cc. Within-group data on frequency of UI frequency ratio from 0.7 at baseline to mean 0.57 during treatment ($P > 0.000$). Within-group data on volume of UI: small significant differences in the mean volume over the 14 data collection periods ($t = 2.60$, $P < 0.005$)	12 weeks assessment and evaluation procedures implemented by research staff. PURT implemented by usual care staff following 4 hours of education/ training. It took staff 2.5 minutes longer per resident to toilet than to change them	Individualised scheduled toileting 24 hours/day for 12 weeks combined with staff education, feedback and encouragement	Mean volume of incontinence per individual per 24 hours based on pad weighing + frequency of UI measured over 24-hour periods at 3 week intervals for 36 weeks based on hourly checks – enhanced by data logger	Attrition of 25: Gp 1: 12; Gp 2: 13. 88/113 completed the study. Reasons for attrition: death and illness	Staff adhered to protocol 61% of the time

Researchers' reflections: 'Introducing and maintaining programmes, such as PURT, in nursing homes are complex undertakings. First, there must be careful selection of which residents should receive a particular type of urinary incontinence management. Second, UI management should be taught to new aides, and the practice of experienced aides teaching new aides should be questioned as it leads to reinforcing the status quo. Many of the nursing staff preferred to maintain their current routines rather than adjust to individual patient needs which may have occurred partly because it took staff an average of 2.5 minutes longer per resident to toilet than to change them when they were wet. Thus, nursing aides did not experience a benefit from toileting residents, especially those who were quite immobile. Further, some commented that unless the resident could be trained to be completely continent, it was not worth toileting them. Other reasons given for not following the toileting programme: were too hard to change routines; it is better to change residents than to bother them with toileting; they are too difficult or too demented to be toileted. Finally, a few aides expressed resentment about the project being imposed on them by administration and outsiders. These comments raise the question: who *does* make specific patient care decisions?'

E. Colling, J., Owen, T.R., McMcreedy, M. & Newman, D. (2003) The effects of a continence programme on frail community dwelling elderly persons. *Urologic Nursing*, 23 (2), 117–31.

Participants	Methods	Intervention	Outcomes	Resource requirements	Intervention implementation strategies	Assessment and evaluation methods	Attrition and reasons	Adherence to protocol
n = 102 home-based family caregivers and their care recipient (many with cognitive impairment)	RCT	Individualised scheduled toileting for 6 weeks versus deferred patterned-urge response toileting (PURT)	Frequency of UI: Gp 1: (32) mean = 4.0 episodes/24 hours (SD 2.82) Gp 2: (24) mean = 3.43 episodes/24 hours (SD 1.93) UI frequency reduced by an average of 0.9 per 24-hour period from baseline (*P* = 0.02). Volume of UI: Gp 1: (32) mean = 292 cc 24 hours (SD 202 cc), Gp 2: (24) mean = 193 cc 24 hours (SD 233 cc) Average volume of UI volume decreased from 480 cc at baseline to 292 cc at the end of treatment (*P* = 0.04). Other outcomes: skin health, UTI and caregiver burden	Research staff home visits: (6 visits per participant) and weekly F/U phone calls. Temperature-sensitive thermister (used to detect UI episodes) connected to an electronic data logger. Ultrasound bladder scanner		3 weeks assessment and evaluation procedures implemented by caregivers and research staff, involving 2-hourly wet checks for 24 hours/day for 3 days × 6 times	Attrition rate 28/106 Reasons for attrition: illness, death, caregivers declined to continue, unavailable	'A lack of consistency was noted in some caregivers' protocol adherence. The data logger confirmed voiding diary recording discrepancies'

Appendix continues

Appendix 12.1 continued

Participants	Methods	Intervention	Outcomes	Resource requirements	Intervention implementation strategies	Assessment and evaluation methods	Attrition and reasons	Adherence to protocol
			Skin health: within-group reduction in incidence of skin rash (17.7% at baseline to 9.4% at conclusion of treatment period). Within-group reduction in incidence of skin breakdown (11.6% at baseline to 2.3% at conclusion of treatment period) ($P = 0.05$) versus non-significant increase in skin breakdown for control group. UTI: *E. coli* at 3 weeks Gp 1: [5] Gp 2: [2] then 1–2 for study duration. Caregiver burden: total reduction from 30% to 18% of caregivers who felt unprepared to care for their care recipient's incontinence. Pre-intervention – incontinence management 3rd most frequent stressor Post-intervention – incontinence management 6th most frequent stressor					

Researchers' reflections: 'The use of the electronic voiding recorder uncovered a number of voiding diary recording discrepancies; therefore its use to monitor compliance is superior to relying on voiding diaries alone. The authors note the difficulty of recruiting an appropriate sample and, further that retention in studies is problematic among frail elders and their caregivers.'

F. Gaitsgori, Y., Gruenwald, I., Zarmi, S. & Michalak, R. (1998) Individual timed voiding as a long-term treatment modality for demented patients in nursing homes. Abstracts from the 28th Annual Meeting International Continence Society, Jerusalem, Israel. *Neurourology and Urodynamics,* 17 (4), 323–4.

Participants	Methods	Intervention	Outcomes	Resource requirements	Intervention implementation strategies	Assessment and evaluation methods	Attrition and reasons	Adherence to protocol
$n = 35$ 'demented' patients from 2 nursing homes	Before and after study with a single group	10 days of individualised toileting schedule + medication	94% of patients improved: 15 (43%) totally dry and 18 (51%) dry during the day. 6% failed treatment	Usual care staff	Frequent re-evaluation and adjustments were made during intervention period. A full explanation on this modality and its aims was given to caregivers and to most patients	Baseline: 3 days of 1 hourly checks to identify the patients optimal voiding times. Evaluation at 10 months	No data	No data

Researchers' reflections: 'This protocol initially demands instance and persistence and requires more attention and care from the part of the staff. The protocol finally becomes a part of daily routine in the nursing home and is rewarding. Success is due to the tailored individuals' scheme and particularly depends on the constant supervision of the nursing staff.'

Appendix continues

Appendix 12.1 continued

G. Jirovec, M.M. (1991) Effect of individualized prompted toileting on incontinence in nursing home residents. *Applied Nursing Research*, 4 (4), 188–91.

Participants	Methods	Intervention	Outcomes	Resource requirements	Intervention implementation strategies	Assessment and evaluation methods	Attrition and reasons	Adherence to protocol
n = 14 elderly in long-term care – average age 86.9 years	Quasi-experimental pretest – post-test design	6 weeks of individualised PV	No significant difference in incontinence when all subjects were compared before and after the toileting programme. *t*(13) = 0.35, *P* > 0.05. Unit A: had significantly less UI post-test *t*(5) = 3.46, p < 0.02 (M = 3.66, SD = 2.16 before; M = 1.66, SD = 1.86 after). Unit B: no significant differences post-test *t*(7) = −1.69, *P* > 0.05 (M = 1.62, SD = 1.06) and after (M = 2.75, SD = 1.16	Research staff conducted clinical assessments. Nursing aides conducted baseline and evaluation checks and implemented the intervention with education/ support from research staff	The nurse aides were instructed to toilet residents at the identified times, indicate on the forms the results of each toileting episode as well as indicating times and approximate amounts of wet episodes. A new form was posted each day and forms were reviewed on a weekly basis and the residents' voiding times adjusted accordingly	1-hourly checks from 07.00 to 22.00 hours – duration is unreported	No data	In Unit B where no significant change in incontinence occurred, the toileting procedure was poorly implemented

Researchers' reflections: 'Inconsistencies in the staffing environment and the individualised toileting programme in Home B actually resulted in a greater degree of incontinence after the program.' 'The average nursing home with its shortages of professional nursing staff would have difficulty implementing a similar programme unless competent nursing supervision was available to incorporate individualized toileting procedures within other routine activities on the floor.'

H. Jirovec, M.M. & Templin, T. (2001) Predicting success using individualised scheduled toileting for memory-impaired elders at home. *Research in Nursing and Health*, 24 (1), 1–8.

Participants	Methods	Intervention	Outcomes	Resource requirements	Intervention implementation strategies	Assessment and evaluation methods	Attrition and reasons	Adherence to protocol
n = 118 community-dwelling elders with cognitive impairment	RCT	6 months of individualised scheduled toileting + education on bladder function versus socialisation support	Baseline UI frequency: Exp gp: M = 0.43, SD 0.23 versus Con gp: M = 0.47, SD = 0.31. 6-month UI frequency: Exp gp: M = 0.37, SD 0.28 versus Con gp: M = 0.49, SD = 0.36. 28/44 in treatment group and 15/30 in control group showed a decrease in incontinence	Assessment conducted by nurses with expertise in continence. Support visits/education provided by research staff. Protocol implemented by home-based caregivers with research staff overseeing	Home visits by research staff. Voiding schedule developed in consultation with caregiver. Monthly phone calls to both groups. Fluid patterns discussed and recommendations provided re. fluid intake. Contextual home stimuli manipulated	Week-long voiding records pre- and post-intervention kept by caregivers	44/118 (37%) attrition Reasons: 2 elders got sick, 14 reported it was too burdensome or were unable to be contacted at second data collection point, 9 died and 19 were admitted to a nursing home	'Caregivers in both groups found keeping a week-long record burdensome: thus more frequent measurement of degree of incontinence was not thought to be feasible. Caregivers in the treatment group did not normally keep a record of incontinent episodes.'

Researchers' reflections: 'Several more severely cognitively impaired elders successfully participated in the program – most were uncooperative with the toileting protocol and resisted attempts to toilet them.' 'Caregivers are the best judges as to whether the cognitively impaired elder can be toileted on a regular basis.'

Appendix continues

Appendix 12.1 continued

I. King, M.R. (1980) Treatment of incontinence. *Nursing Times*, June, 1006–10.

Participants	Methods	Intervention	Outcomes	Resource requirements	Intervention implementation strategies	Assessment and evaluation methods	Attrition and reasons	Adherence to protocol
15 elderly women from psychogeriatric wards	Before and after study with a single group	HRT	Urinary incontinence: 2 patients were completely cured and 2 were almost cured, 10 patients improved, one patient improved moderately. Faecal incontinence of 13 incontinent at baseline: 6 were cured, 3 considerable improvement, 2 some improvement, 2 no improvement	Usual care staff conducted baseline checks and implemented intervention and provided feedback for evaluation. Medical care: 2 weekly MSUs and rectal examinations	Nurses were made aware that the success or failure of the project would be attributed to them	1 month observation period, hourly recording of continence	No data	No data.

J. Saltmarche, A., Pringle, D.M., Reid, D.W. & Zorzitto, M. (1991) Habit retraining: an incontinence study that leaked. *Neurourology and Urodynamics*, 10 (4), 413–14.

Participants	Methods	Intervention	Outcomes	Resource requirements	Intervention implementation strategies	Assessment and evaluation methods	Attrition and reasons	Adherence to protocol
40 elderly males (age not stated) residing in a long-term care facility	RCT	9 weeks' duration/Gp 1 : 4 weeks of HRT then 4 weeks with no formal monitoring and 1 week of follow-up. HRT included individualised toileting, positive social reinforcement, adequate fluid intake and a colour-coded dot chart to record information versus delayed treatment	Experimental group did not improve significantly compared with baseline over the study period. Control group deteriorated in continence status over the study period	Research medical staff conducted clinical assessments. Research associate monitored intervention. Nursing staff implemented individualised toileting regime and social reinforcement and recorded data on colour-coded dot chart	Nursing staff education workshops. Full-time research associate utilised manipulation checks for the application of the intervention	Urological review (consent for cystoscopy and urodynamics were requested for each subject). 'Standardised indices' used to assess cognitive and functional levels	No data.	Although the study was well designed using conventional methodology and monitored closely by a full-time research associate utilising manipulation checks for the application of the intervention, the analysis indicated that the Habit Retraining intervention had not been consistently implemented

Researchers' reflections: Lack of control of the environment, coupled with nursing shortages, use of relief staff, bed closures and patient relocation are factors negatively impacting upon intervention research. The heterogeneity of the population and the changes in a number of important variables over this period of time brings into question the use of conventional research design methods, such as randomised controlled studies.

13 What Makes a Good Midwife?

Lynn Nicholls and Christine Webb

Introduction

In this chapter we discuss an integrative review designed to answer the question: 'What makes a good midwife?'. The underlying motivation for the review was that we could not find a research-based definition of a good midwife that could be used in research and curriculum development. We give an overview of the review, including the protocol and search methods, how we appraised the studies included, and the methodological issues in these studies. We then report the review findings and discuss issues arising when conducting the review. Finally, we draw some conclusions for future integrative reviews and for midwifery care.

Background

Few studies have been reported that relate directly to our review question. Kennedy (1995, 2000) in the USA carried out a study to define an 'exemplary midwife' – an equivalent term to 'good' in this context. She concluded that three themes were vital to exemplary midwifery care: (1) the midwife in relationship with the woman; (2) orchestration of an environment of care; and (3) the effects or outcomes of care, called 'life journeys', for the woman and midwife. However, midwifery practices and cultures differ widely between countries and Kennedy's findings may not be internationally applicable.

Tonks (2002) tried to identify the characteristics of a good doctor and how one is produced, and came up with the requirement to demonstrate compassion, understanding, empathy, honesty, competence, commitment, humanity and, less predictably, courage, creativity, a sense of justice, respect, optimism and grace. Her conclusion was that: 'Good doctors are not just better than average at their job. They are special in some other way too: extra dedicated, extra humane or extra selfless' (Tonks, 2002:712).

'Competence' is a term often used to describe fitness to practise in health care, but this is also a contested concept and there is little agreement on how competence could be assessed and whether a quantitative (Calman et al., 2002) or qualitative (Webb et al., 2003) approach is appropriate (for a review of this literature, see McMullan et al., 2003). All midwives should be competent at the point of registration, but women's reports of their experiences make it clear that there is a 'value added' factor that distinguishes a 'good' midwife from one who is merely competent (Hodnett, 2002).

Overview of the review

Protocol and search methods

A full protocol was written for the review and is summarised in Box 13.1. After implementing the

---

Box 13. 1   Summary of review protocol.

Objectives

(1)   To identify research studies relevant to determining what makes a good midwife
(2)   To analyse and appraise the studies
(3)   To synthesise the findings of the studies to contribute towards answering the research question

Inclusion and exclusion criteria

Papers to be included if they were:

(1)   Published in English
(2)   Investigated a topic relevant to being a 'good' midwife
(3)   Had a clear methodological stance, although the actual method was unimportant
(4)   Empirical research reports
(5)   High-quality studies, assessed in terms of their rigour, validity and reliability

   Papers to be excluded if they were:

(1)   Anecdotal papers
(2)   Discussion papers
(3)   Narrative reviews
(4)   Without an explicitly stated methodology

Search strategy

Databases and keywords

- Databases to be searched: MEDLINE, CINAHL, Cochrane, BNI, HMIL, AMED, PSYCHOINFO, ASSIA, Caredata, EMBASE, Eric and MIDIRS. A hand search will be undertaken of midwifery texts commonly used in midwifery programmes
- Initial keywords used: 'midwi*', 'nurse-midwi*' and 'good'
- Searches in texts rather than as keywords because these terms are unlikely to appear as keywords in published papers

Limits

Publications from 1993 to 2005, i.e. after publication of 'Changing childbirth' (Department of Health, 1993) in the UK.

Data extraction and analysis

- Appraisal using the Critical Appraisal Skills Programme (CASP) format (Public Health Research Unit, 1993)
- Synthesis based on a comparison table using the headings: author, year, topic, sample, rationale for sample, sample size, data collection method, method of analysis and quality

---

search methods and applying the inclusion and exclusion criteria, 38 studies remained. Reading of the abstracts revealed that these included both quantitative and qualitative studies, and therefore an integrative approach would be required. This meant that we needed to use an appraisal scheme that could be applied to both types of reports.

Appraising the studies

We therefore decided instead to use the Critical Appraisal Skills Programme (CASP) system (Public Health Research Unit, 1993) as this has different appraisal formats for different methodologies; however, these are similar enough to allow comparisons

Is there a clear focus for the survey/questionnaire? *What was being surveyed?* *Who was taking part in the survey?*	
Is a survey/questionnaire appropriate? *Does the research try to gain a broad view/perspective* *of the quality/quantity of the topic area?*	
Sampling strategy *Is the sampling strategy well explained?* *Is the sample likely to be representative of the population?* *Does the sample need to be representative of the population?* *Was the sample size justified?*	
Data collection tool *Was the questionnaire piloted?* *Were alterations made as a result of the pilot study?* *How were the questions constructed?* *Were other experts asked about question construction?* *Were possible subjects asked about question construction?* *Were any tests of internal validity carried out on the* *questionnaire?* *Was an existing questionnaire that had been tried before* *used in the study? Were there closed and open questions?* *Were any forms of quantification used, e.g. Likert scales?*	
Data collection *How was the questionnaire administered?* *Postal, telephone, face-to-face, etc. Was method of data* *collection appropriate for the research topic?* *What was the reponse rate?* *Were reminders sent?*	
Data analysis *Was the method of analysis well described and appropriate* *for the type of data?* *Were computer packages used in the analysis?* *What method was used to analyse qualitative data?* *What tests of significance were used to analyse* *quantitative data?* *Was account taken of non-responders and efforts made to* *trace them?*	
Effects of the researcher on the research *Was there a degree of reflexivity in the research?* *Is possible researcher bias taken into account?* *Could there be any Hawthorne effect?*	
Results/Findings *Are the results and/or findings clearly set out and easy to* *understand?* *Is appropriate use made of tables and graphs?*	
Are the results/findings linked to previous or existing research on the topic? *Is theory used to help to explain the results/findings?* *Does the research confirm or refute existing* *research/practice?*	
How relevant is the research? *Should the research by used to alter practice?* *Does the research contribute something new to the* *topic area?*	

Figure 13.1   Grid for survey/questionnaire analysis, based on Critical Appraisal Skills Programme (CASP) approach.

across the papers. Perhaps surprisingly, CASP did not have a tool for surveys, and we therefore constructed one using the CASP format (Figure 13.1).

The appraisal was initially carried out by one person (L.C.N.) and a random sample of 20% of the papers was appraised independently by a second person (C.W.). A high level of agreement was obtained and minor differences eliminated by consensus discussion.

Conducting this appraisal gave insight and depth of understanding of each article, which was helpful in the subsequent synthesis process and could be compared with becoming immersed in the data or comprehending the data (Mays & Pope, 1995) when reading and re-reading transcripts of primary research. Five of the 38 articles appraised were not considered appropriate for the synthesis because they were not sufficiently focused on the research question. Thus, the final review included 33 studies.

There are no universally agreed and empirically reliable criteria for evaluating qualitative studies for use in meta-syntheses (Sandelowski & Barroso, 2003). Therefore studies were not excluded based on quality. The justification for this is that it is possible that valuable insights and perspectives of study participants could be lost if papers were excluded on the grounds of quality (Sandelowski et al., 1997).

In appraising the papers, they were summarised in table form, showing the reference, methodology or design, sample, rationale for sample, sample size, data collection method, method of analysis and quality assurance (Table 13.1). This was to facilitate synthesis of methodologies and methods. Further details of the methods are given in Nicholls & Webb (2006).

Analysing the findings of the included studies

A thematic analysis was conducted of the findings of the included studies. This involved several 'rounds' of identifying themes that were common to one or more studies, constructing tables to illustrate which themes appeared in each paper, and then amalgamating these to produce the final key concepts. This process parallels that of thematic content analysis as a data analysis method in qualitative research (Polit & Hungler, 1999). Two

examples of these tables are shown in Box 13.2 and Table 13.2. Box 13.2 lists the papers mentioning preliminary themes, and Table 13.2 shows in more detail how these were identified in the papers.

Methodological issues in the included studies

The focus of the 33 studies varied enormously, but all included some contribution to answering the research question: 'What makes a good midwife?' The two with the most closely related research questions were those of Fraser (1999) in a paper titled 'Women's perceptions of midwifery care: a longitudinal study to shape curriculum development', and Pope et al. (1998) in 'Aspects of care: views of professionals and mothers'. Both studies were conducted in the UK.

Sampling differences

Study participants included midwives, midwifery students, nurse-midwives, supervisors of midwives, pregnant women, low-income pregnant women, postnatal women, nurses, health visitors, doctors and fathers. Thus, a wide variety of opinions was sampled and all participants would have had direct experience or knowledge of midwives.

Sample sizes varied from 6 to over 1000. Of the studies where sample size was important for the purposes of statistical testing (e.g. randomised controlled trials) only one (Morrell et al., 2000) used a power calculation to confirm that the sample was appropriate for the inferential statistical calculations used. In qualitative studies a relatively small sample size can be acceptable; for example, the phenomenological studies of Hildingsson & Haggstrom (1999) and Stewart (1999), each had sample sizes of seven.

Several types of sample selection were used. Eleven studies used convenience samples, which were also described as self-selected, opportunistic or networked, and this is considered the weakest form of sampling. Twelve studies used samples that were described as 'all' who were eligible within a given time frame. For example, 'all first-time mothers in Powys (n = 445) who delivered during the ten-month period' (Churchill & Benbow, 2000:42).

Table 13.1 Summary of papers included in the review (adapted from and reproduced with permission from Nicholls, L. & Webb, C. (2006) What makes a good midwife? An integrative review of methodologically-diverse research. *Journal of Advanced Nursing*, 56 (4), 414–29).

Author and date	Methodology/ design	Sample	Rationale for sample	Sample size	Data collection method	Method of analysis	Quality assurance**
Begley (1999)	Phenomenology	Student midwives	'All students' p. 265; convenience	$n = 125$ Diary keeping = 19 Interviewed = 31 Focus groups = 125	Individual and group interviews, diary keeping and questionnaires	Descriptive and inferential statistics; the Ethnograph Phenomenological approach; Dutch School	Respondent verification
Berg et al. (1996)	Phenomenology	Postnatal women	Convenience	$n = 18$ 6 primiparous 12 multiparous	Tape-recorded interviews	Phenomenological approach; meaning units; themes; essential structure of phenomenon	Not discussed
Berggren (1996)	Survey (mainly quantitative data)	Midwives	Convenience	$n = 146$ Response rate 74%, $n = 118$	Survey postal questionnaire	Descriptive statistics; average adoption scores; percentages	Pilot study; Cronbach's alpha calculated
Bewley (2000)	Survey (mainly qualitative data)	Midwives	Convenience; self-selected	$n = 184$	Postal survey; questionnaire 10 interviews	SPSS thematic analysis	Based on previous study
Butterworth & Bishop (1995)	Survey (mainly quantitative data)	Nurses, midwives and health visitors	Expert respondents identified by nurse executives	$n = 2006$ Response rate 61%, $n = 1221$	Delphi study; postal survey; questionnaire	Descriptive statistics; categories, coding	Non-responders followed up by phone; inter-rater reliability tested by modified Kappa test
Churchill & Benbow (2000)	Survey (mainly qualitative data)	First time mothers; 3 months post-partum	To control extraneous variables from previous experience of childbirth	$n = 445$ 49.9% response of which 48.3% were eligible, $n = 215$	Postal questionnaires	Qualitative and quantitative data; descriptive statistics	Questionnaire was piloted

Study	Design	Population	Sampling	Sample	Data collection	Analysis	Rigour
Clement et al. (1996)	Randomised controlled trial	Pregnant women	At low risk, booked before 22 weeks gestation, understood English or one of seven other languages	$n = 2893$ Response rate of 71%, $n = 1882$	Maternity Antenatal Questionnaire	Chi-square statistics; P values; Logistic regression; Fisher's exact test	Use of validated tool (EPDS and questions from OPCS survey); pilot study undertaken
Crawford & Kiger (1998)	Grounded theory	Student midwives	Convenience sample	$n = 10$	Interviews	Grounded theory approach	Researcher involvement discussed
Earle (2000)	Grounded theory approach	Pregnant women	Convenience sample of primigravidae	$n = 19$	Repeated in-depth interviewing	Modified grounded theory; QSR NUD.IST	Not discussed
Fleming (1998)	Grounded theory	Midwives and clients	Representative of the criterion being discussed; theoretical sampling	$n = 250$ midwives $n = 219$ clients	Unstructured interviews	Grounded theory; constant comparative analysis; codes and categories	Data and analysis presented to clients and midwives not involved in the study for critique
Fraser (1999)	Descriptive, longitudinal	Child-bearing women	Opportunistic sample	$n = 41$ in total $n = 41$ antenatally $n = 28$ immediately after birth $n = 39$ postnatally	Interviews; maternity records	Textbase Alpha; similar to grounded theory; constant comparative method	Second person checked the analysis
Halldorsdottir & Karlsdottir (1996)	Phenomenology	Mothers	Through networking; must have had caring and uncaring encounters with a midwife	$n = 10$	Dialogues; interviews	Phenomenology; coding, categorisation, thematic analysis, constant comparison	Two researchers did the analysis

Table continues

Table 13.1 continued

Author and date	Methodology/design	Sample	Rationale for sample	Sample size	Data collection method	Method of analysis	Quality assurance**
Hallgren et al. (1995)	Interpretive qualitative	Pregnant women	Convenience; women undertaking childbirth education classes, expecting first child	n = 11	Tape recorded interviews at 27 and 36 weeks' gestation and 1–3 weeks after birth.	Thematic; interpretative	Analysis by more than one researcher; consensus discussion where necessary; related to Antonovsky's concept sense of coherence
Hancock et al. (2000)	Indeterminate	Midwives	Self-selected	Over 60 midwives were approached. 24%, n = 14 in sample	Pre- and post-intervention questionnaires, self-administered	Demographic data; content analysis; inductive analysis, themes and constructs	Not discussed
Hicks (1995)	Experimental	Midwives	Random selection from population of 54 midwives attending post-registration courses	n = 30	Different subject experimental questionnaire	Questionnaire; following the setting of a scenario relating to personality traits; unrelated t-tests; probability	Recognition of 'design flaws' (p. 83)
Hildingsson & Haggstrom (1999)	Phenomenology	Midwives	Quasi random selection from population in one geographic area	n = 7	Interviews	Ricoeur's phenomenological hermeneutic method	Consensus achieved between authors; discussion of results in workshops and seminar
Hodnett (2000)	Systematic review	Controlled trials	Cochrane Pregnancy and Childbirth Group trials register	n = 2	From database	Analysis and synthesis of trials	Cochrane methodology used
Kabakian-Khasholian-Khasholian et al. (2000)	Descriptive, longitudinal	Child-bearing women	Any parity, normal delivery in last 3 months; three geographic areas	n = 117	Semi-structured interviews	Descriptive statistics; manual analysis, themes identified following interview guideline	Interviewers trained, practice interviews conducted

Lugina et al. (2002)	Grounded theory approach	Nurse-midwives	Quasi-random selection from list of all eligible midwives in the area of the study (n = 80) continued until saturation reached	n = 49	Focus groups	Modelled on grounded theory	Participant verification
Morgan et al. (1998)	Survey (mainly quantitative data)	Child-bearing women and case notes	All women in two group practices over 10-month period	n = 340 antenatally (72% response). n =327 postnatally (68% response)	Postal questionnaires; review of case notes	Chi squared; Mann–Whitney U test; logistical regression analysis	Not discussed
Morrell et al. (2000)	Randomised controlled trial	Child-bearing women	All women who delivered in the recruiting hospital if living in the area, aged 17 or over and understand English	n = 623 Power calculation undertaken	Questionnaire; Short Form 36; EPDS* and DUFSS*; breastfeeding rates	Analysis by intention to treat-tests; Mann–Whitney U test; Chi-square tests. Fisher's exact test; descriptive statistics	Limitations discussed
Norman et al. (2002)	Mixed methods	Nursing and midwifery students; clinical competence assessment tools; clinically related academic assessments	Population of all nursing and midwifery programmes in Scotland, seven programmes were excluded	257 from 482 nursing students (53%). 43 from 55 midwifery students (78%). n = 3 nursing programmes, n = 3 midwifery programmes, n = 4 institutions	Questionnaire; key areas assessment instrumentation; clinical competence assessment tools compared with national competencies; academic assessment results in percentages; entrance qualifications	Scores collected or assessed on two occasions and compared; multivariate and univariate correlation coefficients	Multi-method approach

Table continues

Table 13.1 continued

Author and date	Methodology/ design	Sample	Rationale for sample	Sample size	Data collection method	Method of analysis	Quality assurance**
Oakley et al. (1996)	Survey (mainly quantitative data)	Child-bearing women	Low-risk women receiving antenatal care	$n = 710$ women cared for by obstetricians; $n = 471$ women cared for by nurse-midwives	Questionnaires on four occasions	Bivariate analysis; chi-square tests; Student t-tests; multiple linear regression	Power calculation undertaken
Omar & Schiffman (2000)	Survey (mainly quantitative data)	Rural low-income women receiving antenatal care; maternity and neonatal records	Convenience sample	$n = 60$	Questionnaire using established satisfaction scales; infant outcomes	Kotelchuck's APNCU index ANOVA; two-group t-tests; standard deviations, probabilities	Content validity examined; Cronbach's alpha
Pope et al. (1998)	Mixed methods	Midwives, supervisors, doctors and mothers	National stratified random sample	Midwives, $n = 1100$ (70% rr) Supervisors, $n = 205$ (83% rr) Consultants, $n = 205$ (58% rr) Registrars, $n = 196$ (46% rr) General practitioners, $n = 250$ (65% rr)	Postal questionnaire; semi-structured interviews; interviews	Descriptive statistics; probabilities; qualitative analysis	Assessment by 20 midwife testers and 13 critical readers
Rice & Naksook (1998)	Ethnographic	Thai women living in Australia	Theoretical sampling; saturation reached	$n = 30$	Ethnographic interviews and participant observation	Thematic analysis	Translations checked by English-speaking person
Shallow (2001)	Qualitative	Midwives undergoing integration	Purposive	$n = 6$	Interviews	Grounded theory approach	Not discussed
Stewart (1999)	Phenomenology	Lesbian mothers	Nominated, snowball	$n = 7$	Semi-structured, in-depth interviews	Phenomenological approach; themes, post-coding	Pilot interview

Study	Design	Population	Sampling	Sample	Data collection	Analysis	Quality assurance
Vehvilainen-Julkunen & Liukkonen (1998)	Survey (mainly qualitative data)	Fathers	Non-random	$n = 137$ 81% response rate	Survey using questionnaire	SPSS frequencies percentages and factor analysis; probabilities and t-test	Pilot study; Cronbach's alpha
Wallace et al. (1995)	Mixed methods	Retrospective review of notes and prospective analysis of labour ward consultations over 4-week period	Midwife doctor referrals regarding all women over 4-week period on the hospital labour ward; $n = 377$ women; $n = 259$ requiring doctor	Total, $n = 377$ Prestudy, $n = 129$ Prospective, $n = 280$	Review of case notes and use of study analysis sheet	Percentages; chi squared; probabilities	Preparation of study participants.
Webster et al. (1995)	Survey (mainly quantitative data)	Pregnant women	All women giving birth in a 2-month period	$n = 513$ Response rate 68%	Exploratory survey design; self-administered questionnaire	Percentages; probabilities; Kruskal–Wallis and Wilcoxon rank sum test	Possible bias discussed
Whelan & Lupton (1998)	Qualitative	Breastfeeding women	Women with low income who had breast fed their last baby and delivered in a specific hospital during a 5-month period	$n = 15$	Semi-structured interviews	Codes and categories	Verbatim transcripts; inter-observer reliability assessed
Wiegers et al. (1996)	Survey (mainly quantitative data)	Midwives and women using services	Low-risk pregnancies who had planned to give birth either at home or in hospital	$n = 97$ midwives $n = 1836$ women	Questionnaires and maternity records	Chi squared and Student's t-test	Power analysis conducted; Cronbach's alpha calculated

**If 'Not discussed' appears in the 'Quality assurance' column, this does not mean the study quality was in question. Rather that explicit discussion of quality issues was not made in the article.

*EPDS, Edinburgh Postnatal Depression Scale.

*DUFSS, Duke Functional Social Support.

rr = response rate.

Box 13.2   Initial categories identified in the studies.

(1) International perspective

'Developed world'

Begley 1999, Ireland
Berg 1996, Sweden
Berggren 1996, Sweden
Bewley 2000, UK
Butterworth 1995, UK
Churchill 2000, UK
Clement 1996, UK
Crawford 1998, UK
Earle 2000, UK
Fleming 1998, NZ and UK
Fraser 1999, UK
Halldorsdottir 1996, Iceland
Hallgren 1995, Sweden
Hancock 2000, Australia
Hicks 1995, UK
Hildingsson 1999, Sweden
Hodnett 2000, UK and Australia
Morgan 1998, UK
Morrell 2000, UK
Norman 2002, UK
Oakley 1996, USA
Omar 2000, USA
Pope 1998, UK
Rice 1998, Australia (Thai women)
Shallow 2001, UK
Stewart 1999, UK
Vehvilainen-Julkunen 1998, Finland
Wallace 1995, UK
Webster 1995, Australia
Weigers 1996, Netherlands
Whelan 1998, UK

'Developing world'

Kabakian-Khasholian, 2000, Lebanon
Lugina 2002, Tanzania

(2) Education, training, learning, mentors

Begley 1999
Crawford 1998
Stewart 1999
Norman 2002
Shallow 2001

(3) Provision of care

Antenatal: Clement 1996, Hallgren 1995, Rice 1998, Morgan 1998, Omar 2000
Labour: Berg 1996, Vehvilainen-Julkunen 1998, Wallace 1995, Morgan 1998, Halldorsdottir 1996
Postnatal: Lugina 2002, Whelan 1998, Morgan 1998
Overall: Kabakian-Khasholian 2000, Morrell 2000

(4) Midwives and research, users and researchers

Hancock 2000
Berggren 1996
Hicks 1995

(5) Attributes of a midwife (Hallmarks)

Pope 1998
Shallow 2001

(6) Stakeholders

Hildingsson 1999, Fathers
Vehvilainen-Julkunen 1998, Fathers

(7) Care v. carer (continuity)

Earle 2000
Churchill 2000
Morgan 1998
Hodnett 2000

(8) Midwife and doctor

Omar 2000
Wallace 1995
Webster 1995
Hodnett 2000
Oakley 1996

(9) Communication, relationship

Berg 1996
Stewart 1999
Halldorsdottir 1996
Fleming 1998
Earle 2000
Hildingsson 1999
Fraser 1999
Vehvilainen-Julkunen 1998

Table 13.2 Further development of the thematic analysis.

Title	Personal attributes of a midwife	Education	Research	What a midwife does: antenatal, labour, postnatal	Place of Care v. Carer Continuity Individualised	Midwife and other professionals	Stakeholders, e.g. fathers	International perspective
Begley 1999 Being a student		Learning to be a midwife in Ireland						Ireland
Berg 1996 Care in labour				Labour 'presence' of a midwife	See labouring women as individuals			Sweden
Berggren 1996 Using research			Use of research findings					Sweden
Bewley 2000 Midwives having children	Empathy compassion friendliness openness trust Midwifery skills Knowledge	Educate on how to answer this question Can attitudes be learned or are they innate?						UK
Butterworth 1995 Optimum practice	Innovators Leadership Personal qualities Communication Expertise Multi-disciplinary team	Requirement for optimum practice is to be involved in education	Requirement for optimum practice is the ability to use research				Views of large sample of mixed professionals	UK
Churchill 2000 Informed choice					Continuity of carer provided where possible			UK
Clement 1996 Antenatal visit schedule				Pregnancy antenatal	Frequency of care Not possible to predict satisfaction need to ask women			UK
Crawford 1998 Students' strategies for self assessment		Students' strategies for self-assessment						UK

Table continues

Table 13.2 continued

Title	Personal attributes of a midwife	Education	Research	What a midwife does: antenatal, labour, postnatal	Place of Care v. Carer Continuity Individualised	Midwife and other professionals	Stakeholders, e.g. fathers	International perspective
Earle 2000 Antenatal care in community				Antenatal	Care more important than carer Women as individuals, unique self identity			UK
Fleming 1998 Midwife/women		Model developed that could be used in education		Research-based conceptual model				New Zealand and UK
Fraser 1999 Women's perceptions	Gender list of personal qualities Knowledge Psychology	Research done to inform pre-registration curriculum		Individualised infant feeding Parent education (superficial information)	Care, if not possible to have continuity of carer Individual care important Rules-orientated care Not meeting women's needs	Interprofessional relationship	Women's views	UK
Halldorsdottir 1996 Empowerment disencouragement	Competent Responsible Attentive Deliberate Communicates			Labour	Carer through labour Individual care in labour			Iceland
Hallgren 1995 Childbirth education and labour				Parent education	Information-giving Individual women's needs			Sweden

Study							
Hancock 2000 Midwives accessing research		Use of and attitudes to computerised research findings					Australia
Hicks 1995 Good researcher, poor midwife	Kind Compassionate Reflective	Good researcher, poor midwife					UK
Hildingsson 1999 Midwife supporting women	Advocate		Pregnancy	Individual care		Fathers (absent)	Sweden
Hodnett 2000 Continuity or giver of care				Team midwifery	Midwifery or continuity with midwife		UK and Australia
Kabakian-Khasholian 2000 Women's experiences			Antenatal Labour Postnatal		Want safety of medical care	Women's views	Lebanon
Lugina 2002 Tanzanian midwives' views of their roles			Postnatal				Tanzania
Morgan 1998 Models of continuity				Shared caseload, team caseload	Shared or midwife only		UK
Morrell 2000 Postnatal support workers			Postnatal	Support workers valued but expensive			UK
Norman 2002 Assessing competence	Methods of assessing competence						UK

Table continues

Table 13.2 continued

Title	Personal attributes of a midwife	Education	Research	What a midwife does: antenatal, labour, postnatal	Place of Care v. Carer Continuity Individualised	Midwife and other professionals	Stakeholders, e.g. fathers	International perspective
Oakley 2005 Obstetrician or nurse-midwife						Obstetrician or nurse-midwife		USA
Omar 2000 Prenatal care, rural, low-income women				Antenatal	Tailor care to individual needs	Physician or nurse-midwife		USA
Pope 1998 Views of professionals and mothers	Knowledge Listens Approachable Friendly Pleasant And others, some which are less frequent	Research done to inform post-registration curricula				32/41 preferred midwife over doctor	Midwives Supervisors Doctors Mothers Fathers	UK
Rice 1998 Thai experiences				All aspects antenatal care important	Australia better care than Thailand Thai women not getting adequate information			Australia Thai women
Shallow 2001 Integration and its problems		Apprentice- style training, role modelling			Going into teams and the effect on midwives			UK

				Continuity		
Stewart 1999 Lesbian mothers	Open Sensitive Non-judgemental	Education on minority group Lesbians and sexuality				UK
Vehvilainen-Julkunen 1998 Fathers				Individual families	Fathers' experiences	Finland
Wallace 1995 Midwife medical staff			Labour		Midwife doctor referrals	UK
Webster 1995 Antenatal care in hospital			Antenatal	Hospital or general practitioner shared care Shared care more personal		Australia
Whelan 1998 Breastfeeding in low-income women			Breastfeeding postnatal	More continuity of care gives better breastfeeding rates		UK
Weigers 1996 Home or hospital			Labour	Home or hospital		Netherlands

However, location-specific sampling may limit the transferability of the findings.

Some studies used appropriate methods of sample selection and justified these in the report. For example, Fleming (1998:138) included 'those who were representative of the criterion being studied'. Butterworth & Bishop (1995) selected experts for their Delphi panels; Stewart (1999) used snowball sampling (although her sample size was small); Hicks (1995) used random selection, albeit from a small population; Pope et al. (1998) used a national, stratified, random sample; and Hodnett (2000) selected controlled trials for her systematic review of effectiveness. Hildingsson & Haggstrom (1999:84) stated that: 'The physician in charge of antenatal care was asked to select by lottery seven midwives to represent the five clinics', but it is not clear why a sample of seven was used.

Data collection methods

Data collection methods also varied throughout the 33 studies. Interview type was said to vary among tape-recorded, in-depth, repeated, unstructured, semi-structured or group. There were also dialogues, ethnographic interviews and focus groups. Questionnaires were popular methods of data collection and may have been posted or given to women while in hospital. Some contained satisfaction scales or established scales, such as the Edinburgh Postnatal Depression Scale (Cox et al., 1987). One report mentioned diary-keeping and another participant observation. Maternity records or case notes were accessed in two studies, and Hodnett (2000) took data from original studies.

Data analysis

There were also many methods of data analysis. Quantitative studies used descriptive and/or inferential statistics. Qualitative studies mentioned ethnographic, phenomenological (in one case specifically Ricoeur's approach) and grounded theory approaches. Other terms used were themes, categories, codes, interpretative, content, and inductive and constructs. Three computer programs were used: SPSS, NUD.IST and Textbase Alpha. The methods used in each study appeared to be ap-propriate, although few reports commented on the methodological aspects of the research.

Summary of review findings

Eight key themes were derived from the included studies:

- Attributes of a midwife
- Education
- Research
- What a midwife does
- Care organisation
- Other professionals
- Partners
- International perspective.

Although the review included studies with very diverse methodologies, the findings were mainly consistent. However, there were some differences of opinion, for example, about whether 'continuity of care' was better 'than continuity of carer'; here, conflicting evidence was apparent but writers on each side justified their views.

The personal attributes of a good midwife emerged from three studies, and are summarised in Table 13.3. Having good communication skills made the major contribution to being a good midwife, being mentioned in some form in most of the papers. The elements of being compassionate, kind and supportive (affective domain), knowledgeable (cognitive domain) and skilful (psychomotor domain) also made major contributions. Being involved in education and research were also necessary requirements for a good midwife. With regard to what a midwife does, the overriding features were the abilities to treat women as individuals, adopt a caring approach, have good communication skills, and 'be there' for women. Care-delivery systems are important, but a good midwife can compensate for poor management systems. Women should be able to choose the professional who provides their care, and good midwives will include partners in the care they provide.

Being 'good' is different from being competent. It is very difficult to define or quantify, as it is multi-faceted and subjective, but the key features seem to be communication skills, compassion, kindness, being supportive, knowledgeable and skilful. Some of these (communication skills, knowledge and

Table 13. 3   Positive and negative personal attributes of a midwife (reproduced with permission from Nicholls, L. & Webb, C. (2006) What makes a good midwife? An integrative review of methodologically-diverse research. *Journal of Advanced Nursing*, 56 (4), 413–29).

Authors	Positive attributes	Negative attributes
Fraser (1999)	Communication skills Personable Friendly Smiling Cheerful Caring Outgoing	Unhelpful Insensitive Lacking intuition Rushed Abrupt Officious Miserable Rude
Pope et al. (1998)	Knowledgeable Good listener Approachable Friendly Pleasant Non-critical Non-judgemental Has time for the mother Good communicator	Not listening Giving conflicting advice Lack of concern
Halldorsdottir & Karlsdottir (1996)	Professionally competent Skilful Responsible Attentive Co-operative Communicating caringly Nurturing Kind Respectful	Insensitive Rough when giving care Not taking the initiative Lacking understanding Lacking flexibility Thoughtless

skills) are taught in midwifery curricula, but others (compassion, kindness and being supportive) are either present in a person prior to midwifery education or should be developed during the programme through clinical experience and self-awareness.

Issues arising from the review process

Conducting integrative reviews

Many authors comment on the innovation and complexity of systematic reviews and meta-synthesis (Dixon-Woods & Fitzpatrick, 2001a). This is so when dealing with qualitative evidence alone (Pearson, 2004) and also when the review includes qualitative and quantitative research (Thomas et al., 2004).

The techniques are still developing rapidly and are outlined in Popay (2006), including methods to synthesise solely qualitative research (Pearson, 2004; Attree, 2005). There are also developments in synthesising quantitative and qualitative research (Thomas et al., 2004; Oliver et al., 2005). However, in view of the fact that our review was of papers using a very diverse group of methodologies, we considered that a descriptive synthesis was most appropriate to take account of the individuality of each paper.

Writing the protocol

Writing the protocol was a challenge, as there were no ideal pre-existing formats on which to base this. The one we adopted was based on that used by Woodward & Webb (2001). The protocol was intended to be a guiding not proscriptive document, and covered the stages of search, appraisal and synthesis. Some of the parts of the protocol were adapted as the review process went along and these adaptations are discussed below.

The search

The search for articles was intended to be thorough and comprehensive because this is one of the hallmarks of a systematic review (Sutton et al., 1998; Higgins & Green, 2005, Glanville, 2006). However, carrying out the search was not easy because not all databases allow searching on the keyword 'qualitative research'. For example, we began the work in 2002 and 'qualitative research' was only included as a MeSH term in 2003 (http://www.nlm. nih.gov.mesh/MBrowser.html (accessed 17 March 2003)). As Dixon-Woods & Fitzpatrick (2001b:130) say: 'Searching for and identifying appropriate material remains frustrating and difficult, and it can be difficult to demonstrate that searches have been systematic and exhaustive.'

This can lead to searches becoming very complex, for example that reported by Jones (2004). However, Egger et al. (2003) conclude that the time and money spent on tracing reports that are difficult to find via the main bibliographic databases may not be well spent, as such work is usually of low methodological quality. Although their work concerned trials, the principle may well translate to qualitative work, and the omission of minor papers is unlikely to have a significant effect on the overall outcome of the synthesis.

In addition, as this was not a medically based enquiry, MeSH terms (Medical Subject Headings) were not helpful. In 2001 Dixon-Woods et al. stated that MEDLINE did not as yet include 'qualitative' as an MeSH term. However, this was introduced in 2003 (National Library of Medicine, 2006). The MeSH list includes 'nurse-midwives' as a subject heading, but not midwi*. There are some adjectives which are MeSH terms, for example 'superior' in relation to anatomy (superior vena cava), but 'good' is not an MeSH term.

'Good' is not likely to be used as a keyword, which meant that the whole text of papers had to be searched, inevitably leading to a large number of false positives. These were papers that contained the word 'good' (and midwi* or nurse-midwi*) but did not focus on being a good midwife.

While there were many false positives, there may also have been false negatives. These are papers that could contribute to answering the research question but did not contain the keywords searched. In order to investigate this, the search was repeated using other keywords: 'exemplary' (used by Kennedy, 2000), 'excellent' and 'superb' as synonyms for 'good' and the antonym 'bad'. This revealed several hundred more papers which were reduced to eight relevant ones, but none of these added significantly to the themes.

Appraisal

When appraising papers for inclusion in a systematic review, a numerical scoring system may be use – a technique in line with the epistemology of quantitative research (Higgins & Green, 2005). There have been some attempts to translate the use of a scoring appraisal system to qualitative studies (Spencer et al., 2003). However, this is at odds with the methodology of qualitative research.

In our review, appraisal was undertaken with the initial intent of determining whether the papers were of sufficient quality to be included. However, it was soon apparent that, because there is no definitive method on which to base this judgement (Dixon-Woods et al., 2001), using appraisal in this way was not feasible.

Therefore, we did not use the appraisal process to judge the value of the papers, other than their ability to contribute to answering our research question. Rather, a structured format was used to gain a deep understanding and knowledge of the papers by becoming immersed in them, in a similar way to the analysis of primary qualitative research (Strauss & Corbin, 1998).

Synthesis

After reading and re-reading the papers and compiling the two comparison tables, themes and key concepts were identified, as described above. The research question itself led almost automatically towards some categories, notably 'attributes', and the primary researchers' own research questions also led to obvious themes. For example, Hicks'

(1995) paper entitled 'Good researcher, poor midwife: an investigation into the impact of central trait descriptions on assumptions of professional competencies' led to the theme of 'good midwife and research', and then the other papers were analysed to identify material contributing to this theme. The same process followed with Begley's (1999) article on 'Student midwives' views of "learning to be a midwife" in Ireland' provoking the theme 'good midwife and education' and then other articles contributed to this theme.

Conclusion

The review findings suggest that a good midwife must be more than technically skilled in terms of physical care. A safe pregnancy and labour for both woman and baby are fundamental outcomes. However, the 'value added' by 'good' midwives is the psychological safety that results from 'being there' for women and showing kindness and compassion. This is the element that may be missing in medicalised healthcare systems and that is at risk when services are under-resourced. Our evidence-based identification of the factors constituting a good midwife could be used in service development and evaluation, as well as curriculum development to offer more woman-centred care. It could also be used as an operational definition for further research into what makes a good midwife. The review findings could be used to inform midwifery education, both at pre- and post-registration levels, and to encourage students and practitioners to assess and develop their own practice against the key concepts identified. The findings could also be used in service development and quality assurance projects in midwifery practice.

With regard to methodological issues, the principal issues remain how to choose keywords to ensure that all the relevant studies are included, which approach to use for appraising the included studies, and whether to include or exclude qualitative studies that are judged to be methodologically rigorous. In the absence of definitive guidance in the literature, we had to make pragmatic decisions about how to conduct the review. We hope that, by sharing this process, we can contribute to the ongoing development of the methodology for integrative reviews.

References

Attree, P. (2005) Low-income mothers, nutrition and health: a systematic review of qualitative evidence. *Maternal and Child Nutrition*, 1, 227–40.

Begley, C.M. (1999) Student midwives' views of 'learning to be a midwife' in Ireland. *Midwifery*, 15 (4), 264–73.

Berg, M., Lundgren, I., Hermansson, E. & Wahlberg, V. (1996) Women's experience of the encounter with the midwife during childbirth. *Midwifery*, 12 (1), 11–15.

Berggren, A. (1996) Swedish midwives' awareness of, attitudes to and use of selected research findings. *Journal of Advanced Nursing*, 23 (3), 462–70.

Bewley, C. (2000) Feelings and experiences of midwives who do not have children about caring for childbearing women. *Midwifery*, 16 (2), 135–44.

Butterworth, T. & Bishop, V. (1995) Identifying the characteristics of optimum practice: findings from a survey of practice experts in nursing, midwifery and health visiting. *Journal of Advanced Nursing*, 22 (1), 24–32.

Calman, L., Watson, R., Norman, I., Redfern, S. & Murrells, T. (2002) Assessing practice of student nurses: methods, preparation of assessors and student views. *Journal of Advanced Nursing*, 38, 516–23.

Churchill, H. & Benbow, A. (2000) Informed choice in maternity services. *British Journal of Midwifery*, 8 (1), 41–7.

Clement, S., Sikorski, J., Wilson, P., Das, S. & Smeeton, N. (1996) Women's satisfaction with traditional and reduced antenatal visit schedules. *Midwifery*, 12 (3), 120–8.

Cox, J., Holden, J. & Sagovsky, R. (1987) Detection of postnatal depression: development of the 10-item Edinburgh Postnatal Depression Scale. *British Journal of Psychiatry*, 150, 782–6.

Crawford, M.W. & Kiger, A.M. (1998) Development through self-assessment: strategies used during clinical nursing placements. *Journal of Advanced Nursing*, 27 (1), 157–64.

Department of Health (1993) *Report of the Expert Maternity Group: 'Changing Childbirth'*. Department of Health, London.

Dixon-Woods, M. & Fitzpatrick, R. (2001a) Including qualitative research in systematic reviews: opportunities and problems. *Journal of Evaluation in Clinical Practice*, 7 (2), 125–33.

Dixon-Woods, M. & Fitzpatrick, R. (2001b) Qualitative research in systematic reviews has established a place for itself. *British Medical Journal*, 323 (7316), 765–6.

Dixon-Woods, M., Fitzpatrick, R. & Roberts, K. (2001) Including qualitative research in systematic reviews: opportunities and problems. *Journal of Evaluation in Clinical Practice*, 7 (2), 125–33.

Earle, S. (2000) Pregnancy and the maintenance of self-identity: implications for antenatal care in the community. *Health and Social Care in the Community*, 8 (4), 235–41.

Egger, M., Juni, P., Bartlett, C., Holenstein, F. & Sterne, J. (2003) How important are comprehensive literature searches and the assessment of trial quality in systematic reviews? Empirical study. *Health Technology Assessment*, 7 (1), 1–76.

Fleming, V. (1998) Women-with-midwives-with-women: a model of interdependence. *Midwifery*, 14 (3), 137–43.

Fraser, D. (1999) Women's perceptions of midwifery care: a longitudinal study to shape curriculum development. *Birth*, 26 (2), 99–107.

Glanville, J. (2006) Available at website http://www.york.ac.uk/inst/crd/pdf/crd4_ph3.pdf (accessed 21 August 2006).

Halldorsdottir, S. & Karlsdottir, S. (1996) Empowerment or dis-encouragement: women's experience of caring and uncaring encounters during childbirth. *Healthcare for Women International*, 17, 361–79.

Hallgren, A. K.M., Norberg, A. & Forslin, L. (1995) Women's perceptions of childbirth and childbirth education before and after education and birth. *Midwifery*, 11 (3), 130–7.

Hancock, H., Emden, C., Schubert, S. & Haller, A. (2000) They were different and few: an Australian study of midwives' attitudes to research and computerised research findings. *Australian College of Midwives Incorporated Journal*, 13 (1), 7–13.

Hicks, C. (1995) Good researcher, poor midwife: an investigation into the impact of central trait descriptions on assumptions of professional competencies. *Midwifery*, 11 (2), 81–7.

Higgins, J.P.T. & Green, S. (eds) (2005) *Cochrane Handbook for Systematic Reviews of Interventions 4.2.5*. Available at website http://www.cochrane.org/resources/handbook/hbook.htm (accessed 31 May 2005).

Hildingsson, I. & Haggstrom, T. (1999) Midwives' lived experiences of being supportive to prospective mothers/parents during pregnancy. *Midwifery*, 15 (2), 82–91.

Hodnett, E.D. (2000) Continuity of caregivers for care during pregnancy and childbirth. In: *The Cochrane Database of Systematic Reviews Issue 1 (2004)*. John Wiley, Chichester.

Hodnett, E.D. (2002) Pain and women's satisfaction with the experience of childbirth: a systematic review. *American Journal of Obstetrics and Gynaecology*, 186 (5), 160–72.

Jones, M. (2004) Application of systematic review methods to qualitative research: practical issues. *Journal of Advanced Nursing*, 48 (3), 271–8.

Kabakian-Khasholian-Khasholian, T., Campbell, O., Shediac-Rizkallah, M. & Ghorayeb, F. (2000) Women's experiences of maternity care: satisfaction or passivity. *Social Science and Medicine*, 51 (1), 103–13.

Kennedy, H.P. (1995) The essence of nurse-midwifery care. *Journal of Nurse Midwifery*, 40 (5), 410–17.

Kennedy, H.P. (2000) A model of exemplary midwifery practice: results from a Delphi study. *Journal of Midwifery and Women's Health*, 45 (1), 4–19.

Lugina, H.I., Johansson, E., Lindmark, G. & Christensson, K. (2002) Developing a theoretical framework on postpartum care from Tanzanian midwives' views of their role. *Midwifery*, 18 (1), 12–20.

Mays, N. & Pope, C. (1995) Rigour and qualitative research. *British Medical Journal*, 311, 109–12.

McMullan, M., Endacott, R., Gray, M. et al. (2003) Portfolios and assessment of competence: a review of the literature. *Journal of Advanced Nursing*, 41 (3), 283–94.

Morgan, M., Fenwick, N., McKenzie, C. & Wolfe, C.D. (1998) Quality of midwifery led care: assessing the effects of different models of continuity for women's satisfaction. *Quality Health Care*, 7 (2), 77–82.

Morrell, C.J., Spiby, H., Stewart, P., Walters, S. & Morgan, A. (2000) Costs and benefits of community postnatal support workers: a randomised controlled trial. *Health Technology Assessment*, 4 (6), 1–276.

National Library of Medicine (2006) Medical subject headings. Available at website http://www.nlm.nih.gov/mesh/MBrowser.html (accessed 17 March 2006).

Nicholls, L. & Webb, C. (2006) What makes a good midwife? An integrative review of methodologically-diverse research. *Journal of Advanced Nursing*, 56 (4), 414–29.

Norman, I.J., Watson, R., Murrells, T., Calman, L. & Redfern, S. (2002) The validity and reliability of methods to assess the competence to practise of pre-registration nursing and midwifery students. *International Journal of Nursing Studies*, 39 (2), 133–45.

Oakley, D., Murray, M.E., Murtland, T. et al. (1996) Comparisons of outcomes of maternity care by obstetricians and certified nurse-midwives. *Obstetrics and Gynaecology*, 88 (5), 823–9.

Oliver, S., Harden, A., Rees, R. et al. (2005) An emerging framework for including different types of evidence in systematic reviews for public policy. *Evaluation*, 11 (4), 428–46.

Omar, M.A. & Schiffman, R.F. (2000) Satisfaction and adequacy of prenatal care utilisation among rural low-income women. *Outcomes Management for Nursing Practice*, 4 (2), 91–6.

Pearson, A. (2004) Balancing the evidence: incorporating the synthesis of qualitative data into systematic reviews. *Joanna Briggs Institute Reports*, 2, 45–64.

Polit, D. & Hungler, B. (1999) *Nursing Research. Principles and Methods*. Lippincott, Philadelphia.

Popay, J. (2006) *Moving Beyond Effectiveness in Evidence Synthesis: Methodological Issues in the Synthesis of Diverse Sources of Evidence*. National Institute for Health and Clinical Excellence, London.

Pope, R., Conney, M., Graham, L., Holliday, M. & Patel, S. (1998) Aspects of care 4: views of professionals and mothers. *British Journal of Midwifery*, 6 (3), 144–7.

Public Health Research Unit (1993) *Critical Appraisal Skills Programme (CASP)*. Public Health Research Unit, Oxford.

Rice, P.L. & Naksook, C. (1998) The experience of pregnancy, labour and birth of Thai women in Australia. *Midwifery*, 14 (2), 74–84.

Sandelowski, M. & Barroso, J. (2003) Writing the proposal for a qualitative research methodology project. *Qualitative Health Research*, 13 (6), 781–820.

Sandelowski, M., Docherty, S. & Emden, C. (1997) Qualitative metasynthesis: issues and techniques. *Research in Nursing and Health*, 20, 365–71.

Shallow, H. (2001) Competence and confidence: working in a climate of fear. *British Journal of Midwifery*, 9 (4), 237–44.

Spencer, L., Ritchie, J., Lewis, J. & Dillon, L. (2003) Quality in qualitative evaluation. Government Chief Social Researcher's Office. Available at website http://www.policyhub.gov.uk/docs/qqe_rep.pdf (accessed 23 November 2006).

Stewart, M. (1999) Lesbian parents talk about their birth experiences. *British Journal of Midwifery*, 7 (2), 96–101.

Strauss, A. & Corbin, J. (1998) *Basics of Qualitative Research. Techniques and Procedures for Developing grounded Theory*. Sage, Thousand Island, California.

Sutton, A.J., Abrams, K.R., Jones, D.R., Sheldon, T.A. & Song, F. (1998) Systematic reviews of trials and other studies. *Health Technology Assessment*, 2 (19), 1–276.

Thomas, J., Harden, A., Oakley, A. et al. (2004) Integrating qualitative research with trials in systematic reviews. *British Medical Journal*, 328 (7446), 1010–12.

Tonks, A. (2002) What's a good doctor and how do you make one? *British Medical Journal*, 325, 711–15.

Vehvilainen-Julkunen, K. & Liukkonen, A. (1998) Fathers' experiences of childbirth. *Midwifery*, 14 (1), 10–17.

Wallace, E.M., Mackintosh, C.L., Brownlee, M., Laidlaw, L. & Johnstone, F.D. (1995) A study of midwife–medical staff interaction in a labour ward environment. *British Journal of Obstetrics and Gynaecology*, 15, 165–70.

Webb, C., Endacott, R., Gray, M.A., Jasper, M.A., McMullan, M. & Scholes, J. (2003) Evaluating portfolio assessment systems: what are the appropriate criteria? *Nurse Education Today*, 23, 600–9.

Webster P., Ulmer, B., Mann, J. et al. (1995) As good as anyone: antenatal shared care at an inner Sydney hospital. *Australian Health Review*, 18 (4), 95–104.

Whelan, A. & Lupton, P. (1998) Promoting successful breast feeding among women with a low income. *Midwifery*, 14 (2), 94–100.

Wiegers, T.A., Keirse, M.J.N.C., Zee, J.v.d. & Berghs, G.A.H. (1996) Outcome of planned home and planned hospital birth in low risk pregnancies: a prospective study in midwifery practice in the Netherlands. *British Medical Journal*, 313, 1309–13.

Woodward, V. & Webb, C. (2001) Women's anxieties surrounding breast disorders: a systematic review of the literature. *Journal of Advanced Nursing*, 33 (1), 29–41.

14 Older People and Respite Care

Rachel McNamara and Chris Shaw

Introduction

The importance of carers who care for frail and disabled older people has been acknowledged over recent years. It is also recognised that as the population ages the issue of care for older people will become increasingly important. It is projected that in the UK the number of people over pensionable age will increase to over 15 million by 2040, compared to nearly 4.5 million in 2002 (Population Trends, 2003). This has the potential to have a significant impact on health and social care systems, as nearly half of people over the age of 75 years report having a limiting long-standing illness (Office of National Statistics, 2002).

Prior to the focus on community care in the early 1990s, carers were considered a 'resource', with formal care provided to disabled people only in the absence of informal carers (Pickard, 2001). However, by the late 1990s a number of policy statements were published promoting active support for informal carers. The National Strategy for Carers (Department of Health, 1999) consisted of three elements: information, support and care for carers. As part of this strategy a document was published called *Caring about Carers* (Department of Health, 1999), the central principle of this being the provision of short-term breaks or respite care to support carers and improve their health and well-being, thus ensuring that caring can continue within the informal framework in the community. In this chapter we describe the methodological issues surrounding an integrative review of quantitative and qualitative research to assess the evidence for effectiveness of respite care in improving the well-being of carers and the extent to which informal care enables care in the community.

Who are carers and what impact does their role have on them?

Many informal carers of the frail and elderly are themselves in mid to late life, being spouses, siblings or adult children of care recipients. In 2001 nearly 2.8 million people in England and Wales, who were themselves aged 50 years and over, provided unpaid care for family members, friends or neighbours, and 24% of carers in the 50–60 age group spent 50 hours/week or more on caring activities (Office of National Statistics, 2001, 2002). Women are more likely than men to be carers, and have a heavy caring commitment of over 20 hours/week. About one-third of carers are the only means of support for the care recipient, and nearly half have been in a caring role for at least 5 years. The majority of help provided is of a practical nature, such as help with meal preparation, shopping and household tasks. More than half provide social support or report that they just 'kept an eye' on the care recipient. Around a quarter to a third carry out more personal activities, such as personal hygiene or helping with mobility problems (Office of National Statistics, 2002).

Such long-term and continuous commitments can have significant impacts on both the physical and mental health of carers. They report consistently poorer health than their non-caring peers and this is related to the number of hours spent caring. Psychosocial effects may include restrictions on social activity, lack of privacy, impaired sleep, feelings of stress, dissatisfaction with the caregiving relationship, and effects on family and job. Carers frequently feel that poor health such as musculoskeletal problems can be directly attributable to their caring role, with additional complaints of tiredness, depression, loss of appetite, stress and short temper. These types of complaint are higher in those who provide care for an older person living in the same household, as opposed to those living elsewhere. This probably reflects the number of hours spent caring and the level of care provided (Ashworth & Baker, 2000; Office of National Statistics, 2002; Wimo et al., 2002). It may also result from the greater difficulty of taking a break from caring when the care recipient is living with the carer. While there may be direct effects on health and well-being, there may also be indirect effects through lower earnings and/or increased costs involved in caring. All these factors together have been conceptualised as 'carer burden'. However, research has demonstrated that carer burden is complex and it is not the case that carers of the most impaired care recipients are those experiencing greatest burden: there are a number of mediating factors. Female caregivers experience greater burden than males, and white caregivers have been reported to experience greater burden than African Americans (Dunkin & Anderson-Hanley, 1998). Other factors include caregiver support, carer health status, coping abilities, the type of problems experienced by the care recipient and the quality of the prior relationship with the care recipient. Although the experience of burden varies between different subgroups of carers, carer burden is a stronger predictor of institutionalisation than patient variables (Dunkin & Anderson-Hanley, 1998); this points to the importance of carer support if frail elders are to continue being supported in the community.

Respite care and evidence for its effectiveness

One strategy for supporting the well-being of carers is to provide temporary short-term breaks in care. Such respite care can be provided in a number of different ways, including as an in-patient in a care home or hospice (typically for 1 or 2 weeks), day care, or in-home and sitting services. Night sitting services are another possibility. Care may be provided by voluntary services, social services or healthcare providers. Evidence of the effectiveness of respite care has tended to focus on outcomes for carers, although it is increasingly being recognised that the impact of respite care on care recipients is also important (Nolan & Grant, 1993).

There have been several previous systematic reviews of services for carers, but these have tended to focus on care recipients having specific problems such as dementia and mental health problems, and not all focus specifically on respite care (Arksey, 2003; Lee & Cameron, 2004). Other reviews have addressed respite care for carers of mixed age groups of care recipients or frail elders as well as palliative care, but the results remain unclear (Forster et al., 1999; McNally et al., 1999; Zarit et al., 1999; Sorensen et al., 2002; Ingleton et al., 2003; Stoltz et al., 2004). Because of the nature of the intervention, few randomised controlled trials (RCTs) have been undertaken, and in non-randomised studies effect sizes are frequently small. The evidence, therefore, is mixed, with some positive and some negative effects. Although respite is designed to maintain the independence of the older person, some studies suggest that there is an increased risk of institutionalisation after respite care. The evidence to date does point to the need to take into account factors that might act as confounders, such as type of respite care, type of care received by control groups and type of carer (Zarit et al., 1999).

Another finding reported in the literature is a reluctance by some carers to take up services, despite an expressed need for this type of support (Brodaty et al., 2005), for a number of reasons, such as a lack of knowledge of available services, concern about the quality of care and services being inappropriate or inconvenient. Much of this literature uses qualitative methods, but none of the systematic reviews to date have attempted to synthesise the qualitative evidence. Any discrepancy between expressed need and take-up of services must be explored before heavy investment is made in this type of service provision.

Overview

Review aims

The aims of the systematic review were to:

(1) Appraise, summarise and synthesise the quantitative literature on the effectiveness and cost-effectiveness of services providing temporary breaks in caring for informal carers of older people, i.e. those over the age of 65 years
(2) Appraise, summarise and synthesise the qualitative literature on:
   (a) Carer and/or care recipient views of respite care
   (b) Reasons for non-uptake of respite services
   (c) Expressed need for respite care
   (d) Impact of respite care on carer and/or care recipient

The review built on previous reviews by giving a more comprehensive account of the literature pertaining to respite care, which includes a wider range of care recipients, i.e. those with both mental and physical disabilities, as well as those undergoing palliative care at the end of life. Previous reviews have also pointed to the need to consider the context of respite care, and so the synthesis will focus, where possible, on each of the different service options, i.e. institutional care, day care, home care and mixed services (Parker et al., 2002). The literature also suggests that carers' experiences differ according to the underlying condition of the care recipient (Colvez et al., 2002) and so the different characteristics of care recipients will be considered separately if feasible, e.g. mental impairment, physical disability, palliative care and mixed problems.

The aims of the review were to describe outcomes, both positive and negative, for both carers and care recipients, as well as service outcomes such as institutionalisation. The outcomes for carer and care recipient have the potential to be at odds for, although the aim of respite care is to benefit carers, there is a possibility of adverse outcomes for care recipients. For example, being exposed to an institutional environment may pose a high risk of infection and accidental injury, or may disrupt the routine of cognitively frail individuals and result in an increase in difficult behaviours.

Methodology

While we adopted standard systematic review methods, this presented a number of challenges. The overall challenge was to integrate information from three different perspectives: a review of quantitative literature, a review of qualitative studies, and a cost-effectiveness review. In the quantitative review, studies were heterogeneous as no exclusions were based on methodology, thus including observational studies as well as randomised and non-randomised trials. Scoping studies of the literature also revealed that few data were available on the cost-effectiveness of respite care, and this was confirmed on more detailed searching. There was also little information available on the constituent elements of respite interventions to allow costing of different types of respite care. The aim was, therefore, to develop a potential model for cost analysis and the requirements of future research in populating such a model. Despite the obvious differences in these three areas of the review, the aim was to maintain a standard methodological approach where possible. For the purposes of this chapter, we focus on the methods used in the quantitative and qualitative aspects of this review and how data were collected to allow the syntheses to be complementary.

The process of the review included a number of stages, as follows:

(1) Development of a search strategy to incorporate literature relevant to both quantitative and qualitative components of the review
(2) Reference search on all major online databases
(3) Identification of included and excluded articles for qualitative and quantitative studies separately – first, based on titles, followed by abstracts and, finally, the full article should the abstract be unclear
(4) Development of data extraction sheets and processes for each aspect of the review
(5) Data extraction
(6) Data synthesis

Methodological issues

The following section details the review methodology, and highlights particular methodological challenges relating to devising an appropriate search strategy and adequate inclusion criteria, and the design of appropriate data extraction and quality assessment tools for the quantitative and qualitative syntheses.

Devising an appropriate search strategy

The remit of the review was very broad. Therefore, designing a search strategy with appropriate sensitivity and specificity was a challenge. Respite care might feasibly occur within community and institutional settings, and across many different conditions (e.g. dementia, palliative care, stroke). Moreover, interventions or services designed to give caregivers a break from their caring role might not be explicitly labelled as respite care. Therefore, the specificity of the search was sacrificed to some degree to maximise sensitivity.

The search strategy comprised three distinct blocks: the first set of terms were designed to capture all relevant literature related to respite care, while the remaining two sets were intended to limit articles retrieved to those within older populations and those specifically mentioning carers, respectively. Words and phrases within each set were combined using the Boolean 'OR' operator; the three sets were then combined using the 'AND' operator. Possible search terms were trialled initially on MEDLINE, mapping words and phrases to indexed medical subject headings, and also searching for key terms within the title, abstract and subject heading (using the .mp operator). Input and opinion on the appropriateness and comprehensiveness of the search terms were sought from an information specialist, all co-applicants (covering specialist expertise in geriatric medicine, evaluation of health services for the elderly and health economics) and user representatives from two UK organisations. The finalised MEDLINE search strategy is shown in Table 14.1.

The list of terms in Table 14.1 was used as a template for searching all other databases. Keywords and the use of subject headings were adapted as appropriate to each database. A total of 24 online databases were searched (from the earliest possible date to the end of 2005) and are listed in Table 14.2.

The final search yielded a total of 12 992 hits, once all references had been transferred to reference management software and duplicates removed. There was a significant degree of overlap between databases: taking four electronic databases as an example, the majority of references (64%) came from MEDLINE, original citations on EMBASE accounted for a further 24%; PSYCHINFO for 11%; BNI for just 1% (see Figure 14.1).

Assessment of study quality

Assessment of study quality formed an integral part of the review, and the methods used for assessing quality of both quantitative and qualitative studies are outlined in the following sections.

Quality assessment for quantitative studies

Tools for formally assessing the quality of randomised trials are numerous: at least 25 are currently in use to differing degrees (Moher et al., 1995). However, a MEDLINE search from 1990 to 1997 failed to identify any such tools for the assessment of cohort and case-control studies (Downs & Black, 1998). A brief review of the literature to the end of 2005 indicated that this situation has changed little since the late 1990s. Given the inclusive nature of the review, it was necessary to identify a tool that could be used to assess the quality of various quantitative designs, including randomised trials, cohort and case-control studies.

Two quality checklists were identified from the literature (Downs & Black, 1998; Kmet et al., 2004)

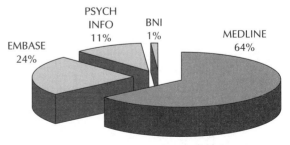

Figure 14.1 Overlap between electronic databases. Values have been approximated to the nearest % and are for 2005 only.

Table 14.1   MEDLINE search strategy.

No.	Search history	
1	respite$.af.	Block 1
2	(community care$ or community nurs$).mp.	Search terms to
3	exp Community Health Services/[1] or community health service$.mp.	identify any study
4	(community health nurs$ or community mental health).mp.	that might include
5	exp Community Psychiatry/ or community psychiat$.mp.	respite care
6	(community healthcare$ or community health care$).mp.	
7	(home care$ or home health care$).mp.	
8	home nurs$.mp.	
9	health service$ for the ag$.mp.	
10	informal care$.mp.	
11	(day centre$ or day center$).mp.	
12	(day care$ or daycare$).mp.	
13	night care$.mp.	
14	(night sitt$ or night service$).mp.	
15	domiciliary.mp.	
16	holiday$.mp.	
17	(short break$ or break$ in car$).mp.	
18	old age assistance.mp.	
19	temporary care$.mp.	
20	exp Nursing Homes/ or nursing home$.mp.	
21	exp Residential Facilities/ or residential facilit$.mp.	
22	home$ for the ag$.mp.	
23	(residential home$ or residential care$).mp.	
24	(cancer care$ or oncologic$ care$).mp.	
25	palliative$.mp.	
26	exp Terminal Care/ or terminal care$.mp.	
27	terminal$ ill$.mp.	
28	end of life.mp.	
29	dying$.mp.	
30	hospice$.mp.	
31	exp Aged/ or aged.mp.	Block 2
32	exp Aging/ or aging.mp.	Search terms to limit
33	ageing.mp.	the search to
34	old$.mp.	the frail elderly group
35	elder$.mp.	
36	frail$.mp.	
37	senior$.mp.	
38	veteran$.mp.	
39	(geriatric$ or gerontolog$).mp.	
40	psychogeriatric$.mp.	
41	exp Dementia/ or dementia$.mp.	
42	alzheimer$.mp.	
43	(caregiver$ or care giver$).mp.	Block 3
44	carer$.mp.	Terms to limit to carers
45	or/1–30	
46	or/31–42	
47	or/43–44	
48	45 and 46 and 47	
49	limit 48 to humans	

Keywords using the '.mp' operator were used either in addition to MeSH headings, or in place of, when they produced the same, or additional, hits.

Table 14.2 List of online databases searched.

Medical	MEDLINE (including in-progress and non-indexed citations)
	EMBASE
	Allied and Complementary Medicine (AMED)
	PubMed Cancer Citations Only (maintained by NCI/NLM – formerly CancerLit)
Nursing research	Cumulative Index to Nursing and Allied Health Literature (CINAHL)
	British Nursing Index (BNI)
Social science and social care	Applied Social Sciences Index and Abstracts (ASSIA)
	PSYCHINFO
	BIDS International Bibliography of the Social Sciences (IBSS)
	Social Care Online (previously CareData)
	Sociological Abstracts
	Web of Science (including Social Science Citation Index)
	Scopus
Databases of reviews	Database of Abstracts of Reviews of Effects (DARE)
	Cochrane Database of Methodology Reviews
	Cochrane Database of Systematic Reviews (CDSR)
	Health Technology Assessment Database (HTA)
Ongoing research databases	National Research Register (NRR)
	Computer Retrieval of Information on Scientific Projects (CRISP)
Economics	NHS Economic Evaluation Database
	EconLit
Others	Cochrane Methodology Register (CMR)
	Cochrane Register of Controlled Trials (CENTRAL)
	Health Management Information Consortium (HMIC – including the King's Fund database)

which contained useful elements relevant to the review. Downs & Black (1998) developed a tool to assess study quality of both randomised and non-randomised designs. The resulting checklist gives an overall score of study quality, and contains 27 items related to the appropriateness and adequate description of the study hypothesis, design, intervention, main outcomes under study and methods of analysis. The authors demonstrated good inter-rater reliability using their checklist, although it was suggested that further development and testing would be required. Kmet et al. (2004) also developed a checklist for assessing quality of both randomised and non-randomised studies, following a review of the available instruments and discussion of issues central to internal validity. This checklist also gives a summary score, although the authors acknowledge that this in itself may introduce bias, and that their assessment of inter-rater reliability was somewhat limited (10 studies scored by 2 reviewers). The checklist of Kmet et al.

(2004) comprised 14 items assessing quality and appropriateness of the study design, intervention, outcome measures and methods of analysis.

For the purposes of the current review, it was considered that both checklists contained useful items but that each had particular disadvantages. The Downs & Black checklist is heavily weighted towards randomised designs, of which there are few in the current review, and is quite long (27 items). In comparison, the Kmet et al. tool contains just 14 items and is less detailed, e.g. *excludes* description of the intervention. Therefore, a single checklist was created, based on the most appropriate items in these two existing tools. The current tool was also developed using the US Preventative Services Task Force (USPSTF) framework (Harris et al., 2001), which is a recommended framework for carrying out a high-quality systematic review. The framework comprises three strata. The first, at the individual study level, relates to quality assessment. The other two strata refer to the quality of the body of evidence for a particular question and the quality of the body of evidence for the review as a whole. We created a set of operational parameters for evaluating the internal validity of five study designs: systematic reviews; randomised controlled trials; case-control; cohort and diagnostic accuracy studies. Rather than giving a quality score, the USPSTF provides an indication of quality based on certain parameters; first the five study designs are organised into a hierarchy (RCT, non-randomised controlled, cohort or case control, etc.) and then designated as 'good', 'fair' or 'poor' according to criteria specific to the particular study design.

The final checklist comprised 18 items (Table 14.3). Three levels were assigned to each item ('good', 'fair', 'poor') and scored from 2 to 0: scores were then summed to produce an overall rating of study quality. The checklist was piloted within the current review and inter-rater reliability assessed (on a subsample of studies) and compared to the reliability of both the Downs & Black and Kmet et al. tools.

Quality assessment for qualitative studies

While assessment of quality is a fairly standard and established activity related to the synthesis of quantitative data in systematic reviews, the use of standardised assessment tools in qualitative reviews is comparatively new. Considerable debate has developed concerning the assessment of methodological quality, as qualitative work is increasingly acknowledged and accepted by the mainstream community of healthcare researchers. It is now accepted as an important method to inform healthcare provision, and is seen as particularly useful in addressing patients' views. Studies using mixed methods are becoming more common and, to some extent, expected.

At the most fundamental level, debate has considered the appropriateness of quality assessment, as some researchers consider that this just serves to stem the interpretive and creative aspects of qualitative study (Dixon-Woods et al., 2004). However, there is substantial consensus that some means of

Table 14.3   Items in the quality assessment checklist for quantitative studies. Each item was scored 0–2 (0, poor; 1, fair; 2, good). Details were given of the definitions of these categories for each item in the complete version of the instrument.

Items
Study aims
1. Is the hypothesis/aim/objective of the study clearly and sufficiently described?
Study design and sample characteristics
2. Is the study design well described and appropriate? *(If study question not given, infer from conclusions)*
3. Is the method of patient/control group selection described and appropriate?
4. Are the characteristics of patient/control group(s) clearly described (i.e. age range, health characteristic/s)?
5. Are caregiver characteristics clearly described (i.e. age, gender, relationship to care recipient, time spent caring)?
6. Were patients/participants randomised to intervention groups?
7. *For RCTs only*: was randomisation/allocation concealed from patients?
8. Have the characteristics of patients lost to follow-up been described?
9. Are intervention(s) clearly described?
10. Are the main outcomes to be measured clearly described in the introduction/method?
11. If possible, was an attempt made to blind those measuring the main outcomes of the intervention?
12. Are population characteristics (if measured and described) controlled for and adequately described?
13. Are the main findings clearly described?
Data analysis
14. Are methods of analysis adequately described and appropriate?
15. Are estimates of variance reported for the main results?
16. In trials/cohort studies, do analyses adjust for different lengths of follow-up, or in case-control studies, is the time between intervention and outcome the same for cases/controls?
17. If appropriate, were data analysed according to ITT (intention to treat) principle?
Conclusions
18. Are the conclusions supported by the results?

assessing quality is required if qualitative research is to be taken seriously (Popay et al., 1998; Mays & Pope, 2000; Fade, 2003). This is, of course, important in the concurrent synthesis of quantitative and qualitative evidence in order to convince readers of the equal weight and importance of the two aspects of the review. The development of a structured tool for quality assessment, similar to those used in quantitative reviews, is crucial in enabling mixed teams of researchers to appraise studies that use methods that may not be within their area of expertise. In our particular study, the team consisted of statisticians, economists and health services researchers who had greater quantitative experience, as well as those who were familiar with qualitative methods.

In order to maintain consistency across the two aspects of the review the aim was to develop a quality tool that was similar in structure to the quantitative assessment tool, while bearing in mind the different aims of qualitative and quantitative research. Quantitative research seeks to eliminate bias in order to render the research results generalisable to a population, whereas qualitative research is context-bound and seeks to expose and discuss bias. For these reasons it has been proposed that a common language may be misleading (Fade, 2003). Alternatives to terms such as internal and external validity, reliability and objectivity have been proposed, e.g. credibility, dependability, transferability and confirmability (Lincoln, 1995). Others, however, feel that issues of validity and relevance are appropriate to qualitative research even though the concepts supporting them may be dissimilar to those pertaining to quantitative research (Mays & Pope, 2000; Fade, 2003). However, it has been pointed out that there is a need to qualify this by ensuring that the different paradigms within qualitative research are acknowledged (Fossey et al., 2002). Qualitative research is not a unitary activity, and aims and methods will vary according to the philosophical underpinning and the requirements of the study. This could be considered to be similar to the varied approaches in quantitative research with the resultant difficulty of establishing a quality assessment tool that is appropriate to all types of study. However, a number of concepts are of relevance across study types, if interpreted somewhat differently. In order to identify items for inclusion in the assessment tool, a review was undertaken of

articles that either presented a checklist for quality assessment or a narrative account of quality assessment. Although this review was not carried out systematically, it followed a similar approach to that used by Walsh & Downe (2005), who adopted a scoping method designed to assess commonalities between quality assessment tools and eliminate redundant items. The review by Walsh & Downe was based on seven existing checklists and the checklist they developed using this method was included in the present analysis.

This scoping of quality assessment literature revealed considerable overlap and agreement between studies in terms of the relevant criteria for assessing quality. Items to be included in the tool were chosen based on their frequency of occurrence in the articles reviewed, their appropriateness to the requirements of our review, and their generalisability across different qualitative methods. However, the types of study likely to occur in the respite care review mainly involved thematic analysis or occasionally a phenomenological approach. Studies using direct observation, or data collected from sources other than focus groups or interviews were excluded. Some quality assessment checklists were quite broad and vague, although they appeared shorter and more succinct than others. We preferred a more detailed and structured approach in order to have clear definitions to facilitate interpretation and increase inter-rater reliability. Therefore we used a rating format based on the checklist developed by Kmet et al. (2004) for quality assessment of qualitative research. This was also in line with the format used for the quantitative assessment tool (also based on Kmet). The tool was piloted and amended and the items included in the final version are shown in Table 14.4. Three levels were assigned to each item in the tool, which were scored from 2 to 0. The scores could then be summed to give an overall quality rating.

Identification of studies and data extraction

In identifying studies for inclusion and exclusion, clear definitions were needed of the various concepts. A preliminary review of a small number of studies emerging from the searches showed respite care components to be difficult to identify within the interventions being assessed. Often the study

Table 14.4   Items in the quality assessment checklist for qualitative studies. Each item was scored 0–2 (0, poor; 1, fair; 2, good). Details were given of the definitions of these categories for each item in the complete version of the instrument.

Items in checklist

Study aims and context
1.   Is the research question sufficiently described?
2.   Is qualitative method appropriate?
3.   Is the setting/context clearly described?

Sampling
4.   Is the sampling strategy clearly described?
5.   Is sampling method likely to recruit all relevant cases? (purposive, theoretical sampling)
6.   Are relevant characteristics of sample given?
7.   Is rationale for sample size (e.g. data saturation) given?
8.   Are methods of data collection clearly described?

Data collection
9.   Is method of data collection appropriate for research question and paradigm?
10.   Has the researcher verified the data (e.g. by triangulation)?

Data analysis
11.   Are data analysis methods clearly described?
12.   Are data analysis methods appropriate?
13.   Are competing accounts/deviant data taken into account?

Reflexivity
14.   To what extent is the researcher reflective?

Interpretation and conclusions
15.   Are the interpretations and conclusions supported by the data?

involved a more active intervention, with respite being an unintended outcome. Ideally it would have been preferable to identify studies in which the respite component was not confounded by other types of intervention. However, this proved difficult, particularly in residential admissions, because, as well as being aimed at providing respite, they also frequently include some medical or nursing review. After discussion in the review team, it was agreed to include studies that explicitly aimed to provide a break from caring and to exclude interventions such as palliative care or hospital-at-home interventions unless a stated aim was to provide respite, or carer outcomes were specifically mentioned. This distinction was of particular relevance to the quantitative review as this was an effectiveness review and, as such, required the reporting of a comparison between respite and no respite care (or some other type of intervention). This comparison varied considerably between studies and occasionally the respite intervention was, in fact, presented as the control for a more active intervention. However, as well as studies that reported a between-group analysis, regression analyses were also included in which respite was a predictor of carer outcomes, such as carer burden. Within-group longitudinal comparisons were also included that reported carer outcomes before and after the delivery of the respite intervention.

The definition of respite care was particularly difficult to operationalise in the literature on palliative care. Medical or nursing input was more prominent in this context, as symptom control is a major aspect of any palliative care admission. In addition, descriptions of interventions generally tended to be very poor, and it was frequently difficult to ascertain the exact nature of the intervention and its constituent components. These types of issues were not as pertinent to the qualitative review as inclusion was not dependent on participation in respite care but on the reporting of views of *either* carers or care recipients about respite services, respite needs or reasons for non-uptake.

The definition of frail elderly can also be problematic, but in this case it was constrained by how the population was likely to be defined in the literature. An age threshold of 65 years and over was identified and, although other arbitrary cut-offs could be argued for, the majority of studies categorised samples as under or over 65 years. The definition of 'frail' was based on the fact that we were examining carer outcomes and the contention was that any person over the age of 65 years who also required a carer was either physically or mentally frail. The definition of frail elderly applied across both the quantitative and qualitative reviews.

In the quantitative review we aimed not to exclude studies on the basis of language. However, limited resources required us to focus this approach and to include the foreign language papers that appeared to contribute most substantially to the review. This decision was based on the number of papers available in a particular language and the similarity and relevance of the study context to the healthcare system in the UK. The qualitative review, however, excluded all foreign language papers as the issue of translation and interpretation would have greater potential impact on the findings. In the data extraction stage of the qualitative review the language of the original data collection was noted, even in studies reported completely in English, in order to identify those that had undergone an additional stage of interpretation.

Included papers were identified first by sifting titles to exclude the obvious, e.g. reports of respite for carers of children rather than frail elderly, second by review of abstracts, and finally by reading of the complete article in cases where inclusion could not be discerned from the abstract. The numbers of articles included at each stage are summarised in Table 14.5.

The qualitative and quantitative papers were handled together at this stage as frequently studies used mixed methods and so could report both quantitative and qualitative data. However, because of the wider remit and less stringent inclusion and

exclusion criteria adopted in the qualitative review, a larger number of qualitative papers were identified for possible inclusion at the abstract stage than originally anticipated. This was due partly to the wider remit of the qualitative review, and partly to the reliance on qualitative methods in an area in which it is difficult to carry out controlled trials for ethical and practical reasons. It was difficult to identify inclusions and exclusions from the abstracts of papers that focused on the impact of caring. In these studies respite needs were often mentioned, but were a small part of the findings and so were not always described in the abstract. To ensure reliability of the process, all inclusion/exclusion decisions were carried out by a minimum of two people. Full papers were retrieved if either of the reviewers nominated a study as eligible for inclusion at the abstract screening stage. If, on reading the full article, there was still disagreement between two reviewers on eligibility, then the paper was discussed by the wider team. These types of disagreement were generally a result of the need to clarify definitions, and occurred most frequently at the beginning of the study.

Data extraction was carried out as a two-stage process in both reviews. Initially, study methods were extracted, including information about the intervention, characteristics of carers and care recipients and the types of outcome measured. This was followed by extraction of statistical data by the statisticians in the team. Data extraction was carried out directly into a database to avoid the need for an additional stage of transcribing data from paper to electronic format. This also aided consistency of data extraction by allowing only certain types of options to be entered, thus ensuring that data were categorised in a similar way by all data extractors. The qualitative review followed a similar pattern, with an initial meta-methods analysis in which data were extracted to a summary

Table 14.5   Numbers of included articles at each stage of the review.

Sift stage	Number of articles
Initial search (duplicates removed)	12 992
Irrelevant titles excluded	8042
Included articles following abstract sift	1227
Included articles following full-paper retrieval	91 + 67 qualitative

table as described in the following section. A meta-data-analysis was then carried out on a subsample of papers: the findings from the qualitative studies were extracted into a software package specifically designed for qualitative analysis (NUD.IST version 6).

Analysis plan and data synthesis

Methods of analysis and approaches to data synthesis are outlined in the following sections for the quantitative and qualitative components of the review.

Quantitative synthesis

Where appropriate and possible, quantitative results from individual studies were synthesised using meta-analysis techniques, taking due account of statistical, clinical and methodological heterogeneity (Sutton et al., 2000a). To account for the variety of ways in which some outcomes, such as quality of life and satisfaction, were measured, standardised effect sizes were used.

A total of 91 quantitative studies (Table 14.6) met the inclusion criteria for the review: of these, 7 were fully randomised designs (RCTs), and 18 were classified as quasi-experimental (longitudinal studies with experimental and control conditions). However, only 6 RCTs and 12 quasi-experimental studies were suitable for inclusion in the meta-analysis, as key data were insufficient or missing from the 7 excluded studies (e.g. mean values not given at follow-up). Therefore, a total of 18 studies were included in the meta-analysis. In terms of respite setting, the majority of evaluations were carried out within day-care or mixed services (see Table 14.7).

Initially, between-study heterogeneity was investigated within RCTs and quasi-experimental studies; studies where intervention group members served as their own controls (i.e. 'before and after' studies) were analysed separately ($n = 10$). Cross-design/Generalised Evidence Synthesis methods were used to model the effectiveness of interventions across study types (e.g. RCT, quasi-experimental), making due allowance for the potential biases and confounding that might be present in non-randomised studies (Abrams & Jones, 1995; Prevost

Table 14.6   Included quantitative studies by design.

Study design	Number included and extracted	Number appropriate for synthesis
Randomised controlled trial	7	6
Quasi-experimental	18	12
Before and after	10	10
Longitudinal observational	15	15*
Cross-sectional	41	41*
Total	91	84

*Narrative synthesis only.

Table 14.7   Respite setting.

	Day care	Home care	Institutional	Mixed
RCT dementia	1	–	1	1
RCT frail elderly	3 (1 UK)	–	–	–
RCT total (6)	4 (1 UK)	–	1	1
Quasi dementia	3 (1 UK)	1	1	4 (1 UK)
Quasi frail elderly	1	1 (UK)	–	1
Quasi total (12)	4 (1 UK)	2 (1 UK)	1	5 (1 UK)

RCT, randomised controlled trial; UK, United Kingdom.

et al., 2000; Sutton & Abrams, 2001; Spiegelhalter et al., 2003). In addition, evidence from RCTs and quasi-experimental studies was considered separately.

Meta-regression techniques were applied, using a range of study-level covariates such as intervention (e.g. location of care) and population (e.g. cognitive impairment or frailty) as well as study quality (Lambert et al., 2002). Outcomes for carers were the primary focus of the meta-analysis, and all included studies tended to assess a similar set of outcomes (e.g. burden, depression, anxiety, positive affect, physical health). Once effect sizes for these various outcomes were established, patient outcomes were assessed relative to these effects to determine whether a beneficial effect of respite on burden, for example, had a measurable negative impact on care recipients. This was considered an important step, as the qualitative data indicated that a common reason for non-uptake of services was concern on the part of carers that respite would somehow be detrimental to care recipients. Level of publication bias was investigated using a variety of methods, and sensitivity analyses performed to assess its impact on the results of the review (Sutton et al., 2000b).

Observational studies included in the review ($n = 56$) formed the basis of a narrative synthesis, with particular reference to rate of institutionalisation amongst those accessing respite as compared to non-users. However, much of the observational work in the area tended to focus on use of respite as a generic, dichotomous outcome, and so differentiating between the effects of diverse respite settings (i.e. home care, day care) was problematic.

Qualitative analysis

The methods used to review the qualitative literature followed those used in carrying out primary qualitative research and were based on the methods of meta-synthesis described by Paterson et al. (2001) and Noblit & Hare (1988). The synthesis aimed to be both interpretive, in order to provide further explanation of research findings in the quantitative review, and aggregative, in order to identify the extent of the literature and gaps that need to be addressed. To do this a two-stage process was adopted by, first, carrying out a meta-method analysis and, second, a meta-data-analysis.

Meta-method analysis assesses both the quality of the research methods of the primary research papers and the ways in which the methodological context may have influenced the study findings (Paterson et al., 2001). Each paper was summarised into a table under the headings shown in Table 14.8.

Separate tables were constructed, depending on the country in which the research was conducted, and the factors influencing study findings could then be explored. For example, as well as differences in sampling procedures, variation in data collection methods might have an impact on study findings, e.g. data collected by face-to-face interview versus focus groups. Such tables may also

Table 14.8 Table headings for summary of qualitative studies included in the review.

Table heading	Detail of content under table headings
First author (date) and country	
Study design	Sample and setting. If the provision of respite care was a part of the study, the type of respite would be included here
Sampling and type of interview	e.g. Purposive sampling and semi-structured interview
Sample characteristics	Number in sample, age, gender, relationship to care recipient
Focus of the study	Whether the study's main aim addressed respite care issues or whether data on needs and/or uptake of services were additional to intended aims
Theoretical framework and/or type of analysis	e.g. Grounded theory or thematic analysis
Quality rating	Total score on the quality assessment tool
Summary of the study findings	Study authors' interpretations of findings

provide information about the generalisability of findings if consistent results are found across samples and contexts, such as place of care, extent of the literature and gaps for future research. The listing of sampling procedures could reveal the types of carers and care recipients whose views were not sought, giving an indication of the representativeness of the findings. These tables also give a view of the literature over time, as preferred methods have changed and developed, and how the field of research is likely to develop in the future.

Because of the large number of studies identified in the qualitative literature search, a purposive sampling technique was used in the meta-data analysis stage. At the outset of the study we had intended to sample according to type of respite provision (e.g. institutional care, day care, home care) and characteristics of the care recipients (e.g. dementia, physically impaired, palliative care). However, such categorisations were not possible as the majority of studies reported a mix of respite use and often a mix of care recipients. We therefore decided to focus, in the first instance, on the organisational context of studies and relevance to UK policy. Accordingly, all UK studies were included. Although there were a substantial number of studies carried out in the UK, studies carried out in the USA were also prominent and tended to be of higher quality, with a more direct focus on respite care issues. We considered that the concerns of carers of older people in the USA would be similar, within the Medicare system, to those of carers in the UK and so these too were included, along with all studies conducted in Canada, where the healthcare system is more similar to that in the UK.

This stage of the analysis was carried out using similar methods to those used in primary qualitative studies. The findings from each study (as reported by the authors) were extracted and a coding frame developed, using a hierarchical coding framework to identify main and sub-themes. Synthesis of the data involved reciprocal translational synthesis and refutational synthesis, as described by Noblit & Hare (1988). This refers to the identification of similarities and differences in the findings of the primary studies. As in primary qualitative research, discrepant cases were sought in order to expand the proposed explanatory theory to account for the findings in a broad range of contexts. By exploring relationships between codes across the different studies, a theory of recipients' and carers' experiences of respite care was developed. Comparison was made between studies on the basis of characteristics of care recipients, methodological quality rating, date of study and country. It was also important to assess the similarities and differences between UK, USA and Canadian studies to explore any fundamental differences related to the different settings.

These findings were then compared to the findings of the quantitative review. One important feature was to identify whether the outcomes addressed in the quantitative study were consistent with those identified in the qualitative studies as being important for both care recipients and carers. Any outcomes not addressed in the quantitative studies were highlighted. Another important consideration was how far the quantitative studies addressed both positive and negative outcomes. Discrepancies in the findings of the quantitative and qualitative reviews were explored and explanations sought within the qualitative data.

Lessons for future reviews

The aim of this study, to carry out complementary syntheses of quantitative and qualitative literature, raised a number of methodological issues. First, it is important to consider the role of the qualitative synthesis in relation to the quantitative review because this will inform the order in which they should be undertaken. This process follows the same principles as in primary research, where a qualitative study can direct the design of a quantitative study, e.g. to identify relevant outcomes, or alternatively be conducted concurrently or after the quantitative study to aid interpretation of results. In this review one of the purposes of the qualitative review was to shed light on the appropriateness of the outcomes assessed in quantitative studies, although it could not have influenced the pre-determined outcomes included in these quantitative studies. It was notable, however, that the outcomes measured in the quantitative studies were fairly restricted and homogeneous, and so left little choice for the selection of outcomes from the qualitative studies. It did, however, inform the analysis by highlighting the importance of assessing care recipient outcomes in relation to carer outcomes.

It is also important to consider the research question of the qualitative review in relation to the quantitative review. As in this study, it is likely that the qualitative research purpose will be much broader and, although it will be more resource effective to have common definitions and a single comprehensive search strategy, close scrutiny is required to ensure that the methods fulfil the requirements for both reviews. How best to define the review topic also needs careful consideration, and reviewers should be aware that different definitions may yield different results. For example, in the current review, respite was defined quite specifically as an intervention designed to give carers a break from caring, and services with a largely medical focus for recipients (e.g. rehabilitation) were excluded. If we had chosen a broader categorisation of respite, the nature of the papers retrieved, and therefore the results of the review, might have been quite different.

It is worth remembering that there are likely to be more qualitative studies than anticipated, particularly in difficult-to-research areas such as respite care, where RCTs are often methodologically and ethically difficult. A sufficiently flexible time frame for scoping searches should be factored into the review timetable, as the number of papers retrieved on full search (both qualitative AND quantitative) may be much greater than originally anticipated. Also, in terms of data extraction, qualitative studies may be more time-consuming if papers are not available in electronic format, as large sections of text must be typed into the analysis software. Study costings should allow for appropriate clerical resources to support this. Qualitative studies can also be more difficult to screen for inclusion/exclusion, as relevant findings may be reported as a subsidiary theme and may not be highlighted in the abstract.

While combinations of different types of qualitative research based on different theoretical frameworks proved challenging in this study, there was little heterogeneity in methodological approach. The majority of studies used some form of thematic analysis, many based on a constant comparative approach. However, at the outset of the review we considered that varying research approaches would not preclude thematic analysis and synthesis of the findings.

Furthermore, the quality of reporting of qualitative studies causes problems for this type of systematic review. Generally, quantitative studies were more rigorous in identifying participant characteristics and describing of the research context, whereas in qualitative studies these were often only partially reported or not reported at all. It was, therefore, often difficult to identify whether care recipients were elderly or not, or whether carers had received respite services. Inclusion criteria had to be a little more flexible and assumptions made about characteristics of participants. For example, reports could give the age of carers but not care recipients, but by extrapolating from the relationship of carer to care recipient, an estimate of care recipients' age could be made. Finally, given the relative scarcity of RCTs in this area, the current review also highlights the need to consider less rigorous types of quantitative evidence (e.g. cohort studies) in order to make appropriate recommendations for further research.

Conclusion

While offering some methodological challenges, a multi-method approach to systematic literature reviews is a useful means of improving and expanding the evidence base for healthcare interventions. This is of particular relevance in areas where, for various reasons, little good-quality quantitative evidence is available. However, even in the presence of good-quality RCTs, a qualitative synthesis will aid interpretation and provide insight into the relevance of the quantitative synthesis to participants themselves. This approach has the potential to provide a more comprehensive involvement of user views when carried out in conjunction with the inclusion of selected user representatives on the project management team. The inclusion of qualitative studies in rigorously conducted systematic reviews may also provide an impetus to improve the quality of reporting of qualitative research.

The aim of this systematic literature review was to assess the effectiveness of respite care for carers of frail older people, but the complexities involved in synthesising the evidence on this type of service intervention are representative of many service areas related to nursing practice. It is often difficult to identify which of the constituent elements of a service are responsible for the effects seen in RCTs. When assessing the evidence concerning service interventions with the intention of applying them in a different setting this must be borne in mind, along with a consideration of user views as illustrated in the qualitative element of this review. In the context of this particular study the quantitative synthesis will demonstrate the level of effectiveness of interventions, but this is meaningless to practitioners if account is not taken of why carers do not take up these services.

From a methodological perspective, future researchers must seek to perfect and standardise qualitative syntheses of evidence, and explore how to combine studies that have used different theoretical frameworks. Methods, other than thematic analysis (e.g. discourse analysis), could also be applied to identify the underlying attitudes of the authors of individual studies in a review, which might shed further light on the reasons behind discrepant findings. From the perspective of provision of respite care, our review highlighted that the main focus of research was on carers of dementia sufferers, with least research in the area of palliative care. In the few studies that had been carried out in palliative-care settings, it demonstrated that concerns and issues of these carers are somewhat different, and further research is required to determine how the needs of carers of dying patients may be met. The qualitative synthesis suggested a number of barriers to respite care, all of which could be addressed in future service provision and future research, including low awareness and knowledge of services, concerns about quality, and the importance of flexibility. Perhaps the most important findings was that 'one size does not fit all', and that carers benefited most from provision of a variety of different types of respite, depending on their individual circumstances. Finally, an issue for further exploration is the distinction between a physical and a mental break from caring, which were not always synonymous, and how carers may best be helped to achieve the mental break that appeared to be most beneficial to their well-being.

Acknowledgements

This chapter is based on a systematic review of respite care for frail elderly funded by the UK Department of Health through its Health Technology Assessment Programme, and carried out under the direction of project lead Dr Chris Shaw. The work is subject to Crown Copyright. The opinions expressed here are those of the authors and do not necessarily reflect those of the UK National Health Service or the Department of Health.

References

Abrams, K.R. & Jones, D.R. (1995) Meta-analysis and the synthesis of evidence. *IMA Journal of Mathematics Applied to Medicine and Biology*, 12, 297–313.

Arksey, H. (2003) Scoping the field: services for carers of people with mental health problems. *Health and Social Care in the Community*, 11 (4), 335–44.

Ashworth, M. & Baker, A.H. (2000) 'Time and space': carers' views about respite care. *Health and Social Care in the Community*, 8 (1), 50–6.

Brodaty, H., Thomson, C., Thompson, C. & Fine, M. (2005) Why caregivers of people with dementia and memory loss don't use services. *International Journal of Geriatric Psychiatry*, 20, 537–46.

Colvez, A., Joël, M.E., Ponton Sanchez, A. & Royer, A.C. (2002) Health status and work burden of Alzheimer patients' informal caregivers. Comparisons of five different care programs in the European Union. *Health Policy*, 60, 219–33.

Department of Health (1999) *Caring about Carers: A National Strategy for Carers*. Department of Health, London.

Dixon-Woods, M., Shaw, R.L., Agarwal, S. & Smith, J.A. (2004) The problem of appraising qualitative research. *Quality & Safety in Health Care*, 13 (3), 223–5.

Downs, S.H. & Black, N. (1998) The feasibility of creating a checklist for the assessment of the methodological quality both of randomised and non-randomised studies of health care interventions. *Journal of Epidemiology and Community Health*, 52, 377–84.

Dunkin, J.J. & Anderson-Hanley, C. (1998) Dementia caregiver burden: a review of the literature and guidelines for assessment and intervention. *Neurology*, 51 (1), S53–S60.

Fade, S.A. (2003) Communicating and judging the quality of qualitative research: the need for a new language. *Journal of Human Nutrition and Dietetics*, 16 (3), 139–49.

Forster, A., Young, J., Langhorne, P., on behalf of the Day Hospital Group (1999) Systematic review of day hospital care for elderly people. *British Medical Journal*, 318, 837–41.

Fossey, E., Harvey, C., McDermott, F. & Davidson, L. (2002) Understanding and evaluating qualitative research. *Australian and New Zealand Journal of Psychiatry*, 36 (6), 717–32.

Harris, R.P., Helfand, M., Woolf, S.H. et al. for the Methods Work Group, Third U.S. Preventive Services

Task Force (2001) US Preventive Services Task Force framework 2001. Current Methods of the U.S. Preventive Services Task Force. A Review of the Process. *American Journal of Preventive Medicine*, 20 (3S), 21–35.

Ingleton, C., Payne, S., Nolan, M. & Carey, I. (2003) Respite in palliative care: a review and discussion of the literature. *Palliative Medicine*, 17, 567–75.

Kmet, L.M., Lee, R.C. & Cook, L.S. (2004) *Standard Quality Assessment Criteria for Evaluating Primary Research Papers from a Variety of Fields*. Heritage Foundation for Medical Research, Edmonton, Canada.

Lambert, P.C., Sutton, A.J., Abrams, K.R. & Jones, D.R. (2002) A comparison of summary patient-level covariates in meta-regression with individual patient data meta-analysis. *Journal of Clinical Epidemiology*, 55 (1), 86–94.

Lee, H. & Cameron, M. (2004) Respite care for people with dementia and their carers. *The Cochrane Database of Systematic Reviews, Issue 1*. John Wiley & Sons, Chichester.

Lincoln, Y. (1995) Emerging criteria for quality in qualitative and interpretive research. *Qualitative Inquiry*, 1, 275–89.

Mays, N. & Pope, C. (2000) Qualitative research in health care: Assessing quality in qualitative research. *British Medical Journal*, 320, 50–2.

McNally, S., Ben-Schlomo, U. & Newman, S. (1999) The effects of respite care on informal carers' well-being: a systematic review. *Disability and Rehabilitation*, 21 (1), 1–14.

Moher, D., Jadad, A.R., Nichol, G., Penman, M., Tugwell, P. & Walsh, S. (1995) Assessing the quality of randomized controlled trials: an annotated bibliography of scales and checklists. *Controlled Clinical Trials*, 16 (1), 62–73.

Noblit, G.W. & Hare, R.D. (1988) *Meta-ethnography: Synthesizing Qualitative Studies*. Sage Publications, London.

Nolan, M. & Grant, G. (1993) Service evaluation: time to open both eyes. *Journal of Advanced Nursing*, 18, 1434–42.

Office of National Statistics (2001) Census 2001. Available at website http://www.statistics.gov.uk/census2001/ (accessed June 2005).

Office of National Statistics (2002) *General Household Survey 2002. Living in Britain, results from the 2001 General Household Survey*. Office of National Statistics, London.

Parker, G., Bhakta, P., Lovett, C.A. et al. (2002) A systematic review of the costs and effectiveness of different models of paediatric home care. *Health Technology Assessment*, 6, 35.

Paterson, B., Thorne, S.E., Canam, C. & Jillings, C. (2001) *Meta-Study of Qualitative Health Research. A Practical Guide to Meta-Analysis and Meta-Synthesis*. Sage Publications, London.

Pickard, L. (2001) Carer break or carer blind? Policies for informal carers in the UK. *Social Policy and Administration*, 35 (4), 441–58.

Popay, J., Rogers, A. & Williams, G. (1998) Rationale and standards for the systematic review of qualitative literature in health services research. *Qualitative Health Research*, 8 (3), 341–51.

Population Trends (2003) *PT III*. National Statistics, Crown Copyright, London.

Prevost, T.C., Abrams, K.R. & Jones, D.R. (2000) Hierarchical models in generalised synthesis of evidence – a breast cancer screening example. *Statistics in Medicine*, 19 (24), 3359–76.

Sorensen, S., Pinquart, M., Habil, D. & Duberstein, P. (2002) How effective are interventions with caregivers? An updated meta-analysis. *The Geronotologist*, 42 (3), 356–72.

Spiegelhalter, D.J., Abrams, K.R. & Myles, J.P. (2003) *Bayesian Approaches to Clinical Trials and Health-care Evaluation*. Wiley, Chichester.

Stoltz, P., Uden, G. & Willman, A. (2004) Support for family carers who care for an elderly person at home – a systematic literature review. *Scandinavian Journal of Caring Science*, 18, 111–19.

Sutton, A.J. & Abrams, K.R. (2001) Bayesian methods in meta-analysis and evidence synthesis. *Statistical Methods in Medical Research*, 10 (4), 277–303.

Sutton, A.J., Abrams, K.R., Jones, D.R., Sheldon, T.A. & Song, F. (2000a) *Methods for Meta-Analysis in Medical Research*. Wiley and Sons, Chichester.

Sutton, A.J., Song, F., Gilbody, S.M. & Abrams, K.R. (2000b) Modelling publication bias in meta-analysis: a review. *Statistical Methods in Medical Research*, 9 (5), 412–45.

Walsh, D. & Downe, S. (2005) Meta-synthesis method for qualitative research: a literature review. *Journal of Advanced Nursing*, 50 (2), 204–11.

Wimo, A., von Strauss, E., Norberg, G., Sassi, F., Johansson, L. (2002) Time spent on informal and formal care giving for persons with dementia in Sweden. *Health Policy*, 61, 255–68.

Zarit, S.H., Gaugler, J.E. & Jarrott, S.E. (1999) Useful services for families: research findings and directions. *International Journal of Geriatric Psychiatry*, 14, 196–8.

15 Use of Physical Restraint

David Evans

Introduction

The past few decades have seen a growing volume of research literature addressing the use of physical restraint in health care. A major focus has been the identification of strategies that help minimise the use of restraining devices in health care. However, drawing conclusions about this body of literature has been challenging because of the diversity of the research. Yet, given the importance of this topic, a comprehensive and reliable summary of the research was urgently needed.

A review was therefore undertaken to summarise the physical restraint research. Given the nature of the topic and type of research to be summarised, a systematic review approach was not appropriate. Therefore a broader review that focused on six specific aspects of physical restraint was conducted. The review method was based on that used during systematic reviews, but modified to suit the broader nature of review questions. On completion of the review, the six review areas formed the comprehensive summary of restraint research.

Focusing the review

The first activity in preparing to undertake the review was to determine its focus. This entailed a preliminary review of the literature and develop-

ment of the review protocol. The purpose of this preliminary review was to become familiar with the literature and to identify the key concepts and definitions of the topic, the populations that have been investigated and the scope of the existing physical restraint research.

Key concepts and definitions

In developing the review protocol it was necessary to define the concept of restraint. This was an important activity as it provided the first step in determining the boundaries of the review. For example, there was literature addressing restraint in the context of law enforcement, chemical restraint and physical restraint. The major interest for this review was physical restraining devices, such as those that stop a person leaving their bed, chair or room. While restraint has been defined many different ways in the literature, the definition that was selected provided a broad description of physical restraint:

> any device, material or equipment attached to or near a person's body and which cannot be controlled or easily removed by the person and which deliberately prevents or is deliberately intended to prevent a person's free body movement to a position of choice and/or a person's normal access to their body (Retsas, 1998:186).

The preliminary review of the literature also highlighted that investigation of harm secondary to the use of physical restraint was a component of some studies. Harm, like physical restraint, is a concept that is quite nebulous and difficult to define. After investigating the nature of harm reported in research, two definitions were developed for the review:

Direct injury   Physical injury caused as a direct result of external pressure from the restraining device, and including such examples as lacerations, bruising or strangulation.

Indirect injury   Injury or adverse outcome related to the enforced immobility of a person, and including such variables as increased mortality rate, development of pressure ulcers, falls or failure to be discharged home.

It was also noted that psychological injury may occur as a consequence of the use of physical restraint. This aspect of restraint has received only limited attention in the literature and so, for the review, harm was defined only in terms of physical injury. However, one component of the review focused on the impact of physical restraint and it was therefore anticipated that psychological harm would be explored from this perspective.

Population

Physical restraint has been investigated in a number of different settings and with a range of unique populations. In terms of settings, restraint has been investigated in acute, residential and mental health care. Given the large volume of literature on this topic, a pragmatic decision was made to limit the setting to acute and residential care. Acute and residential were selected for the review populations because of the similarities in the use of restraint across the two settings.

Scope of research

As previously noted, the physical restraint literature is very diverse, addressing many different aspects of restraint. In addition, while some studies had a single focus such as injury, others focused on a range of issues. The intent of the review was to provide a comprehensive summary of this research, its scope extending beyond effectiveness. Following the preliminary review of the literature, six broad areas of interest were identified to provide a clear focus for summarising the research. These areas were:

- How restraint is used
- Who is restrained
- Reasons for using restraint
- Injury associated with the use of restraint
- Experience of being restrained
- Restraint minimisation

Review questions were then developed for each of these six areas (see Table 15.1). The questions provided the basis for development of the selection criteria that were used to help determine which research should be included in the review.

This approach to the review topic provided a framework for the inclusion of a diverse body of literature in a single review. Research was included in the review when it could contribute to one of the six areas of interest, and some studies contributed to more than one area. This approach overcame the difficulty encountered during integrative reviews of how to summarise and synthesise the findings from both quantitative and qualitative research to produce a coherent and useful report.

Selection criteria

Selection of studies for inclusion in the review should be based on sound scientific reasoning (Petitti, 1994). To ensure this, selection criteria are used that define the characteristics of interest, such as study participants, intervention, outcomes and type of study design. Given the complex nature of the physical restraint review, the inclusion criteria were much broader than those used in systematic reviews of effectiveness. Careful selection of these criteria was important because they provided the framework and boundaries for the review.

Participants

Only studies that involved adults in an acute care or residential care institution were included in the

Table 15.1 Review questions.

Use of restraint	• What proportion of patients and residents are physically restrained? • What is the duration of the physical restraint of patients and residents? • What physical restraint devices are used in the acute and residential care setting?
Who is restrained	• What specific patient or resident characteristics increase the likelihood of the use of physical restraint?
Reasons for restraint	• Why do healthcare workers restrain people in their care?
Injury and restraint	• What injuries do physical restraint devices cause? • What proportion of people suffer a restraint-related injury? • What injuries are caused by the specific restraint devices, such as vests, wrist restraints and bedrails?
Experience of restraint	• How do patients and residents describe their experience of being restrained in an acute or residential care facility? • How do people describe the experience of having a relative physically restrained in an acute or residential care facility?
Restraint minimisation	• Do restraint minimisation programmes reduce the use of physical restraint devices in the acute and residential care setting? • Is there an increase in adverse events following the restraint minimisation?

review. Studies involving children were excluded because reports of restraint involving children in hospital focused on short periods of restraint, such as during invasive or unpleasant procedures. Studies in the mental health setting were excluded because they were considered to differ in a number of aspects from those in acute or residential care settings. All studies involving custodial or community restraint were considered to be beyond the scope of the review.

Intervention

The nature of restraint was previously described in the review definitions and this section listed specific restraining devices. These devices included waist and chest restraints, wrist and leg ties, mitts, straps, belts and bedrails. Special restraining chairs and lapboards were also included as restraining devices.

Outcomes

The protocol described the outcomes of interest to the review. However, given the six areas of restraint being investigated, multiple outcomes were used. There were specific outcomes for each of the six areas of interest:

Use of restraint Studies were included in the review if the outcome related to the use of physical restraint, prevalence, duration of restraint or the specific devices used.

Who is restrained Studies were included if they collected data related to the characteristics of people who had been subject to physical restraint, through observation or inspection of healthcare records. These outcomes included such variables as age, gender and mental status. Studies were excluded from the review if they investigated the characteristics of people subject to restraint using questionnaires or surveys of healthcare workers, as this was seen to reflect perceptions of use rather than the actual use of restraint.

Reasons for restraint Studies were included if they reported the reasons cited or documented by healthcare workers for initiating physical restraint.

Injury and restraint Studies were included if outcomes were those related to direct and indirect injury. Examples of direct injury outcomes included fractures, death, strangulation, cuts and bruises. Indirect injury included adverse outcomes such as changes in duration of hospitalisation, infection rates or mental status.

Experience of restraint Studies that explored the impact of restraint and reported descriptions of the experience of people subject to restraint or their families were included in the review.

Restraint minimisation Studies were included in the review if they reported descriptions of restraint minimisation programmes, or outcomes related to the evaluation of effectiveness of these programmes.

Types of studies

Given the nature of the review topic, a broad range of study designs provided relevant information. Optimal study designs were identified for each of the six areas of interest.

Use of restraint A preliminary review of the literature suggested that most of the evidence related to how restraint is used would come from descriptive studies. These descriptive studies would provide a series of snapshots across many different clinical settings. A number of observational studies also reported findings related to the use of physical restraint. Experimental studies, by their very nature of controlling all variables, would not contribute useful information to this component of the review.

Who is restrained Observational studies were considered to provide the most valid information because they typically compared the characteristics of restrained people to similar populations who were not subject to restraint. However, descriptive studies also provided some information on the characteristics of restrained patients and residents, but lacked the comparison groups.

Reasons for restraint A preliminary review of the literature suggested that descriptive and observational studies reported reasons why physical restraint was used. The common approach in these studies was via surveys of healthcare workers.

Injury and restraint The restraint-related injury literature was the most diverse. Descriptive studies have reported injuries that have occurred in residential and acute care settings. There have been a number of studies investigating documents such as coroners' reports. Observational studies have compared injuries and health outcomes between restrained and unrestrained people. A number of case study reports provided important descriptions of single episodes of injury related to specific devices. A preliminary search of the literature suggested that clinical trials have rarely been used to evaluate any aspect of restraint and so be would unlikely to provide any information for this component of the review.

Experience of restraint Qualitative studies were considered to provide the best evidence on the experience of being restrained or having a relative restrained. However, again the preliminary search of the literature suggested that this approach had rarely been used for investigation of restraint in acute or residential care settings. However, descriptive studies were also considered appropriate for providing simple descriptions on the impact of physical restraint.

Restraint minimisation Descriptive studies and case reports were considered to provide useful descriptions of restraint minimisation strategies but, in terms of the effectiveness of restraint minimisation, the randomised controlled trial was considered to provide the best evidence. However, as previously noted, few clinical trials have investigated issues related to physical restraint, with the pre-post research design being the most common approach identified during the preliminary search of the literature.

Search strategy

Given that database searches for clinical trials fail to identify many published studies (Dickersin *et al.*, 1994), a comprehensive search strategy was developed to increase the likelihood of finding all relevant studies. This strategy included electronic databases, bibliographies, hand searching key journals and contacting experts on the review topic. During the preliminary phase, a limited search of MEDLINE and CINAHL was undertaken to obtain a sample of articles addressing physical restraint. The terms used in the titles and abstracts of these articles, and those used by the electronic databases were analysed to identify common terms specific to physical restraint articles. As part of this preliminary work, databases were also inspected to determine which would be likely to produce relevant articles.

The second phase of the strategy involved a comprehensive search of selected databases using all the key search terms. The databases searched included CINAHL, MEDLINE, Current Contents, Dissertation Abstracts International, PSYCHINFO, EMBASE and the Cochrane Library. The three major search terms used were restrain*, bedrails, siderail* and cotside*. The final phase involved a search for those articles missed during the electronic database searches. This entailed a search of the reference lists of identified articles and hand searching key journals. A small number of experts in the area of physical restraint were also contacted to help identify additional papers or to supply missing data.

The majority of studies were identified through database and bibliography searches. Hand searching journals proved to be very time-consuming and only produced a few studies not previously identified.

Critical appraisal

Critical appraisal was challenging, given the diverse nature and the many research designs included in the review. It was planned to critically appraise all randomised controlled trials (RCTs) using criteria based on the four most common sources of bias (Higgins & Green, 2005). However, only a single RCT was identified during this review and so this was not done. The most common research design used to evaluate restraint-related interventions was the before-and-after design. Given the limitations of this design, studies were only included in the review to help document restraint minimisation strategies and not to determine the effectiveness of these strategies. There is a lack of agreement on how best to critically appraise qualitative research (Evans & Pearson, 2001). To address this, simple criteria were developed for the review (Evans & FitzGerald, 2002a):

- The research design was appropriate for the question
- Adequate information was given about the method
- Adequate description was given of participants
- There were supporting data for themes, categories and labels

However, like with the RCT, there have been few qualitative investigations of issues related to physical restraint in acute or residential settings. For descriptive research, criteria similar to those used for qualitative studies were used. The aim of this appraisal was to ensure a homogeneous group of studies, and pooling data from studies would be appropriate (Evans & FitzGerald, 2002a).

Data extraction

To extract data from individual study reports, it is common practice to use a data extraction form (Higgins & Green, 2005). Therefore a data collection tool was developed to record demographic information, the research processes and results. These data extraction forms enabled a succinct summary of each study to be generated, which formed the basis of the analysis.

Data synthesis

The aim of the synthesis was to pool the findings from individual studies. However, given the broad nature of the review, this was a complex process. The synthesis was achieved by grouping studies according to the six areas of interest that were identified in the review questions. The review synthesis was therefore a series of smaller syntheses, pooling the data that addressed each area of interest.

Use of restraint   Data related to the type, duration and prevalence of restraint were summarised in tables and graphs, and when possible mean values and range calculated.

Who is restrained   When possible, data on characteristics that increased the likelihood of restraint obtained from observational studies were pooled in a meta-analysis, using odds ratios and 95% confidence intervals.

Reasons for restraint   Content analysis has been used to generate objective descriptions of different communication media (Nandy & Sarvela, 1997), and so was used to categorise reasons cited by healthcare workers for using physical restraint.

Injury and restraint   When possible, data on restraint-related injury obtained from observational studies were pooled in a meta-analysis, using odds ratios and 95% confidence intervals. In addition, information on injury from descriptive studies and case reports were summarised using narrative.

Experience of restraint   A range of different approaches has been recommended or used to synthesise the findings from qualitative research (Noblit & Hare, 1988; Jensen & Allen, 1996), and data on the experience of restraint were synthesised using a simple qualitative synthesis process.

Restraint minimisation   When possible, data on the effectiveness of restraint minimisation programmes obtained from randomised controlled trials were pooled in a meta-analysis, using odds ratios and 95% confidence intervals. In addition, descriptions of restraint minimisation programmes were summarised using narrative and tables.

Results

The presentation of findings of this review was challenging due to its broad focus. The aim was to provide a meaningful summary of the research that would inform practice, policy and research. Results were presented according to the six areas of interest of the review. Some studies contributed to more than one area of interest; for example, a study might report information on the use of restraint and reasons why restraint devices were used. Studies were then grouped into acute care or residential care for the analysis. In terms of the practical aspects of undertaking the review, these six areas of interest provided a clear framework for the analysis and reporting of results.

Use of physical restraint

The first area of interest, use of restraint, investigated how restraining devices were used in acute and residential care facilities. The specific issues addressed were the proportion of people subject to restraint, duration for which they were restrained and the devices that were used in the two settings. The research that contributed to this section included surveys of clinical practice and observational studies.

Descriptive studies and surveys are often excluded from systematic reviews, being rated as low-level evidence. However, they are able to provide valid information about the use of restraint. The findings from these studies were summarised using a tabular summary of data on the proportions of patients subject to restraint (Table 15.2).

This approach allowed the differences across settings to be evaluated and the variation in practice identified. The data summary showed that 27% of those in residential care were subject to physical restraint during the period of study, compared to only 10% of patients in the acute care setting.

A similar approach was taken to summarise data on the duration of physical restraint, although only four studies reported on this outcome. Table 15.3 shows the range and mean duration of restraint according to the two settings. This tabular presentation of data allowed for easy comparison of results. Data in this table clearly highlight the great variation present in clinical practice.

In evaluating the type of restraining devices identified by studies, a different approach to data summary was used. First, findings from individual studies were grouped according to the different restraint devices, such as wrist or chest restraints (Table 15.4). These findings also highlight great variability in practice. Mean values for restraining devices across studies were calculated and findings from both settings were plotted to identify commonly used devices and differences in practices in acute and residential care (Figure 15.1).

Summary of findings

This component of the review demonstrates that there is great variability in practice of using restraint in acute and residential care facilities. The use of restraint is clearly more common in residential care and, based on the findings of a single study, some residents spend extended periods of time restrained. In terms of the restraining devices used, acute care most commonly uses wrist restraints and bedrails while residential care is more likely to use waist and chest restraint devices.

In terms of the contribution of this review, while descriptive studies are commonly considered to be low-level evidence, they serve to highlight a number of issues of concern that are worthy of further investigation.

Table 15.2   Proportion of people restrained in acute and residential care facilities (reproduced with permission from Evans, 2001:283).

Citation	Percentage restrained	Number restrained
Residential care		
Tinetti et al., 1991	30.7	122 of 397
Karlsson et al., 1996	24	312 of 1325
Burton, 1992	47.8	209 of 437
Magee, 1993	32	55 of 173
Lever, 1994	12	44 of 367
Koch, 1993	26.4	428 of 1620
Total restrained		1170 of 4319 (27%)
Acute care		
Frengley & Mion, 1986	7.4	95 of 1292
Robbins et al., 1987	17	37 of 222
Mion, 1989	13	35 of 278
Lever, 1994	21	91 of 437
Lofgren, 1989	6	102 of 1661
Whitehead et al., 1997	12.5 (this figure includes chemical restraints)	–
Roberge & Beausejour, 1988	25	43 of 171
Minnick, 1998	3.4	–
Total restrained		403 of 4061 (10%)

Table 15.3   Duration of restraint for acute and residential care patients (reproduced with permission from Evans, 2001:284).

Citation	Restraint duration (days; mean)	Restraint duration (days; range)
Acute care		
Frengley & Mion, 1986	2.7	1 to 13
Robbins et al., 1987	3	1 to 35
Mion, 1989	4.5	1 to 18
Mean duration across the three studies	3.4	
Residential care		
Tinetti et al., 1991	86.5	1 to 350

Characteristics of restrained people

The second area investigated by the review concerned the characteristics of people subject to physical restraint. Identification of these characteristics may provide a means to predict which patients or residents are at greatest risk of being restrained and so allow alternative strategies to be implemented. The aim of this section of the review was to determine which characteristics of restrained patients or residents differed from the characteristics of those who were not restrained.

This component of the review focused on observational studies, such as case control or cohort studies, which are able to investigate this type of difference between groups (Schneider et al., 2003). These studies have investigated the relationship between restraint and variables such as age, cognitive status, mobility, incontinence and visual impairment. The findings from these studies were combined for individual characteristics in a meta-analysis, using odds ratios. An example of one of these meta-analyses, for cognitive impairment, is presented graphically in Figure 15.2.

Table 15.4   Type of restraints used in acute care settings, summary table (reproduced with permission from Evans 2001:285).

Citation	Percentage of total number of restrained	Number restrained (number of devices and total number restrained)
Wrist restraints		
Minnick, 1998	59	471 of 799
Frengley & Mion, 1986	13	12 of 95
Robbins et al., 1987	72	27 of 37
Mion, 1989	40	14 of 35
Lofgren, 1989	14	14 of 102
Total		538 of 1068 (mean = 50%)
Vest and chest restraints		
Minnick, 1998	16	128 of 799
Frengley & Mion, 1986	26	24 of 95
Robbins et al., 1987	51	19 of 37
Whitehead et al., 1997	17	8 of 45
Mion, 1989	40	14 of 35
Lofgren, 1989	61	62 of 102
Lever, 1994	5	5 of 91
Total		260 of 1204 (mean = 22%)
Leg or ankle restraints		
Minnick, 1998	3	24 of 799
Frengley & Mion, 1986	5	5 of 95
Mion, 1989	9	3 of 35
Total		32 of 929 (mean = 3%)
Waist/pelvic/belt restraints		
Frengley & Mion, 1986	30	28 of 95
Robbins et al., 1987	31	11 of 37
Mion, 1989	57	20 of 35
Lever, 1994	15	14 of 91
Whitehead et al., 1997	9	4 of 45
Total		77 of 303 (mean = 25%)
Gerichair		
Frengley & Mion, 1986	2	2 of 95
Lever, 1994	7	6 of 91
Total		8 of 186 (mean = 4%)
Bedrails		
Whitehead et al., 1997	52	23 of 45
Lever, 1994	53	48 of 91
O'Keeffe et al., 1996 (assessed bedrail use only)	8.4 (of the total hospital population)	
Total		71 of 136 (mean = 52%)

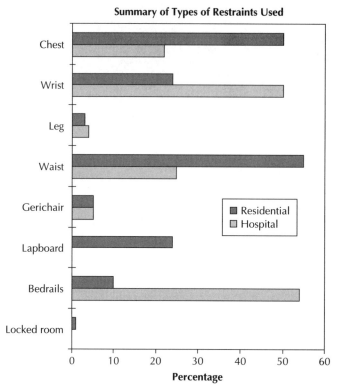

Figure 15.1 Type of restraints used in acute care settings (reproduced with permission from Evans, 2001:286).

Comparison: 04 Aged Care Setting – Predictors of Physical Restraint
Outcome: 02 Cognitive Impairment

Study	Treatment n/N	Control n/N	OR (95% CI Fixed)	Weight %	OR (95% CI Fixed)
Burton	122/209	94/228		46.0	2.00 [1.37, 2.93]
Karlsson	291/312	523/1013		20.4	12.98 [8.20, 20.56]
Tinetti	61/122	89/275		33.6	2.09 [1.35, 3.23]
Total (95% CI)	477/643	706/1516		100.0	4.27 [3.40, 5.35]

Chi-square 48.04 (df = 2) P: 0.00 Z = 12.56 P: <0.00001

.01   .1   1   10   100

Restrained   Unrestrained

Figure 15.2 Cognitive impairment and physical restraint (reproduced with permission from Evans, 2001:289).

Summary of findings

The findings from this component of the review suggested that in acute care, having a psychiatric diagnosis or cognitive impairment, being bedridden or at risk of falling were associated with an increase in the likelihood of being physically restrained. In residential care, incontinence and being unable to perform activities of daily living independently were linked to a greater likelihood of being restrained. In terms of the contribution of this component of the review, summary of the findings of these

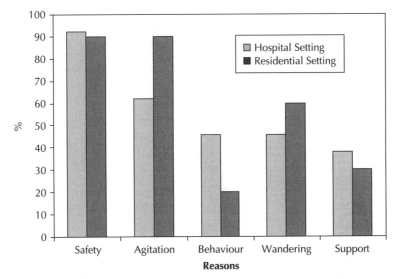

Figure 15.3   Patient-oriented reasons for using restraints as identified in different studies (Evans & Fitzgerald, 2002b: 739, reprinted from the *International Journal of Nursing Studies*, vol. 39, 'Reasons for physically restraining patients and residents', © 2002 with permission from Elsevier.)

observational studies provides another perspective on the use of physical restraint. This evidence gives an opportunity to develop strategies for restraint-free care of these special groups of people.

Reasons for restraining people

The third component of the review investigated reasons for restraining patients and residents. A number of descriptive studies, surveys and observational studies have reported the reasons cited by healthcare workers, and these became the focus of this section of the review. Content analysis was used for the analysis of this data because it is a method that can be used to obtain simple descriptions of different types of communication (Cavanagh, 1997). The reasons cited for restraining people were identified and grouped into common themes, and then reported according to the number of studies in which they were cited. For example, patient safety was cited as a reason for restraint in 92% (12 of 13) of studies. These reasons were presented graphically according to the two settings (Figure 15.3).

Summary of findings

This section of the review provided a detailed description of the reasons cited by healthcare workers for using physical restraint. These findings help identify those situations where alternative strategies to physical restraint are needed. They also highlight practices of concern, such as the use of restraint to allow staff to complete work schedules or as a form of punishment.

Injury and physical restraint

The fourth section of the review, restraint-related injury, was challenging because it is an area that has not been well investigated or reported. An additional challenge was that the injury-related information that has been reported in the literature takes many different forms. For example, injury data are reported from observational and descriptive studies, from audits of coroners' records and from case studies. However, regardless of their form, these data all provide valuable information on restraint-related injuries.

For the synthesis, studies were grouped according to the nature of injury investigated, direct injuries such as cuts and lacerations, or indirect injury such as prolonged hospitalisation or increased mortality. In addition, findings were categorised according to the restraining device that caused the injury. Data from observational studies were summarised in tables and pooled in a meta-analysis. The

Table 15.5 Details of observational studies reporting restraint-associated injury (reproduced with permission from Evans et al., 2003:276).

Author	Setting	Population	Findings
Burton, 1992	8 residential care facilities	Residents – restrained n = 209 – unrestrained n = 228	Residents admitted with moderate to no cognitive impairment experienced greater cognitive decline if restrained No difference for severely cognitively impaired residents
Capezuti et al., 1996	Residential care	Residents – restrained n = 119 – unrestrained n = 203	Restraint was not associated with a significantly lower risk of falls or injuries in confused ambulatory residents
Folmar & Wilson, 1989	Residential care	Residents – never restrained n = 81 – always restrained n = 21	More non-social behaviour observed in restrained residents Highest level of social behaviour observed in unrestrained residents
Frengley & Mion, 1986	General medical wards of acute care hospital	Patients – unrestrained n = 1197 – restrained n = 95	Increased length of hospitalisation of restrained compared to unrestrained patients Restrained had higher mortality rate than unrestrained patients
Lofgren, 1989	General medical wards of acute care hospital	Patients – restrained 4 or fewer days n = 67 – restrained >4 days n = 35	More new pressures sores and nosocomial infections in patients restrained >4 days
Mion, 1989 – Study I	Acute medical ward	Patients – restrained n = 35 – unrestrained n = 243	Higher mortality in restrained patients compared to unrestrained patients Increased length of stay in restrained compared to unrestrained patients More falls, nosocomial infections and immobility-related complications in restrained compared to unrestrained
Mion, 1989 – Study II	Acute care medical rehabilitation ward	Patients – restrained n = 49 – unrestrained n = 143	No difference in length of hospitalisation between groups More falls, nosocomial infections and procedure-related complications in retrained group
Mosley, 1997	Residential care	Residents – restrained n = 740 – unrestrained n = 4333	Restraint was associated with disorientation, and greater dependency for both the activities of daily living and walking
Robbins et al., 1987	Acute care hospital	Medical and surgical patients – restrained n = 37 – unrestrained n = 185	Higher mortality rate for restrained patients Increased length of stay for restrained patients
Stiebeling et al., 1990 (abstract so minimal data provided)	Residential care	Residents – restrained n = not stated – unrestrained n = not stated	Restrained residents had more bladder and bowel incontinence, pressure ulcers and reduced mobility
Tinetti et al., 1992	12 skilled nursing facilities	Residents – restrained n = 122 – unrestrained n = 275	Higher fall-related injury rate for restrained compared to unrestrained residents
Werner et al., 1989	Residential care	Residents with high level of agitation and cognitive impairment – restrained n = 22 – never restrained n = 2	Significantly more strange noises and movement when residents restrained More agitation when resident was restrained compared to when not restrained Higher rates of agitation immediately following application of restraint

Table 15.6   Indirect injury and the use of restraint in acute care settings (reproduced with permission from Evans et al., 2003:278).

Study	Restrained	Unrestrained	Odds ratio (95% CI)
Failure to be discharged home			
Mion, 1989 (medical)	20 of 37	22 of 185	8.72 (3.98–19.11)
Robbins et al., 1987	24 of 35	46 of 428	18.12 (8.34–39.39)
Pooled results			12.42 (7.16–21.52)
Death during hospitalisation			
Frengley & Mion, 1986	11 of 95	13 of 1197	11.93 (5.19–27.43)
Mion, 1989 (medical)	5 of 35	3 of 243	13.33 (3.03–58.62)
Robbins et al., 1987	9 of 37	6 of 185	9.59 (3.17–29.01)
Pooled results			11.24 (6.07–20.83)
Nosocomial infection			
Mion, 1989 (rehabilitation)	29 of 49	31 of 94	2.95 (1.44–6.02)
Mion, 1989 (medical)	8 of 35	13 of 243	5.24 (1.99–13.78)
Pooled results			3.46 (1.93–6.22)
Fall during hospitalisation			
Mion, 1989 (rehabilitation)	28 of 49	18 of 94	5.63 (2.62–12.09)
Mion, 1989 (medical)	6 of 35	3 of 243	16.55 (3.93–69.75)
Pooled results			6.79 (3.44–13.39)

characteristics and findings of observational studies that reported restraint-related injury were summarised in a table (Table 15.5). Data from these studies were pooled in a meta-analysis, using the odds ratio (Table 15.6). The findings demonstrated consistently poorer outcomes for people subject to physical restraint.

In terms of other types of reports of restraint-related injuries, findings were categorised by type of restraining device and summarised by narrative. For example, vest restraints have been implicated in a number of deaths (Katz et al., 1981; Dube & Mitchell, 1986; Miles & Irvine, 1992; Langslow, 1999). Reports commonly describe the person being able to partially climb out of the bed or chair, resulting in the vest being caught around their neck (DiMaio et al., 1986; Langslow, 1999). Alternatively, the description related to the person partially leaving the bed and being left suspended from the bed, with the vest around their chest and so impairing breathing (Miles & Irvine, 1992). From a different perspective, while wrist restraints are commonly used in hospitals, only a single paper reported injury related to these devices (Ruben et al., 1993).

Summary of findings

The findings from this component of the review demonstrated that the use of physical restraint brings with it a degree of risk. However, the nature of included studies meant that it was not possible to determine the magnitude of this risk. Despite this, it is clear that the use of physical restraint is associated with poorer health outcomes and physical injury.

The experience of restraint

A perspective that is excluded from most reviews of health interventions is that of the consumer. Therefore the aim of this section of the review was to attempt to incorporate that perspective into the summary of the research. There were two differing perspectives included in this summary: the experience of being restrained in a healthcare institution and the experience of having a relative restrained in a healthcare institution. Descriptions of the experience of physical restraint were sought from descriptive and qualitative research.

Table 15.7   Summary of studies addressing the impact of restraint and identified themes relating to the experience of restraint (reproduced with permission from Evans & FitzGerald, 2002a:129).

Citation	Population	Original themes from studies	
Patients			
Stumpf, 1988	Medical patients who had been restrained ($n = 20$)	Anger Fear Resistance Humiliation Demoralisation	Discomfort Resignation Denial Agreement
Hardin, 1993	Restrained patients ($n = 25$)	Positive feelings Negative feelings Neutral feelings	Positive effects Negative effects Neutral effects
Family			
Hardin, 1993	Family of restrained patients ($n = 19$)	Positive feelings	Negative feelings
Kanski, 1996	Family of restrained patients ($n = 25$)	Only listed significant statements	
Newbern, 1994	Wives of restrained male patients ($n = 6$)	Major theme: finality	Minor themes: control; denial; anger; degradation

The first finding of this section was that few studies have investigated this issue. The few studies identified during the search were generally quite limited in method or scope. Despite this, a clear and consistent theme emerged from the findings of these studies. The theme for the people subject to physical restraint was one of anger, fear, humiliation and discomfort. For their relatives, it was anger, disagreement and the finality of restraint. The themes reported in individual studies were summarised in a table (Table 15.7).

Summary of findings

This section of the review clearly demonstrated that restraint was an intervention that was disliked by the people subject to it, and by their families. In terms of the contribution of this information to healthcare policy, the evidence highlights the importance of current efforts to minimise or abolish the use of physical restraint.

Restraint minimisation

The final component of the review was restraint minimisation, to evaluate the effectiveness of these programmes and to determine whether reducing restraint impacted on adverse events. A total of 16 studies were identified; however, only one was an RCT. The most common approach to this evaluation was the before-and-after design. As a result, it was not possible to pool the findings of this group of studies in a meta-analysis. Studies were therefore summarised in tables that listed the nature of the intervention, and its impact on restraint, falls and injury (Table 15.8).

Summary of findings

This tabular and narrative summary of restraint minimisation research provided important information to inform clinical practice and help focus future research. However, the major finding of this

Table 15.8 Restraint minimisation programmes – acute care (reproduced with permission from Evans et al., 2002:618).

Citation	Method	Intervention	Change in restraint rate	Change in fall rate	Change in injury rate
Hanger et al., 1999	Before and after	Policy change to reduce use of bedrails Education	30% to 11%	No change	Reduction in serious injury. No change in minor injury
Lever et al., 1995	Before and after	Education programme. Case conferences	Decreased from 32% to 18% at 6 months. Increased to 54% by 12 months	No change	Not reported
Powell et al., 1989	Before and after	Committee formed. Developed 4 patient stereotypes. Determined alternatives. Changed policies and developed guidelines	From 52 restrained patients per 1000 patient days to 0.3 per 1000 patient days	No change	Not reported

section of the review was the limited nature of restraint minimisation research. Most studies tended to be small, and based on a single centre and methods that were at risk of bias.

Conclusion

Implications for practice

A number of implications for practice emerge from this review, the first being that practice is highly variable. In some facilities, restraint is a common intervention for the management of residents and patients, and some people are subject to long periods of physical restraint. However, the use of restraint is far greater in residential care than in acute care facilities.

The findings of the review suggest that, in acute care, having a psychiatric diagnosis or cognitive impairment, being bedridden or at risk of falling increased the likelihood of being physically restrained. In residential care, incontinence and being unable to perform activities of daily living independently were associated with increased likelihood of physical restraint. These findings

suggest that it is elderly, frail and confused people who are most likely to be subject to physical restraint.

Restraint has been clearly linked to a number of adverse events, including deaths of patients and residents. Ironically, one of the common reasons cited for using physical restraint was to maintain the safety of the patient or resident. Studies investigating the psychosocial impact of restraint have also shown that it has a negative impact on the person and their family, being likened to being tied up like an animal. These findings suggest that physical restraint should only be used as a last resort in health care.

Implications for research

The most important implication for research arising from this review is the urgent need for further research on the use of physical restraint in health care. Most studies identified were from the residential care setting, with few from acute care setting. There has been considerable investigation on how and why restraint is used, but little rigorous research on how to minimise or abolish its use.

Implications for future similar reviews

The major implication for reviews is that this broader approach to reviewing research can provide important information for practice. This review allowed findings to be summarised on a number of different aspects of physical restraint that would normally be excluded from systematic reviews of effectiveness. While some of the research included in the review is at a greater risk of error and bias than the most RCTs, it still makes an informative contribution to practice.

Other more specific implications for conducting this type of complex review can also be identified. The most important one is providing the focus, boundaries and framework for the review. This was achieved by developing six clear areas of interest. These allowed a series of questions to be developed, which in turn provided the framework for determining optimal review methods. This approach allowed a broad body of research to be summarised, while still maintaining the clearly stated review outcomes. This approach helped during the conduct of the review, in that it was more achievable to undertake a series of clearly focused subreviews rather than a single very large and complex review.

However, this broad approach also increased the work of conducting the review. It meant that considerable resources were needed to review all the research on physical restraint. This review was a much greater undertaking than if a review of effectiveness had been conducted.

In terms of the methods used to review the different areas of interest, there is still considerable scope for development. The optimal methods to identify, appraise and synthesise the findings from this diverse body of literature have still not been determined. Until this has been done, some of the principles of systematic reviews can be used – pre-planned, systematic and clear reporting of methods and findings.

References

Burton, L.C. (1992) Physical restraint use and cognitive decline among nursing home residents. *Journal of the American Geriatrics Society*, 40, 811–16.

Capezuti, E., Evans, L., Strumpf, N. & Maislin, G. (1996) Physical restraint use and falls in nursing home residents. *Journal of the American Geriatrics Society*, 44, 627–33.

Cavanagh, S. (1997) Content analysis: concepts, methods and applications. *Nurse Researcher*, 4 (3), 5–16.

Dickersin, K., Scherer, R. & Lefebvre, C. (1994) Identifying relevant studies for systematic reviews. *British Medical Journal*, 309, 1286–91.

DiMaio, V.J., Dana, S.E. & Bux, R.C. (1986) Deaths caused by restraint vests. *Journal of the American Medical Association*, 255, 905.

Dube, A. & Mitchell, E. (1986) Accidental strangulation from vest restraint. *Journal of the American Medical Association*, 256, 2725–6.

Evans, D. (2001) Systematic reviews of nursing research: development of a conceptual framework. PhD Thesis, University of Adelaide, Adelaide.

Evans, D. & FitzGerald, M. (2002a) The experience of physical restraint: a systematic review of qualitative research. *Contemporary Nurse*, 13, 126–35.

Evans, D. & FitzGerald, M. (2002b) Reasons for physically restraining patients and residents: a systematic review and content analysis. *International Journal of Nursing Studies*, 39, 735–43.

Evans, D. & Pearson, A. (2001) Systematic reviews of qualitative research. *Clinical Effectiveness in Nursing*, 5 (3), 111–17.

Evans, D., Wood, J. & Lambert, L. (2002) A review of physical restraint minimisation in the acute and residential care setting. *Journal of Advanced Nursing*, 40 (6), 616–25.

Evans, D., Wood, J. & Lambert, L. (2003) Patient injury and physical restraint devices: a systematic review. *Journal of Advanced Nursing*, 41 (3), 274–82.

Folmar, S. & Wilson, H. (1989) Social behaviour and physical restraints. *Gerontologist*, 29, 650–3.

Frengley, J.D. & Mion, L.C. (1986) Incidence of physical restraints on acute general medical wards. *Journal of the American Geriatric Society*, 34 (8), 565–8.

Hanger, H.C., Ball, M.C. & Wood, L.A. (1999) An analysis of falls in the hospital: can we do without bedrails. *Journal of the American Geriatrics Society* 47, 529–31.

Hardin, S.B., Magee, R., Vinson, M.H., Owen, M., Hyatt, E. & Stratmann, D. (1993) Patient and family perceptions of restraints. *Journal of Holistic Nursing* 11 (4):383–97.

Higgins, J.P.T. & Green, S. (eds) (2005) *Cochrane Handbook for Systematic Reviews of Interventions* 4.2.5. The Cochrane Library, Issue 3. John Wiley & Sons, Chichester.

Jensen, L.A. & Allen, M.A. (1996) Meta-synthesis of qualitative findings. *Qualitative Health Research*, 6 (4), 553–60.

Kanski, G.W., Janelli, L.M., Jones, H.M. & Kennedy, M.C. (1996) Family reactions to restraints in an acute care setting. *Journal of Gerontological Nursing* 22 (6):17–22, 48–9.

Karlsson, S., Bucht, G., Eriksson, S. & Sandman, P.O. (1996) Physical restraints in geriatric care in Sweden: prevalence and patient characteristics. *Journal of the American Geriatrics Society*, 44 (11), 1348–54.

Katz, L., Weber, F. & Dodge, P. (1981) Patient restraint and safety vests. *Dimensions of Health Service*, 58, 10–11.

Koch, S. (1993) Restraining nursing home residents. *Australian Journal of Advanced Nursing*, 11 (2), 9–14.

Langslow, A. (1999) Safety and physical restraint. *Australian Nurses Journal*, 7 (2), 34–5.

Lever, J.A. (1994) The use of physical restraint and their relationship to medication use in patients in four different institutional settings. *Humane Medicine*, 10 (1), 17–27.

Lever, J.A., Molloy, D.W., Bedard, M. & Eagle, D.J. (1995) Reduction of restraint use through policy implementation and education. *Perspectives* 19, 3–8.

Lofgren, R.P. (1989) Mechanical restraints on the medical wards: are protective devices safe. *American Journal of Public Health*, 79 (6), 735–8.

Magee, R. (1993) Institutional policy: use of physical restraints in extended care and nursing homes. *Journal of Gerontological Nursing*, 19 (4), 31–9.

Miles, S.H. & Irvine, P. (1992) Deaths caused by physical restraint. *Gerontologist*, 32 (6), 762–6.

Minnick, A.F. (1998) Prevalence and patterns of physical restraint use in the acute care setting. *Journal of Nursing Administration*, 28 (11), 19–24.

Mion, L. (1989) A further exploration of the use of physical restraints in hospitalised patients. *Journal of the American Geriatrics Society*, 37, 949–56.

Moseley, C.B. (1997) The impact of restraints on nursing home resident outcomes. *American Journal of Medical Quality*, 12 (2), 94–102.

Nandy, B.R. & Sarvela, P.D. (1997) Content analysis re-examined: a relevant research for health education. *American Journal of Health Behaviour*, 21 (3), 222–34.

Newbern, V.B. & Lindsey, I.H. (1994) Attitudes of wives toward having their elderly husbands restrained. *Geriatric Nursing: American Journal of Care for the Aging* 15 (3):135–8.

Noblit, G.W. & Hare, R.D. (1988) *Meta-ethnography: Synthesizing Qualitative Studies*, Vol. 11. Sage Publications, Newbury Park.

O'Keeffe, S., Jack, C.I.A. & Lye, M. (1996) Use of restraints and bedrails in a British hospital. *Journal of the American Geriatrics Society*, 44 (9), 1086–8.

Petitti, D.B. (1994) *Meta-analysis, decision analysis and cost-effectiveness analysis*. Oxford University Press, New York.

Powell, C., Mitchell-Pedersen, L., Fingerote, E. & Edmund, L. (1989) Freedom from restraint: consequences of reducing physical restraints in the management of the elderly. *Canadian Medical Association Journal* 141, 561–4.

Retsas, A.P. (1998) Survey findings describing the use of physical restraints in nursing homes in Victoria, Australia. *International Journal of Nursing Studies*, 35 (3), 184–91.

Robbins, L.J., Boyko, E., Lane, J., Cooper, D. & Jahnigen, D.W. (1987) Binding the elderly: a prospective study of the use of mechanical restraints in an acute care hospital. *Journal of the American Geriatric Society*, 35 (4), 290–6.

Roberge, R. & Beausejour, R. (1988) Use of restraints in chronic care hospitals and nursing homes. *Canadian Journal of Ageing*, 7 (4), 377–81.

Ruben, B.S., Dube, A.H. & Mitchell, A.K. (1993) Asphyxial death due to physical restraint: a case series. *Archives of Family Medicine*, 2, 405–8.

Schneider, Z., Elliott, D., Beanland, C., LoBiondo-Wood, G. & Haber, J. (2003) *Nursing Research: Methods, Critical Appraisal and Utilisation*. Mosby, Sydney.

Stiebeling, M., Schor, J., Morris, J. & Lipsitz, L. (1990) Morbidity of physical restraints among institutionalized elderly. *Journal of the American Geriatric Society*, 38, 45A.

Strumpf, N.E. & Evans, L.K. (1988) Physical restraint of the hospitalized elderly: perceptions of patients and nurses. *Nursing Research* 37 (3):132–7.

Tinetti, M.E., Liu, W.L., Marottoli, R.A. & Ginter, S.F. (1991) Mechanical restraint use among residents of skilled nursing facilities: prevalence, patterns and predictors. *Journal of the American Medical Association*, 265 (4), 468–71.

Tinetti, M.E., Liu, W. & Ginter, S.F. (1992) Mechanical restraint use and fall-related injuries among residents of skilled nursing facilities. *Annals of Internal Medicine*, 116 (5), 369–74.

Werner, P., Cohen-Mansfield, J., Braun, J. & Marx, M.S. (1989) Physical restraints and agitation in nursing home residents. *Journal of the American Geriatrics Society*, 37 (12), 1122–6.

Whitehead, C., Finucane, P. & Henschke, P. (1997) Use of restraints in four Australian teaching hospitals. *Journal of Quality in Clinical Practice*, 17, 131–6.

Part 4

Applications and Uses of Reviews

16 Using Systematic Reviews in Health Services

Donna Ciliska, Maureen Dobbins and Helen Thomas

Introduction

Most developed countries have set evidence-based health care as a priority. This has been based on an ethical duty to provide effective care, but also on an economic agenda concerned with not wasting valuable resources in delivering ineffective care. Evidence-based practice integrates the best research evidence with clinical expertise and patient preferences and values in decision-making (Sackett et al., 2000). This definition has been expanded, in nursing, to include healthcare resources in the mix (DiCenso et al., 2005). A similar definition can be put forward for evidence-based policy development: it involves integration of the best research evidence with policy-maker expertise, population preferences, values and expectations and available resources. Fast access to high-quality evidence is necessary to achieve evidence-based decision-making. Systematic reviews can provide a partial solution.

In this chapter we give examples of how systematic reviews have been used in clinical practice, management and policy development. This includes criteria for critically appraising reviews, along with explanation and application of the criteria to an existing systematic review and a clinical scenario. As our experience and our reviews are primarily relevant to public health, our examples will also be public health focused.

The three authors have been involved for over a decade in the Effective Public Health Practice Project (EPHPP). The purpose of this inter-disciplinary, provincial project in Canada is to conduct systematic reviews of effectiveness of public health interventions, to write summary statements of these reviews and of other high-quality reviews that are geared to front-line practitioners and decision-makers in public health, and to engage in activities to promote the transfer and uptake of this knowledge into programme planning and healthy public policy. When a review topic is identified, a review group is constituted to complete the review. The review groups (4–6 members) consist of at least one academic with a cross-appointment in public health who is a methodological expert in systematic reviews, and managers or front-line staff from the other Public Health Research Education and Development programme (PHRED) Health Units, who provide content expertise. The project is located in Hamilton, Ontario, and has been predominantly funded jointly by the Ontario Ministry of Health and Long-term Care, Public Health Branch, and the regional government of Hamilton, Ontario. However, individual reviews have also been funded via contracts and competitive grants. Since 1999, 30 systematic reviews have been conducted on topics such as reducing adolescent risk behavior, obesity prevention in children, prevention of elder abuse, and health promotion interventions in the workplace, and 97 summary statements have been written for these and other high-quality relevant systematic reviews (see http://www.myhamilton.ca/myhamilton/CityandGovernment/HealthandSocialServices/Research/EPHPP/ephpp.htm).

Further, all three authors are also involved in health-evidence.ca (www.health-evidence.ca). This website was designed to provide pre-appraised research evidence from systematic reviews evaluating public health and health promotion interventions, (published since 1985) to public health decision-makers. It offers immense time-saving by searching, screening and rating the systematic review evidence, and then compiling a summary in a searchable online registry.

Shortly after the first reviews were produced, it became apparent that production was not enough. A survey of public health practitioners and decision-makers reported a largely unmet need for research evidence. Respondents considered that systematic reviews had the potential to overcome barriers associated with lack of critical appraisal skills, lack of time to find and appraise research, timeliness and availability of evidence, cost of acquiring evidence and credibility of findings, but not to overcome the barriers associated with the policy climate, authority or resources needed for implementation. Three months after sending out a requested, pertinent systematic review, 71% of respondents reported reading it, while 23% stated that the review played a part in programme planning or decision-making (Ciliska et al., 1999).

Use of systematic reviews in clinical practice/programme planning or service provision

One school in our community had a devastating series of teenaged suicides one spring. Understandably, the entire school community was distraught. The principal asked the local public health department if they would provide suicide prevention programmes in the school, beginning the following autumn term. Fortunately, the programme director took a strong evidence-based approach and, before promising such a programme, suggested that they first look at the literature. The systematic review was completed over the summer months and, first of all, no evidence was found that suicide preven-

tion programmes prevented suicide; secondly, the evidence was weak; and, thirdly, there was some weak evidence of causing more harm to males in that they undertook less adaptive coping after a suicide prevention programme (Ploeg et al., 1996). The review leader met with the Adolescent Programme Director and the school principal to discuss the results. After some deliberations, it was decided that a suicide prevention programme would not be offered, but rather a more comprehensive school approach that would target many issues, including self-esteem, depression and substance use, for all age groups and through a variety of interventions. Included in the plan was a protocol to implement and evaluate this comprehensive school approach. This was a good example of how a systematic review was used to make a decision to not implement a programme. Since this review and a couple of others with similar results have been published, schools have changed their focus regarding suicide prevention programmes. Currently most programmes are directed to teachers and others to whom students may reveal suicide ideation. Schools have developed protocols for dealing with these students, and many school boards have board-wide policies regarding action to prevent adolescent suicide.

In another example, Thomas and colleagues (2002) conducted a review of reviews to evaluate the effectiveness of community-based interventions to improve child mental health. The implications for practice included assuring that early childhood education programmes were of high quality, with a focus on social and cognitive development for pre-schoolers. These results led one region to review their programmes and to enhance their cognitive and social development aspects.

Use of reviews for policy decisions

Early in the life of this review group, the provincial government was considering ending public health nursing visits to postpartum mothers, citing lack of evidence for their effectiveness. In addition, this was one of the largest programmes in the system, and cancelling it would have resulted in large cost savings. However, a systematic review showed that significant social benefits, in the long term, for the mother and child, could be obtained from intensive home visiting by public health nurses, in particular to high-risk mothers (Ciliska et al., 2001). The review was sent to key people, presented at many professional association meetings, and discussed at several key policy meetings. These strategies, along with the support of key champions, and other movements focused on early childhood care, resulted in a reversal of the decision to end public health nursing visits, and instead to increase the intensity of the programme to mothers considered to be at risk.

Further, in 1999, a major provincial policy review of public health programmes was undertaken. Public health consultants, who had been involved in systematic review production, were appointed to each of the five policy review committees in order to find and summarise pertinent research, particularly systematic reviews, of relevance to the committee deliberations. A telephone interview, conducted with committee members after the review process was complete, assessed use of the reviews in developing policy and the extent to which the reviews led to new recommendations for practice. Ninety-six per cent of respondents reported that the systematic reviews had played a part in developing new policy, and 47% indicated that they contributed 'a great deal' to the development of new recommendations for practice (Dobbins et al., 2004).

The results of a recent review on the effectiveness of physical activity enhancement and obesity prevention programmes in children and young people (Thomas et al., 2004) were used in the annual report from the Chief Medical Officer of Health in that year (Basrur, 2004). This report outlines the major public health issues and areas for programme focus for the future. It is widely circulated to all levels of government, to provincial Public Health Units and to others practising health promotion. It outlines recommendations for provincial, national and local governments as well as the food industry, workplaces and schools. These recommendations are then discussed in the various sectors and plans for implementation are developed.

Characteristics associated with using systematic reviews have been identified in several studies: one's position in the organisation, the value the organisation places on research use in decision-making, perceptions that systematic reviews overcome limited critical appraisal skills, training in critical appraisal (Dobbins et al., 2001a, b), relevance to policy decisions, and perceived importance of evidence from systematic reviews in comparison to other sources of information (Dobbins et al., 2004).

Public health decision-makers in Canada have also expressed specific preferences for the ways in which they want to receive research evidence, as well as the type of information they want and need. Initially they want to receive a short summary of a review, with immediate and easy access to the full report if necessary. While many decision-makers want to receive information electronically, a significant proportion likes to receive information in hard copy. They are interested in having a credible and reliable source to inform them of the methodological quality of the review, and to clearly spell out the implications for policy and practice. Finally, they want to be able to let others know what topic areas they are interested in, so that others can take care to ensure that this information is transmitted to them in a timely manner (Dobbins et al., 2004).

Critical appraisal of reviews

In this section we will present commonly accepted criteria for judging the quality of systematic reviews (see Table 16.1) (Ciliska et al., 2005). They will be applied to a real review (Norris et al., 2005) in relation to a clinical scenario.

Clinical scenario

You are a member of a local group of nurses who work either in primary care or public health. The purpose of the group is to conduct joint programmes to improve the health of the local community. The prevalence of type 2 diabetes mellitus is increasing and you are aware that higher weight represents an increased risk for diabetes. The nursing group has considered several possible interventions. You suggested a physical activity and diet intervention programme for adults with prediabetes, defined as impaired glucose tolerance or impaired fasting glucose, but not at the level of diabetes. Your nursing group is interested, and they ask you to see what evidence there is for the effectiveness of such an intervention on weight loss and maintenance, and to report back at the next meeting.

Finding the evidence

Searching is more efficient if a clear question is posed. The PICO formulation (Patients/Population, Intervention, Comparison, Outcomes) helps us to frame a very specific question (Richardson et al., 1995). For this scenario, you identified:

Patient   Adults with prediabetes (impaired glucose tolerance (IGT) or impaired fasting glucose (IFG), but not at values of diabetes).

Intervention   Dietary and/or physical activity interventions.

Comparison   Usual care.

Outcomes   Weight loss and maintenance, improvement in prediabetes measures.

Now that the clinical question is very clear, you begin your search. You are aware of the '4S' hierarchy for finding current best evidence (Haynes, 2005). The top of the pyramid is *systems*, such as portals and guidelines, followed next by *synopses*, as found in the pre-appraised literature, then *syntheses*, as in systematic reviews, and followed at the bottom, by *single studies*. The 4S hierarchy advises that, for the most efficient search for current best evidence, you begin at the top of the hierarchy, the systems level. This level includes clinical practice guidelines. If you are not successful, you go next to the synopses level, to the evidence-based abstracts where articles have been pre-appraised using quality filters. If a relevant article appears in an abstraction journal such as *Evidence-Based Nursing*, then you can have some confidence in the quality of the study methods. If you are still unsuccessful,

you go to syntheses such as the Cochrane Library and, finally, to single studies. For this topic, about weight loss in people with prediabetes, you search the National Guideline Clearinghouse (http://www.guideline.gov), using the terms *weight loss* and *prediabetes* and get six hits. One relevant guideline tells you that there is evidence from randomised trials, for the following recommendations:

- Individuals at high risk for developing diabetes need to become aware of the benefits of modest weight loss and participating in regular physical activity.
- Patients with impaired glucose tolerance (IGT) should be given counselling on weight loss as well as instruction about increasing physical activity (American Diabetes Association, 2005).

This is helpful, but now you are curious to know if any particular interventions have been used for counselling on weight loss and increasing physical activity. You go to the next level of the hierarchy and search *Evidence-Based Nursing*, using *weight loss* and *prediabetes*. You get only one hit, an abstract of a review by Norris and colleagues (2005), which indicated that dietary, physical activity or behavioural strategies induced or maintained weight loss in adults with prediabetes (Review: non-pharmacological interventions induce or maintain weight loss in adults with prediabetes, 2005). This is exactly on the topic you are seeking. It is a Cochrane review and you are aware that generally these are of higher quality than systematic reviews published in journals (Jadad et al., 1998). You decide to go to the Cochrane Library to read the entire review (Norris et al., 2005). But how can you tell if it is actually a good review? Table 16.1 presents a framework for assessing the quality of methods, interpreting

Table 16.1   Users' guide to critical appraisal of a review article (adapted from Ciliska et al., 2005).

Are the results valid?	Did the review address a sensible question?
	Was the search detailed and exhaustive?
	Were the primary studies of high methodological quality?
	Were assessments of primary studies reproducible?
What are the results?	Were the results similar from study to study?
	What were the overall results?
	How precise were the results?
How can I apply the results?	How can I best interpret the results to apply them to patient care/policy decision?
	Were all the important outcomes considered?
	Are the benefits worth the costs and potential risks?

results and applying the results to practice. The criteria will be considered here as they apply to the review by Norris and colleagues (2005).

Critical appraisal

Are the results valid?

Did the review address a sensible question?
The first step is to determine what question the review is answering. Have the authors clearly identified the population, types of interventions and outcomes of interest? In the review by Norris and colleagues (2005), they clearly identified that the overall objective was to assess the effects of dietary, physical activity and behavioural interventions on weight loss or weight control in adults with prediabetes (IFG or IGT). The question of the review is very clear, and addresses the population, intervention and outcomes. Is this a sensible question? Readers need to ask themselves if they would expect similar results across all the patient groups, types of interventions and outcomes. In the Norris example (2005), it certainly makes sense that they separated the prediabetes population from those with diagnosed diabetes, or those without impaired glucose tolerance or impaired fasting glucose. You may argue that the interventions are too broad and varied to include in one review; however, the interventions are often combined in clinical practice and therefore make clinical sense. In summary, the Norris review answers a clearly defined and sensible question.

Was the search detailed and exhaustive?
This criterion establishes if relevant databases were searched, and if there was attention to possible publication bias. The example review searched eight major databases which were highly relevant to the topic, using appropriate MeSH terms and text words. The Cochrane Library and the Cochrane Central Register of Controlled Trials were searched. In order to overcome the possibility of incorrect indexing, and therefore missing articles in the electronic search, the authors also hand searched five key journals related to this topic area. Reference lists were checked for all retrieved articles. Conference proceedings were searched, but no references were obtained from that source due to insufficient details.

In summary, a very extensive and comprehensive search was done for published studies. However, the review may be subject to publication bias as no unpublished studies were retrieved.

Were the primary studies of high methodological quality?
Non-systematic reviews report on study findings, without consideration of study strengths. This is particularly concerning as results of poorer studies tend to overestimate the effectiveness of interventions (Kunz & Oxman, 1998). Systematic reviews tell us the state of the literature about a particular topic in terms of quality and outcomes. If only lower-quality designs are used when randomised trials are possible, the review gives clear direction for research but not such clear direction for practice. This review example (Norris et al., 2005) only included randomised trials with a time frame of at least 12 months after randomisation. Nine trials met the inclusion criteria. Only one report stated how the randomisation sequence was generated; no studies documented adequate concealment of allocation; attrition ranged from 4 to 43%. Overall the methodological quality of the primary studies included in the Norris review was high.

Were assessments of primary studies reproducible?
Within randomised trials there are differences in quality of design. This review used two reviewers to assess the quality of the included studies independently, using a standardised template, and they used consensus to deal with disagreements. The template assessed studies in terms of potential selection, attrition and detection bias and was based on the Cochrane Handbook (Clarke & Oxman, 2001), which gives explicit criteria for assessing quality of studies. The authors present a table of included studies, which documents sampling method, randomisation procedure, baseline comparability of groups and attrition. This level of detail would allow a reader to reproduce the quality assessments.

What are the results?

Were the results similar from study to study?
You can get a good sense of the similarity of study results by viewing the graphic display often used

in meta-analyses, known as a 'blobogram'. Each study has a point estimate (usually a square) and confidence interval (horizontal lines), and the summary statistic is usually a diamond with the vertical points on the point estimate and the horizontal points representing the 95% confidence intervals. Norris et al. used the blobogram to show difference in mean weight loss across the nine trials, and separately combined the data in three meta-analyses by length of follow-up (1 year, 2 years and >2 years) (figure 01, Norris et al., 2005:35). When individual study results are examined, all but one study have results that favour the treatment group. The confidence intervals for each study mostly overlap, helping us to decide that the results were somewhat similar. The statistical test for heterogeneity assesses systematic differences between results of studies that cannot be attributed to chance. If the result is statistically significant, it indicates that the results do differ from each other beyond chance. This was the case in the Norris et al. (2005) review; therefore a random effects model was used for the meta-analysis rather than a fixed effects model. The fixed effects model assumes that there is a single treatment effect, reflected most accurately in the study with the largest sample; the random effects model takes into account the heterogeneity in terms of the individual study results and width of the confidence intervals (Freemantle & Geddes, 1998).

Beyond the test for heterogeneity, it is important for the reader to decide if the statistical combination makes clinical sense. In this example, the authors combined results from all interventions by length of follow-up. This is a clinically useful finding. In addition, other pre-planned comparisons were done to show effect of the interventions on different outcomes (body mass index (BMI), % weight loss, glycaemic control and lipids). If the various study populations, interventions or outcomes vary widely, the review team may make a decision to summarise the results narratively, but not to do a meta-analysis; that is, not take the step of statistically combining the results. However, you as the reader need to feel confident that the statistical combination was a reasonable thing to do. The three meta-analyses by differing length of time after randomisation, and the overall meta-analysis of all studies combined, made sense both statistically and clinically.

What were the overall results?

Vote counting, or adding the number of studies that have results favouring the intervention, does not give us an estimate of the magnitude of effect across studies, and it can lead to distortion of the results (Freemantle & Geddes, 1998). For example, a review may find four small before – after studies that favour the intervention, but one large trial that shows no difference. Vote counting would lead to the erroneous conclusion that the intervention works. However, a meta-analysis would show that the intervention is ineffective. For this reason, where possible and clinically meaningful, study results are statistically combined in a meta-analysis. In this review example, the primary outcome of weight loss was reported as a mean difference in weight loss between intervention and control groups. The mean difference at 1-year follow-up was −2.8 kg, at 2 years it was −2.6 kg, and for studies reporting longer than 2 years follow-up, the mean difference was −4.9 kg (Norris et al., 2005:25); thus, in all cases, the intervention was favoured.

How precise were the results?

The confidence intervals around the point estimate of the meta-analysis tell us both if the results are statistically significant, and give us an idea of the precision of the results. As in any primary study, the true effect cannot be known. The confidence intervals tell us the range within which the true effect probably lies. The confidence intervals become more narrow in the meta-analysis as the sample size is increased through the combining of all samples of every study. In the Norris review, the studies that followed participants for more than 2 years had a mean difference in weight loss of −4.9 kg; the 95% confidence intervals were −6.7 to −3.1 kg (Norris et al., 2005:25). This indicates that the results are statistically significant because the confidence interval did not include 0 (no weight loss). In many meta-analyses, the outcomes are dichotomous (for events, such as dead/alive; hospitalised/home; stroke/no stroke); for dichotomous data, the results of the meta-analysis are reported as odds ratios, and to be statistically significant the confidence intervals cannot include 1.

A confidence interval helps clinicians make a decision about using the results. A CI is precise enough if the decision to use or not use an intervention is the same at either end of the CI. In this example, the decision to implement the intervention would probably be the same, even at the lower end of the CI of –3.1.

How can I apply the results?

How can I best interpret the results to apply them to patient care/policy decision?
Just considering the outcome of weight loss for interventions that last for more than 2 years, at both extremes of the confidence intervals, the weight loss is still clinically meaningful. That is, even if the mean weight loss is only 3.1 kg more in the intervention group than the control group, this difference could translate into a reduction in risk factors for diabetes. It is worthwhile investigating further the costs and skills required to offer such a programme.

It is important to make the distinction, with every study, between statistical significance and clinical significance. It is theoretically possible that this review would have resulted in a much smaller, but still statistically significant, difference in weight loss that, based on other research, would have no impact on risk factors for diabetes. For example, a mean weight change of 0.5 kg, could be statistically significant but not produce much impact on risk for diabetes.

Finally, a comparison of the participant characteristics in the analysis with your population is necessary. Are there any reasons to expect that your clients are so different that the results will not be applicable to them? In the Norris example (2005), the participants were 50% female, and mean age of 52 years; this profile, as well as their baseline glycaemic control, fits with the community population of interest.

Were all the important outcomes considered?
The review details many other outcomes related to weight (BMI, % weight loss) and to other risk factors (blood pressure, lipids, glycaemic control). All outcomes favoured the intervention groups, including the lower incidence of diabetes in three of the five studies that examined that outcome at 3–6 years follow-up (Norris et al., 2005). No studies reported on mortality, quality of life or programme costs.

Are the benefits worth the costs and potential risks?
As the programme costs are not identified, the working group in the scenario would have to compute their costs to offer a programme of the intensity in the intervention. There are no known risks of the interventions.

In summary, the review was very well done and, apart from possible publication bias, had a clear, focused question, thorough search, clear predefined inclusion and quality criteria, and reasonable planned comparisons. There were modest, but statistically significant and clinically meaningful findings of advantage of the diet, physical activity and behavioural interventions for weight loss and glycaemic control in people with prediabetes.

Resolution of the scenario

You present the Cochrane review, a brief critique and summary, and some costs estimates of delivering the programme. The nursing group decides to start a pilot intervention in your community as they conclude that the review presents strong evidence of modest results. They access a toolkit of implementation strategies to help them with the practice change (Registered Nurses Association of Ontario, 2002). The group is also confident that they have the expertise and resources (space, time) to offer the intervention, and they believe that their clients value diabetes prevention and that people with prediabetes will attend.

Conclusion

Systematic reviews usually represent a rigorous and intensive process of finding, appraising and synthesising all relevant information on a particular clinical question. They are valuable to nurses, as they allow fast access to a pre-appraised body of work. Sources of high-quality systematic reviews are shown in Table 16.2. However, not all systematic reviews are well done, and practice at using the appraisal criteria above will ensure that you can quickly assess whether or not you can have faith in the findings of a review – faith enough to apply the results to your patient, population or policy decision.

Table 16.2   Finding the evidence: sources of high-quality systematic reviews.

Name of organization	url	Target audience
Agency for Healthcare Research and Quality	http://www.ahrq.gov/	Healthcare providers; policy-makers and consumers
Canadian Agency for Drugs and Technologies in Health	www.cadth.ca	Healthcare providers and decision-makers
Clinical Evidence	http://www.clinicalevidence.com/ceweb/conditions/index.jsp	Healthcare providers; summarises reviews and primary studies
Cochrane Library	http://www.cochrane.org/reviews/	Healthcare providers and decision-makers; consumers
Effective Public Health Practice Project	www.myhamilton.ca/myhamilton/CityandGoverment/HealthandSocialServices/Research/EPHPP/ephpp.htm	Public health practitioners and policy-makers
Health-Evidence.ca	www.health-evidence.ca	Public health practitioners and policy-makers
NHS Health Technology Assessment Programme	http://www.hta.nhsweb.nhs.uk/	Healthcare practitioners and policy-makers
NICE guidelines (National Institute for Health and Clinical Excellence)	www.nice.org.uk	Healthcare providers

References

American Diabetes Association (2005) Standards of medical care in diabetes. IV. Prevention/delay of type 2 diabetes. *Diabetes Care*, 28 (S1), S7–8.

Anonymous (2005) Review: non-pharmacological interventions induce or maintain weight loss in adults with prediabetes [abstract]. *Evidence-Based Nursing*, 8, 110. Abstract of: Norris, S.L., Zhang, X., Avenell, A., Gregg, E., Schmid, C.H. & Lau, J. (2005) Long-term non-pharmacological weight loss interventions for adults with prediabetes. *Cochrane Database Systematic Reviews*, April 18 (2), CD005270.

Basrur, S. (2004) *Healthy Weights, Healthy Lives*. Chief Medical Officer of Health (Ontario) Annual Report. Toronto, Ontario.

Ciliska, D., Hayward, S., Dobbins, M., Brunton, G. & Underwood, J. (1999) Transferring public health nursing research to health-system planning: Assessing the relevance and accessibility of systematic reviews. *Canadian Journal of Nursing Research*, 31 (1), 23–36.

Ciliska, D., Mastrilli, P., Ploeg, J., Hayward, S., Brunton, G. & Underwood, J. (2001) The effectiveness of home visiting as a delivery strategy for public health nursing interventions to clients in the prenatal and postnatal periods. *Primary Health Care*, 2, 41–54.

Ciliska, D., DiCenso, A. & Guyatt, G. (2005) Summarizing the evidence through systematic reviews. In: *Evidence-Based Nursing: A Guide to Clinical Practice* (DiCenso, A., Guyatt, G. & Ciliska D., eds). Mosby, St. Louis.

Clarke, M. & Oxman, A.D. (eds) (2001) *Cochrane Reviewers Handbook*, Vol. 4. John Wiley & Sons, Chichester.

DiCenso, A., Ciliska, D. & Guyatt, G. (2005) Introduction to evidence-based nursing. In: *Evidence-Based Nursing: A Guide to Clinical Practice* (DiCenso, A., Guyatt, G. & Ciliska D., eds). Mosby, St. Louis.

Dobbins, M., Cockerill, R. & Barnsley, J. (2001) Factors affecting the utilization of systematic reviews. A study of public health decision makers. *International Journal of Technology Assessment in Health Care*, 17 (2), 203–214.

Dobbins, M., Cockerill, R., Barnsley, J. & Ciliska, D. (2001) Factors of the innovation, organization, environment, and individual that predict the influence five systematic reviews had on public health decisions. *International Journal of Technology Assessment in Health Care*, 17 (4), 467–78.

Dobbins, M., Thomas, H., O'Brien, M.A. & Duggan, M. (2004) Use of systematic reviews in the development of new provincial public health policies in Ontario. *International Journal of Technology Assessment in Health Care*, 20 (4), 399–404.

Freemantle, N. & Geddes, J. (1998) Understanding and interpreting systematic reviews and meta-analysis. Part 2: Meta-analyses. *Evidence-Based Mental Health*, 1 (4), 102–4.

Haynes, R.B. (2005) Of studies, summaries, synopses, and systems: the '4S' evolution of services for finding current best evidence. *Evidence-Based Nursing*, 8, 4–6.

Jadad, A.R., Cook, D.J., Jones, A. et al. (1998) Methodology and reports of systematic reviews and meta-analyses: a comparison of Cochrane reviews with articles published in paper-based journals. *Journal of the American Medical Association*, 280, 278–80.

Kunz, R. & Oxman, A.D. (1998) The unpredictability paradox: review of empirical comparisons of randomized and non-randomized tirals. *British Medical Journal*, 317, 1185–90.

Norris, S.L., Zhang, X., Avenell, A., Gregg, E., Schmid, C.H. & Lau, J. (2005) Long-term non-pharmacologcial weight loss interventions for adults with prediabetes. *Cochrane Database Systematic Reviews*, April 18 (2), CD005270.

Ploeg, J., Ciliska, D., Dobbins, M., Hayward, S., Thomas, H. & Underwood, J. (1996) A systematic overview of adolescent suicide prevention programs. *Canadian Journal of Public Health*, 87 (6), 411–12.

Registered Nurses Association of Ontario (2002) Toolkit: implementation of clinical practice guidelines. Registered Nurses Association of Ontario, Toronto, Canada. Available at website http://www.rnao.org/Page.asp?PageID=828&ContentID=823 (accessed 30 April 2006).

Richardson, W.S., Wilson, N.C., Nishikawa, J. & Hayward, R.S.A. (1995) The well-built clinical question: A key to evidence-based decisions. *ACP Journal Club*, 123, A12.

Sackett, D.L., Strauss, S.E., Richardson, W.S., Rosenberg, W.M.C. & Haynes, R.B. (2000) *Evidence-Based Medicine: How to Practice and Teach.* Churchill Livingstone, London.

Thomas, H., Boyle, M., Micucci, S. & Cocking, L. (2002) Community-Based Interventions to Improve Child Mental Health: Review of Reviews. *The Effective Public Health Practice Project.* Last accessed March, 2007, http://old.hamilton.ca/phcs/ephpp/ReviewsPortal.asp

Thomas, H., Ciliska, D., Micucci, S., Wilson-Abra, J. & Dobbins, M. (2004) Effectiveness of Physical Activity Enhancement and Obesity Prevention Programs in Children and Youth (Healthy Weights Review). *The Effective Public Health Practice Project.* Last accessed March, 2007, http://old.hamilton.ca/phcs/ephpp/ReviewsPortal.asp

17 Reflections on the Past, Present and Future of Systematic Reviews

Christine Webb and Brenda Roe

Introduction

The purpose of this final chapter is to draw together the practices and lessons learned from earlier chapters and to offer some suggestions on the way forward for systematic reviews.

Systematic reviews of evidence are rapidly increasing in numbers, type and scope, as the earlier chapters in this book have shown. The term 'systematic review' was first applied to reviews of quantitative research reports, and more precisely randomised controlled trials (RCTs), and the general approach has now been applied both to reviews of qualitative research findings and integrative reviews of research based on a mix of methods. Systematic reviews can produce evidence that is a more reliable basis for decision-making than relying on individual studies, and this information is increasingly available and is used by service users as well as providers via the internet.

Before the systematic review approach began to be developed, the traditional form was the narrative review in which a textual summary based on some kind of content analysis was the norm. A narrative review is still probably the most common type appearing in the 'Background' sections of research papers in journals. The Cochrane review rapidly became the gold standard for reviews of quantitative evidence, and this includes meta-analysis where appropriate data are available. From the mid-1970s onwards, various approaches to the synthesis of qualitative data have been developed, and in the 1990s researchers began to develop techniques for integrating both quantitative and qualitative evidence in a systematic way. In particular, issues in the use of reviews of qualitative evidence and of integrative approaches to qualitative and quantitative evidence have been addressed by the National Health Service Health Development Agency (Dixon-Woods et al., 2004) and the National Institute for Health and Clinical Excellence (NICE) (Popay, 2006). The Cochrane Collaboration also extended its work into the qualitative research area, and this work is now based in the Joanna Briggs Institute in Adelaide, South Australia (see http://www.joannabriggs.edu.au/cqrmg/index.html). The development of this variety of approaches to systematic reviews is summarised in Table 17.1 and definitions of the different techniques are given in Table 17.2.

An early approach to the systematic review of qualitative research was the narrative review, which sought merely to aggregate and summarise evidence. Later developments, however, moved beyond this to synthesis; this involved developing a new interpretation based on the findings of all the included studies. In this approach, the original data (or first-order concepts) are not reinterpreted. Rather, the original researchers' (second-order) concepts are reanalysed to give a new third-order

Table 17.1   Development of the systematic review process, with key references.

Systematic reviews		
Quantitative	Qualitative	Integrative (quantitative and qualitative)
Narrative review	Case survey method (Yin & Heald, 1975)	Integrative review (Kirkevold, 1997)
Meta-analysis (Glass et al., 1981; Egger et al., 1997)	Qualitative comparative analysis (Ragin, 1987)	

Cochrane review http://www.cochrane.org/	Meta-ethnography
	  – reciprocal translational synthesis
	  – refutational synthesis
	  – lines-of-argument synthesis (Noblit & Hare, 1988)	

	Aggregation (Estabrooks et al., 1994)	
	Cross-case analysis (Miles & Huberman, 1994)	
	Meta-synthesis (Sandelowski et al., 1997)	

	Meta-study
	  – meta-theory
	  – meta-method
	  – meta-data-analysis (Paterson et al., 2001)	

	Grounded theory approach (Kearney, 2001)	
	Content analysis (Bryman, 2001)	
	Case study approach (Jensen & Rodgers, 2001)	

interpretation or theory development. It should be noted that this is not equivalent to meta-analysis in quantitative reviews, as these involve re-analysis of the original data themselves.

A basic criticism of systematic reviews of qualitative data is that they ignore the focus on context that is a hallmark of qualitative research. However, these reviews lead to wider dissemination of the included studies, help care providers and policy makers to make sense of research findings, and thus contribute to the development of evidence-based practice. They can also identify directions for future research.

Integrative reviews, combining data from both quantitative and qualitative studies, give rise to even more complexity, and this approach is still in the relatively early stages and continues to evolve. The review product is a narrative that combines the various kinds of evidence, and can be criticised for its greater risks of subjectivity and bias and lack of rigour. To counteract these claims, it is important

that the review, as a form of qualitative study, is subject to processes for enhancing the rigour of qualitative research. Thus, the review report should include evidence of the transparency of the review processes and an audit trail showing how decisions were taken throughout the conduct of the review.

Why conduct systematic reviews?

The reviews discussed in this book illustrate the variety of reasons for carrying out systematic reviews. Increasingly policymakers in both health and social care are calling for policy and practice to be evidence-based. We need to be able to predict which interventions are likely to be most effective and how the various client groups may be affected by these interventions. These questions relate not only to delivering care that achieves its intended outcomes for recipients, but also to using scarce resources in the most cost-effective way. As well as

Table 17.2 Definitions of types of review.

Definition of review	Source
Narrative review The informal selection, assembly and summary of studies for review	Dixon-Woods, M., Agarwal, A., Young, B., Jones, D. & Sutton, A. (2004) *Integrative Approaches to Qualitative and Quantitative Evidence.* Health Development Agency, London.
Systematic review Any type of review that has been prepared using strategies to avoid bias and that includes a material and methods section. A systematic review may or may not include meta-analysis	Egger, M., Juni, P., Bartlett, C., Holenstein, F. & Sterne, J. (2003) How important are comprehensive literature searches in the assessment of trail quality in systematic reviews? Empirical study. *Health Technology Assessment*, 7 (1). HMSO, London.
Cochrane review Produced by the Cochrane Collaboration – a subset of systematic reviews of the effects of health care which: ● Are based on randomised controlled trials ● Always involve consumers in their production ● Are produced to the guidelines in the Cochrane Collaboration Handbook ● Are published in the Cochrane Library	Trinder, L. (ed.) (2000) Evidence-based Practice. A Critical Appraisal. Blackwell Science, Oxford.
Meta-analysis A statistical analysis which combines or integrates the results of several independent clinical trials considered by the analyst to be combinable	Egger, M., Juni, P., Bartlett, C., Holenstein, F. & Sterne, J. (2003) How important are comprehensive literature searches in the assessment of trail quality in systematic reviews? Empirical study. *Health Technology Assessment*, 7 (1). HMSO, London.
Meta-study The primary goal of meta-study is to develop midrange theory concerning a substantive body of qualitative research. Meta-study can also generate new or expanded theoretical frameworks and spawn health or social policy. It can support practitioners in their interpretation of qualitative research findings so that this knowledge may be incorporated into practice *Meta-study* involve(s) four distinct components: *Meta-data-analysis* is the study of the findings of reported research in a particular substantive area of inquiry . . . it is an 'analysis of analyses' *Meta-method* is the study of the rigour and epistemological soundness of the research methods used in the research studies *Meta-theory* involves analysis of the underlying structures on which the research is grounded . . . the philosophical, cognitive, and theoretical perspective underlying the research design strategies; the sources and assumptions inherent in emerging theory; and the consideration of the relationships between emerging theory and the larger contexts in which it has been generated *Meta-synthesis* brings back together those ideas that have been taken apart or deconstructed in the three analytic meta-study processes. It represents the creation of a new interpretation of a phenomenon that accounts for the data, methods, and theory by which the phenomenon has been studied by others	Paterson, B.L., Thorne, S.E., Canam, C. & Jillings, C. (2001) *Meta-Study of Qualitative Health Research. A Practical Guide to Meta-Analysis and Meta-Synthesis.* Sage Publications, Thousand Oaks, California.

Table continued

Table 17.2 continued

Definition of review	Source
Meta-ethnography Meta ethnography (sic, i.e. no hyphen) . . . involves induction and interpretation, and in this respect it resembles the qualitative methods of the studies it aims to synthesise. The product of such a synthesis is the translation of studies into one another, which encourages the research to understand and transfer ideas, concepts and metaphors across different studies . . . The method is applicable to studies that are not ethnographies	Britten, N., Campbell, R., Pope, C., Donovan, J. & Morgan, M. (2002) Using meta ethnography to synthesise qualitative research: a worked example. *Journal of Health Services Research and Policy*, 7 (4), 209–15.
Integrative review An integrative review is a specific review method that summarises past empirical or theoretical literature to provide a more comprehensive understanding of a particular phenomenon or healthcare problem . . . an approach that allows for the inclusion of diverse methodologies . . . and has the potential to play a greater role in evidence-based practice for nursing	Whittemore, R. & Knafl, K. (2005) The integrative review: updated methodology. *Journal of Advanced Nursing*, 52, 546–53.

economic imperatives, there are ethical considerations because it would not be ethically acceptable to spend public money on treatments that are ineffective or to mislead service users into thinking that interventions are likely to be effective when the evidence does not confirm this.

Thus, systematic reviews which summarise and evaluate the quality of evidence are of value for policy makers, practitioners and care recipients. They can inform us about the best ways to diagnose and treat conditions, how different groups are likely to respond to interventions, and whether to consider implementing particular interventions in practice settings in the form of clinical guidelines, care pathways, protocols and so on. As well as being useful for practitioners, who may not have the time or skills to review evidence for themselves, they can have the same benefits for healthcare teachers and students in critiquing and summarising the available information. For all these groups, systematic reviews can advance thinking on the particular topic of the review, on research methodology and on the theoretical development of disciplines.

The systematic review process

Systematic reviews may be described as 'research on research' in that they are based on a pre-determined protocol and transparent methods. The structures and processes originally developed for reviews of quantitative data have formed the basis for the later developments summarised in Table 17.1. However, as the previous chapters have illustrated, the methods are still evolving for reviews of all types of evidence.

Although an initial review protocol is written at the planning stage, as for an empirical research study, this is likely to need modification as the study progresses. With Cochrane reviews the protocol is submitted for appraisal before the review is begun, and the need for adaptation may be identified at this stage. This is an early example of the need for teamwork when carrying out reviews, so that peer review can bring a variety of perspectives to bear and minimise the likelihood of error and bias. The result is likely to be a more comprehensive review.

Searching for evidence

Having established the initial review protocol, the next stage is to begin the search process. Even at this early stage, the protocol may need to be changed. Initial searches using the pre-established keywords may raise a number of queries and reveal that the keywords need to be changed and/or added to. In addition to electronic searches, reviewers often carry out hand searches of journals to pick up additional references and publications that are too recent to appear on electronic indexes. These further sources will then be followed up and authors whose names appear may be contacted to check whether any unpublished material is available. The searches may then need to be modified and repeated to include the additional keywords identified.

However, writing about RCTs, Egger et al. (2003) question the value of going beyond a search for English language literature on the main electronic databases:

> We recommend that when planning a review, investigators should consider the type of litera- ture search and the degree of comprehensiveness that are appropriate for the review in question, taking into account budgetary and time con- straints. The findings that trials that are difficult to locate are often of lower quality raises the worrying possibility that rather than preventing bias through extensive literature searchers, bias could be introduced by including trials of low methodological quality. We believe that in situ- ations where resources are limited, thorough quality assessments should take precedence over extensive literature searches and translations or articles (Egger et al., 2003:3−4)

Particular issues arise at the search stage with regard to identifying qualitative research. MeSH (Medical Subject Headings) terms may not include the desired terms or keywords, and even the term 'qualitative research' has only recently been included as a keyword on some databases. Flemming & Briggs (2007) replicated three searches in seven electronic databases and concluded that, for re- search in nursing, CINAHL was the most efficient. Searches on this identified all the papers included when using the other databases. However, this strategy was tested for only one topic – patients' experiences of living with a leg ulcer – and the authors caution that their findings need to be tested for other nursing topics.

Quality assessment of included studies

For all types of review, there is no consensus on the best way to assess the quality of studies to be included in or excluded from the review, and

different assessment tools may lead to different conclusions about study quality. Indeed, in the case of qualitative data, there is even no consensus on whether studies of questionable methodological strength should be excluded.

A major issue is that the quality of a research report may not necessarily reflect the quality of the actual research or give enough information for this to be evaluated. The reasons for this include: word length limitations imposed by journals, different journal policies on how much methodological detail is included in reports, and journal editor or reviewer bias. There is therefore an argument for contacting authors where there is doubt, so that fuller information can be used in the quality assess- ment. However, this has resource implications that may preclude its use.

There is overwhelming consensus, however, that more than one reviewer should carry out the qual- ity assessment. This helps to minimise bias and error, and allows inter-rater reliability of the assess- ment to be calculated. It is qualitative evidence that gives rise to most debate on quality assessment. Despite much being written on this topic, there is still no agreement on whether a checklist of criteria is appropriate, and if so which criteria should be included in the list. Perhaps the most comprehen- sive discussion to date is that by Popay et al. (2006), who traced more than 100 different sets of such criteria. After considering the issues, including the fact that different qualitative research approaches and data collection methods may not lend them- selves to a unified method of quality assessment, they concluded that:

> . . . the problem of non-agreement on quality standards means that it is extremely difficult to select the best, and only the best, qualitative evidence for inclusion, and even more difficult to demonstrate that only the best has been selected (Popay et al., 2006:9)

The only reasonable conclusion seems to be that, for all types of evidence – quantitative data in the form of survey, RCTs, results, etc., or qualitative findings based on phenomenology, grounded theory, interviews, focus groups, etc. – the most appropriate decision is to use criteria most appro- priate to the particular type of data involved.

However, some reviewers question whether data from qualitative research should be excluded even where methodological inadequacies are identified. The argument here is that the data themselves may offer valuable insights, which may increase understanding of the phenomenon under study.

Quality assessment of the quantitative and qualitative studies included in integrative reviews is particularly challenging (see Chapter 10), as different approaches are needed for these two methodologies and reviewers may need to adopt pragmatic solutions when choosing which assessment formats to use, as was the case for the reviews reported in Chapters 13 and 14.

Using systematic reviews

Despite the promise held out by systematic reviews, it can be frustrating for their potential 'consumers' – healthcare users, providers and policy makers – that so often the review concludes that 'more research is needed'. This may be because of lack of research on the topic of interest and/or poor methodological quality of the original studies.

Even where there is evidence on which to base convincing conclusions, review readers need to take a critical stance and to conduct an appraisal of their own rather than taking for granted the rigour of what the reviewers have done when deciding whether the review conclusions are appropriate to their own areas of practice. For example, it may be that the review definitions, search terms or inclusion/exclusion criteria are not relevant or adequate, clinicians and policy makers should not hesitate to communicate with the reviewers on these kinds of issues. We have included in this book some guidance on how review users may carry out such an appraisal (see Chapters 8 and 16). Clearly, reviews need to be updated regularly to incorporate new evidence, and this is a feature of Cochrane reviews. Feedback from consumers can enhance this process by identifying improvements that can be implemented in future iterations of reviews.

Systematic reviewing is an exciting and rapidly evolving approach which can contribute a great deal to evidence-based practice, methodological development in research, and the theoretical advance of healthcare disciplines. Integrative reviews that include quantitative and qualitative evidence are paving the way of the future. Synopses of systematic reviews may also assist with the dissemination of information on related topics or could help to question existing theories underpinning studies and practice and provide direction for future research. For example, a recent synopsis of four Cochrane systematic reviews on bladder training and voiding programmes for the management of urinary incontinence was undertaken (Roe et al., 2007a, b) using meta-study techniques developed by Paterson et al. (2001) for qualitative research, and has provided a useful descriptive narrative to compare and contrast these clinical practices. The synopsis has given an opportunity to revisit the theory underpinning these common clinical practices, which dates back over 30 years, and detected an overlap in operational definitions used within studies. It has made suggestions for the future standardisation of terminology, as well as comments on future more complex research designs, methods and outcomes. We hope that this book will contribute to this evolution and will help nurses in all fields of practice – clinical, management, research and education – to appraise and use reviews in their work.

References

Bryman, A. (2001) *Social Research Methods*. Oxford University Press, Oxford.

Dixon-Woods, M., Agarwal, S., Young, B., Jones, D. & Sutton, A. (2004) *Integrative Approaches to Qualitative and Quantitative Evidence*. Health Development Agency, London.

Egger, M., Davey Smith, G. & Phillips, A. (1997) Meta-analysis: Principles and procedures. *British Medical Journal*, 315, 1533–7.

Egger, M., Juni, P., Bartlett, C., Holenstein, F. & Sterne, J. (2003) How important are comprehensive literature searches and the assessment of trial quality in systematic reviews? Empirical study. *Health Technology Assessment*, 7 (1), iv.

Estabrooks, C.A., Field, P.A. & Morse, J.M. (1994) Aggregating qualitative findings: An approach to theory development. *Qualitative Health Research*, 4, 503–11.

Flemming, K. & Briggs, M. (2007) Electronic searching to locate qualitative research strategies: evaluation of three strategies. *Journal of Advanced Nursing*, 57 (1), 95–100.

Glass, G.V., Smith, M.L. & McGraw, B. (1981) *Meta-analysis in Social Research*. Sage, Beverly Hills, California.

Jensen, J.L. & Rodgers, R. (2001) Cumulating the intellectual gold of case study research. *Public Administration Review*, 61 (2), 236–46.

Kearney, M.H. (2001) Truthful self-nurturing: A formal grounded theory of women's addiction recovery. *Qualitative Health Research*, 8, 495–512.

Kirkevold, M. (1997) Integrative nursing research – an important strategy to further the development of nursing science and nursing practice. *Journal of Advanced Nursing*, 25, 977–84.

Miles, M.B. & Huberman, A.M. (1994) *Qualitative Data Analysis*. Sage Publications, Thousand Oaks, California.

Noblit, G.W. & Hare, R.D. (1988) *Meta-ethnography: Synthesizing Qualitative Studies*. Sage, Newbury Park, California.

Paterson, B.L., Thorne, S.E., Canam, C. & Jillings, C. (2001) *Meta-Study of Qualitative Health Research. A Practical Guide to Meta-Analysis and Meta-Synthesis*. Sage Publications, Thousand Oaks, California.

Popay, J. (ed.) (2006) *Moving Beyond Effectiveness in Evidence Synthesis. Methodological Issues in the Synthesis of Diverse Sources of Evidence*. National Institute for Health and Clinical Excellence, London.

Ragin, C.C. (1987) *The Comparative Method: Moving Beyond Qualitative and Quantitative Strategies*. University of California Press, Berkeley, California.

Roe, B., Milne, J., Ostaszkiewicz, J. & Wallace, S. (2007a) Systematic reviews of bladder training and voiding programmes in adults: a synopsis of findings on theory and methods using metastudy techniques. *Journal of Advanced Nursing*, 57 (1), 3–14.

Roe, B., Ostaszkiewicz, J., Milne, J. & Wallace, S. (2007b) Systematic reviews of bladder training and voiding programmes in adults: a synopsis of findings from data analysis and outcomes using metastudy techniques. *Journal of Advanced Nursing*, 57(1), 15–31.

Sandelowski, M., Docherty, S. & Emden, C. (1997) Qualitative meta-synthesis: Issues and techniques. *Research in Nursing and Health*, 20, 365–71.

Yin, R.K. & Heald, K.A. (1975) Using the case survey method to analyze policy studies. *Administrative Science Quarterly*, 20, 371–81.

Index